SECOND EDITION

Joint Motion, Muscle Length, and Function Assessment

A Research-Based Practical Guide

SECOND EDITION

Joint Motion, Muscle Length, and Function Assessment

A Research-Based Practical Guide

Hazel M. Clarkson, MA., BPT

Formerly Assistant Professor, Department of Physical Therapy,
Faculty of Rehabilitation Medicine, University of Alberta,
Edmonton, Alberta, Canada

Photography by **Jacques Hurabielle,** PhD., **Sandra Bruinsma,** and **Thomas Turner**
Illustrations by **Heather K. Doy,** BA, BFA.,
Joy D. Marlowe, MA., CMI., and **Kimberly Battista**

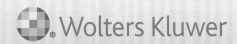 Wolters Kluwer

Philadelphia • Baltimore • New York • London
Buenos Aires • Hong Kong • Sydney • Tokyo

Acquisitions Editor: Matt Hauber
Development Editor: Amy Millholen
Senior Editorial Coordinator: Tim Rinehart
Marketing Manager: Phyllis Hitner
Production Project Manager: Sadie Buckallew
Design Coordinator: Stephen Druding
Art Director, Illustration: Jennifer Clements
Manufacturing Coordinator: Margie Orzech
Prepress Vendor: SPi Global

Second Edition

Cataloging-in-Publication Data available on request from the Publisher

ISBN: 978-1-9751-1224-0

To My Family: my husband, Hans Longerich;
parents, Graham and June Clarkson;
and siblings, Ron Clarkson, Bruce Clarkson,
and Wendy Carter. A family I could not be
more proud and fortunate to be a part of.

George Beneck, MS, PT, OCS
Lecturer
University of California at Long Beach
Long Beach, California

Rachel Diamant, MS, OTR/L, BCP
Associate Professor
Arizona School of Health Sciences
Mesa, Arizona

Suzy Dougherty, MPT
Department of Physical Therapy
Texas State University–San Marcos
San Marcos, Texas

Ruth Freeman, MEd
Program Manager, PTA
Daytona Beach Community College
Daytona Beach, Florida

Nancy Gann, PT, DPT, MS, OCS
Associate Professor
University of Texas Health Science Center
San Antonio, Texas

Mary Hudak, PT, MSPT
Duquesne University
Pittsburgh, Pennsylvania

Joy Karges, PT, EdD, MS, CLT
Assistant Professor and Academic Coordinator
    of Clinical Education
USD SMHS Physical Therapy
University of South Dakota
Vermillion, South Dakota

Kelley Sass, MPT
Associate and Assistant Academic Coordinator
    of Clinical Education
The University of Iowa
Iowa City, Iowa

It is my pleasure to tell you about *new features* of the second edition of *Joint Motion, Muscle Length, and Function Assessment: A Research-Based Practical Guide*. The addition of "Muscle Length" to the title more accurately represents the textbook content. Upon turning the pages, you will see over 600 color photographs and illustrations in the **full color textbook** to enhance ease of use and learning.

The textbook has been **updated** with the latest research findings, distilled and incorporated into the text to continue providing a research-based practical guide for student learning and clinical practice.

Textbook Navigation: Ease of navigating the second edition, to access specific content expeditiously, is important for students, faculty, and clinicians alike in the classroom and clinical settings. To this end, the following features have been incorporated into the design of the book.

Color-Coded Chapters: The chapters are color coded for quick access to these principal parts of the book.

"Quick Find": In addition to the standard Table of Contents located at the beginning of the book, a brief table of contents called "Quick Find" appears on the first page of each Chapter. These "Quick Find"s are just that, listing main content headings, other selected headings, summary tables and figures, and all range of motion (ROM) and muscle length assessment and measurement techniques including the corresponding "Practice Makes Perfect" Summary & Evaluation Forms number for each technique. These Summary & Evaluation Forms are easily accessed either online or in the Appendices of the book.

"Practice Makes Perfect" Summary & Evaluation Forms: The most immediate means of improving reliability in the assessment and measurement of joint ROM is to ensure clinicians are well trained and practiced in the techniques. The importance of practice is reinforced throughout the textbook with "Practice Makes Perfect" reminders and the inclusion of over 100 Summary & Evaluation Forms, specific to each joint ROM and muscle length assessment and measurement technique. These are included to aid the student in practicing and evaluating their proficiency in performing the joint ROM assessment and measurement techniques and may be used as a study tool to review techniques. For faculty, the Summary & Evaluation Forms provide a complete set of practical examination forms to grade student proficiency in the assessment and measurement of joint ROM and muscle length.

My hope is this textbook continues to serve students, faculty, and clinicians as a valuable resource in the classroom and clinical environments to promote a high level of standardization and proficiency in the clinical evaluation of joint ROM and muscle length. I trust the changes incorporated into the second edition of *Joint Motion, Muscle Length, and Function Assessment: A Research-Based Practical Guide* will facilitate enjoyable and productive learning experiences as you pursue the path to achieving professional excellence to the benefit of your patients.

Hazel M. Clarkson

Acknowledgments

I wish to thank all those, even though unnamed, who assisted in the journey to create the publication, *Joint Motion, Muscle Length, and Function Assessment: A Research-Based Practical Guide*.

The visuals created for this textbook would not have been possible without the photographic contributions of Dr. Jacques Hurabielle, Sandra Bruinsma, and Thomas Turner, and models of Troy Lorenson and Ron Clarkson. Kim Battista, Heather Doy, and Joy Marlowe created the unique illustrations to enable the deep anatomy to be "visualized" in the application of the clinical techniques.

Critiques of one's work are essential to promote excellence. I thank all everyone who provided reviews, suggestions, and encouragement. I thank Wendy Brook and Rita Koenig for sharing their perspectives, expertise, and opinions. I am grateful to George Beneck, Rachel Diamant, Suzy Dougherty, Ruth Freeman, Nancy Gann, Mary Hudak, Joy Karges, and Kelly Sass for their reviews of the first edition of this textbook and also to all colleagues who provided more recent reviews that were most helpful in shaping the direction of the second edition.

Thanks to my colleagues at the University of Alberta who supported my work, as well as the Faculty of Rehabilitation Medicine, where the foundation for this work was laid. I am also grateful to the physical therapy and occupational therapy students who I taught and from whom I learned so much regarding teaching and learning.

My thanks are also extended to the team at Wolters Kluwer. This work would not have been possible without them. I have indeed been fortunate to have the opportunity to work with such a highly respected publisher.

I thank, my husband, Hans Longerich for his patience and support during the production of this book and for serving as a model, photography assistant, and artwork reviewer. And last but not least, thanks to my family for the encouragement and support they have given.

Thank you to all,
Hazel M. Clarkson

Contents

SECTION III
Appendices

SECTION I
Principles and Methods

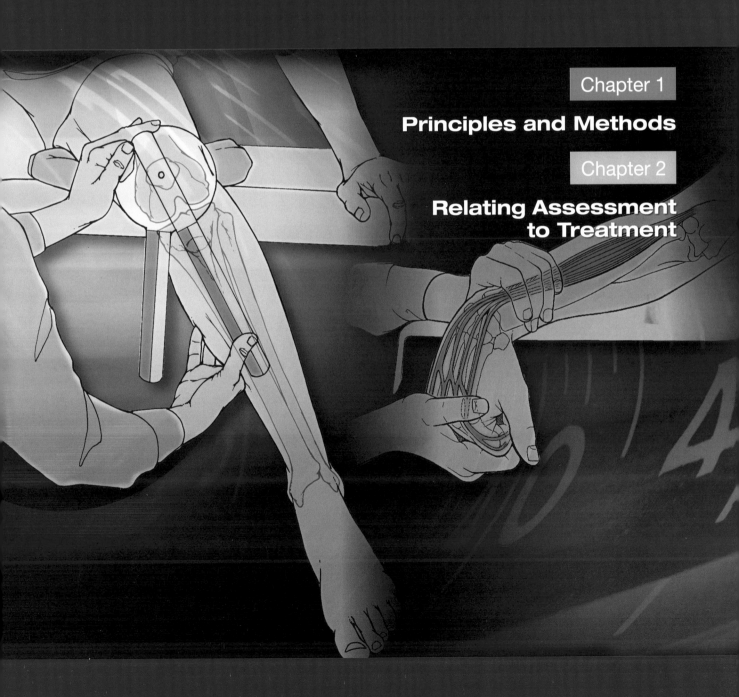

Chapter 1

Principles and Methods

Chapter 2

Relating Assessment to Treatment

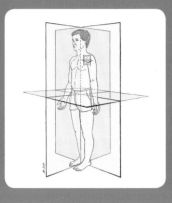

Principles and Methods

1

INTRODUCTION TO PRINCIPLES AND METHODS

A fundamental requisite to the study of evaluation of joint range of motion (ROM) is the knowledge of evaluation principles and methodology. The methods used to assess ROM are based on the principles of assessment, articular function, and movement. This chapter discusses the factors pertinent to the evaluation of joint ROM. A firm foundation in the principles, methods, and associated terminology presented in this chapter is necessary knowledge for the specific techniques presented in subsequent chapters.

Communication

When communicating with the patient:
- Speak slowly
- Use lay terms
- Provide concise and easily understood explanations
- Encourage the patient to ask questions at any time
- Confirm with the patient that she/he understands what has been communicated.

When conducting a physical assessment, explain to the patient the rationale for performing the physical assessment and the component parts of the assessment process as these are carried out.

It is essential that the patient understand the need to do the following:
1. Expose specific regions of the body and assume different body positions for the examination.
2. Communicate any change in his/her signs and symptoms during and after the examination procedures. Inform the patient that she/he might experience a temporary increase in symptoms following an assessment, but the symptoms should subside within a short period.

Visual Observation

Visual observation is an integral part of assessment of joint ROM and muscle strength. The body part being assessed should be adequately exposed for visual inspection. Throughout the initial assessment of the patient, the therapist gathers visual information that contributes to formulating an appropriate assessment plan and determining the patient's problems. Information gained from visual observation includes such factors as facial expression, body posture, symmetrical or compensatory motion in functional activities, muscle contours, body proportions, and color, condition, and creases of the skin.

Palpation

Palpation is the examination of the body surface by touch. Palpation is performed to assess bony and soft tissue contours, soft tissue consistency, and skin temperature and texture. Visual observation and palpation are used to "visualize" the deep anatomy.[1]

Palpation is an essential skill to assess and treat patients. Proficiency at palpation is necessary to perform the following:
- Locate anatomical landmarks needed to align a goniometer, tape measure, or inclinometer correctly when assessing joint ROM.
- Locate bony segments that make up a joint so that one joint surface can be stabilized and the opposing joint surface can be moved to isolate movement at a joint when assessing joint ROM or mobilizing a joint.
- Locate bony anatomical landmarks that are used as reference points to assess limb or trunk circumference.
- Determine the presence or absence of muscle contraction when assessing strength or conducting reeducation exercises.
- Identify bony or soft tissue irregularities.
- Localize structures that require direct treatment.

Proficiency at palpation is gained through practice and experience. Practice palpation on as many subjects as possible to become familiar with individual variations in human anatomy.

Palpation Technique
- Ensure that the patient is made comfortable and kept warm, and the body or body part is well supported to relax the muscles. This allows palpation of deep or inert (noncontractile) structures such as ligaments and bursae.
- Visually observe the area to be palpated, and note any deformity or abnormality.
- Palpate with the pads of the index and middle fingers. Keep fingernails short.
- Place fingers in direct contact with the skin. Palpation should not be attempted through clothing.
- Use a sensitive but firm touch to instill a feeling of security. Prodding is uncomfortable and may elicit tension in the muscles that can make it difficult to palpate deep structures.
- Instruct the patient to contract a muscle isometrically against resistance and then relax the muscle to palpate muscle(s) and tendon(s). Palpate the muscle or tendon during contraction and relaxation.
- Place the tips of the index and middle fingers across the long axis of the tendon and gently roll forward and backward across the tendon to palpate a tendon.

Therapist Posture

Apply biomechanical principles of posture and lifting when performing assessment techniques. Therapist posture and support of the patient's limb are described.

Posture

Stand with your head and trunk upright, feet shoulder width apart, and knees slightly flexed. With one foot ahead of the other, the stance is in the line of the direction of movement. *Maintain a broad base of support* to attain balance and allow effective weight-shifting from one leg to the other. When performing movements that are:

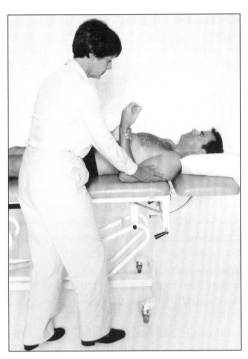

Figure 1-1 Therapist's stance when performing movements parallel to the side of the plinth.

- Parallel to the side of the plinth, stand beside the plinth with the leg furthest from the plinth ahead of the other leg (Fig. 1-1).
- Perpendicular to the side of the plinth, face the plinth with one foot slightly in front of the other (Fig. 1-2).
- Diagonal movements, adopt a stance that is in line with the diagonal movement with one foot slightly ahead of the other.

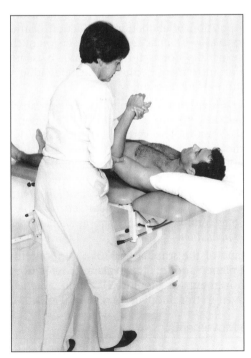

Figure 1-2 Therapist's stance when performing movements perpendicular to the side of the plinth.

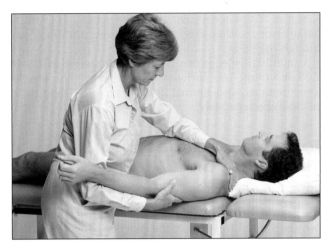

Figure 1-3 The limb supported at the center of gravity using a relaxed hand grasp.

Protect your lumbar spine by assuming a neutral lordotic posture (the exact posture varying based on comfort and practicality) and avoiding extreme spinal flexion or extension.[2] Gain additional protection by the following:

- Keeping as close to the patient as possible.
- Avoiding spinal rotation by moving the feet to turn.
- Using your leg muscles to perform the work by flexing and extending the joints of the lower extremity.

Adjust the height of the plinth to assume a neutral lordotic posture, keep close to the patient, and avoid fatigue.

Supporting the Patient's Limb

To move a limb or limb segment easily, perform the following:

- Support the part at the level of its center of gravity, located approximately at the junction of the upper and middle third of the segment (Fig. 1-3).[3]
- Use a relaxed hand grasp, with the hand conforming to the contour of the part, to support or lift a body part (Fig. 1-3).[3]
- Give additional support by cradling the part with the forearm (Fig. 1-3).
- Ensure that all joints are adequately supported when lifting or moving a limb or limb segment.

JOINT RANGE OF MOTION

Movement Description: Osteokinematics

Kinematics is the term given to the study of movement.[4] *Osteokinematics* is the study of the movement of the bone in space.[4] The movement of the bone is assessed, measured, and recorded to represent the joint ROM. *Joint ROM* is the amount of movement that occurs at a joint to produce movement of a bone in space. To perform *active range of motion (AROM)*, the patient contracts muscle to voluntarily move the body part through the ROM without assistance. To perform *passive range of motion (PROM)*, the therapist or another external force moves the body part through the ROM.

A sound knowledge of anatomy is required to assess the ROM at a joint. This includes knowledge of joint articulations, motions, and normal limiting factors. These topics are discussed separately.

Joint Articulations and Classification

An *anatomical joint* or *articulation* is formed when two bony articular surfaces, lined by hyaline cartilage, meet[5] and movement is allowed to occur at the junction. The movements that occur at a joint are partly determined by the shape of the articular surfaces. Anatomical articulations are classified as described and illustrated in Table 1-1 (Figs. 1-4 to 1-10).

In addition to classifying a joint according to the anatomical relationship of the articular surfaces, a joint may also be classified as a syndesmosis or a physiological or functional joint. A *syndesmosis* is a joint in which the opposing bone surfaces are relatively far apart and joined together by ligaments (Fig. 1-11).[7] Movement is possible around one axis. A *physiological*[5] or *functional*[8] joint consists of two surfaces, muscle and bone (e.g., the scapulothoracic joint) or muscle, bursa, and bone (e.g., the subdeltoid joint), moving one with respect to the other (Fig. 1-12).

Movements: Planes and Axes

Joint movements are more easily described and understood using a coordinate system (Fig. 1-13) that has its central point located just anterior to the second sacral vertebra, with the subject standing in the anatomical position. The *anatomical position* is illustrated in Figures 1-14 through 1-16. The "start" positions for assessing ranges of movement described in this text are understood to be the anatomical position of the joint, unless otherwise indicated.

The coordinate system consists of three imaginary cardinal planes and axes (Fig. 1-13). This same coordinate system can be transposed so that its central point is located at the center of any joint in the body. Movement in, or parallel to, the cardinal planes occurs around the axis that lies perpendicular to the plane of movement. Table 1-2 describes the planes and axes of the body. Many functional movements occur in diagonal planes located between the cardinal planes.

Movement Terminology

Angular Movements

Angular motions refer to movements that produce an increase or a decrease in the angle between the adjacent bones and include flexion, extension, abduction, and adduction (Fig. 1-17).[6]

Flexion: bending of a part so the anterior surfaces come closer together.

Special considerations: Flexion of the thumb—the thumb moves across the palm of the hand. Knee and toe flexion—the posterior or plantar surfaces of the body parts, respectively, come closer together. Ankle flexion—when the dorsal surface of the foot is brought closer to the anterior aspect of the leg, the movement is termed *dorsiflexion*. Lateral flexion of the neck and trunk—bending movements that occur in a lateral direction either to the right or left side.

Extension: the straightening of a part and movement is in the opposite direction to flexion movements.

Special consideration: Ankle extension—when the plantar aspect of the foot is extended toward the posterior aspect of the leg, the movement is termed *plantarflexion*.

Hyperextension: movement that goes beyond the normal anatomical joint position of extension.

Abduction: movement away from the midline of the body or body part. The midline of the hand passes through the third digit, and the midline of the foot passes through the second digit.

Special considerations: Abduction of the scapula is referred to as *protraction* and is movement of the vertebral border of the scapula away from the vertebral column. Abduction of the thumb—the thumb moves in an anterior direction in a plane perpendicular to the palm of the hand. Abduction of the wrist is referred to as *wrist radial deviation*. Eversion of the foot—the sole of the foot is turned outward; it is not a pure abduction movement because it includes abduction and pronation of the forefoot.

Adduction: movement toward the midline of the body or body part.

Special considerations: Adduction of the scapula, referred to as *retraction*, is movement of the vertebral border of the scapula toward the vertebral column. Adduction of the thumb—the thumb moves back to anatomical position from a position of abduction. Adduction of the wrist is referred to as *wrist ulnar deviation*. Inversion of the foot—the sole of the foot is turned inward; it is not a pure adduction movement because it includes adduction and supination of the forefoot.

Shoulder elevation: movement of the arm above shoulder level (i.e., 90°) to a vertical position alongside the head (i.e., 180°). The vertical position may be arrived at by moving the arm through either the sagittal plane (i.e., shoulder flexion) or the frontal plane (i.e., shoulder abduction), and the movement is referred to as *shoulder elevation through flexion* or *shoulder elevation through abduction*, respectively. In the clinical setting, these movements may simply be referred to as *shoulder flexion* and *shoulder abduction*.

The plane of the scapula lies 30° to 45° anterior to the frontal plane,[9] and this is the plane of reference for diagonal movements of shoulder elevation. *Scaption*[10] is the term given to this midplane elevation (Fig. 1-18).

Rotation Movements

These movements generally occur around a longitudinal or vertical axis.

TABLE 1-1 **Classification of Anatomical Articulations**[6]

Ball-and-Socket (spheroidal)	Hinge (ginglymus)	Plane

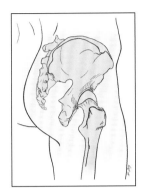

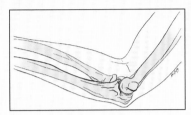

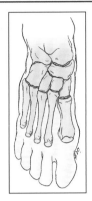

Figure 1-4 Ball-and-socket articulation (hip joint). A ball-shaped surface articulates with a cup-shaped surface; movement is possible around innumerable axes.

Figure 1-5 Hinge articulation (humeroulnar joint). Two articular surfaces that restrict movement largely to one axis; usually have strong collateral ligaments.

Figure 1-6 Plane articulation (intertarsal joints). This articulation is formed by the apposition of two relatively flat surfaces; gliding movements occur at these joints.

Ellipsoidal	Saddle (sellar)	Bicondylar

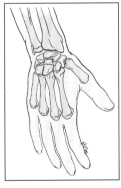

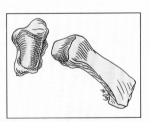

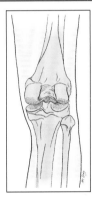

Figure 1-7 Ellipsoidal articulation (radiocarpal joint). This articulation is formed by an oval convex surface in apposition with an elliptical concave surface; movement is possible around two axes.

Figure 1-8 Saddle articulation (first carpometacarpal joint). Each joint surface has a convexity at right angles to a concave surface; movement is possible around two axes.

Figure 1-9 Bicondylar articulations (femorotibial joint). Formed by one surface having two convex condyles, the corresponding surface having two concave reciprocal surfaces; most movement occurs around one axis; some degree of rotation is also possible around an axis set at 90° to the first.

Pivot (trochoid)

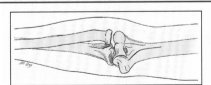

Figure 1-10 Pivot articulation (superior radioulnar joint). Formed by a central bony pivot surrounded by an osteoligamentous ring; movement is restricted to rotation.

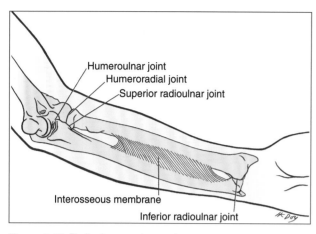

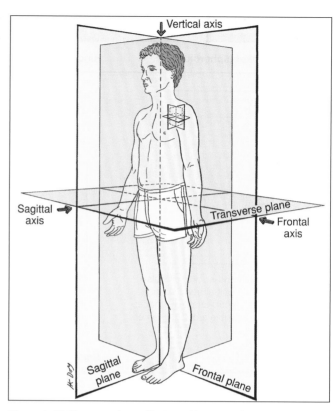

Figure 1-11 Radioulnar syndesmosis.

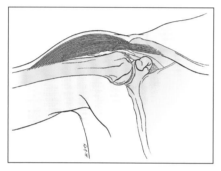

Figure 1-12 Physiological or functional joint (subdeltoid joint).

Figure 1-13 Planes and axes illustrated in anatomical position.

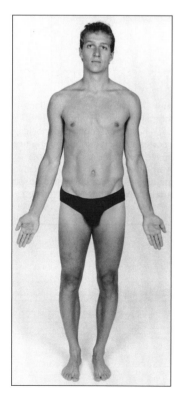

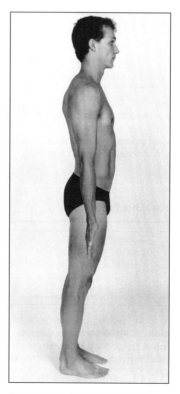

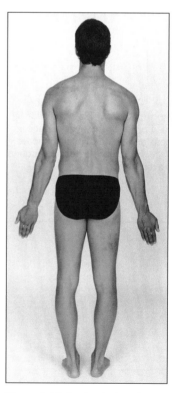

Figure 1-14 Anatomical position—anterior view. The individual is standing erect with the arms by the sides, toes, palms of the hand, and eyes facing forward and fingers extended.

Figure 1-15 Anatomical position—lateral view.

Figure 1-16 Anatomical position—posterior view.

TABLE 1-2 Planes and Axes of the Body

Plane	Description of Plane	Axis of Rotation	Description of Axis	Most Common Movement
Frontal (coronal)	Divides body into anterior and posterior sections	Sagittal	Runs anterior/posterior	Abduction, adduction
Sagittal	Divides body into right and left sections	Frontal (transverse)	Runs medial/lateral	Flexion, extension
Transverse (horizontal)	Divides body into upper and lower sections	Longitudinal (vertical)	Runs superior/inferior	Internal rotation, external rotation

Internal (medial, inward) rotation: turning of the anterior surface of a part toward the midline of the body (Fig. 1-17).

Special consideration: Internal rotation of the forearm is referred to as *pronation*.

External (lateral, outward) rotation: turning of the anterior surface of a part away from the midline of the body (Fig. 1-17).

Special consideration: External rotation of the forearm is referred to as *supination*.

Neck or trunk rotation: turning around a vertical axis to either the right or left side (Fig. 1-17).

Scapular rotation: described in terms of the direction of movement of either the inferior angle of the scapula or the glenoid cavity of the scapula (Fig. 1-19).

Medial (downward) rotation of the scapula—movement of the inferior angle of the scapula toward the midline and movement of the glenoid cavity in a caudal or downward direction.

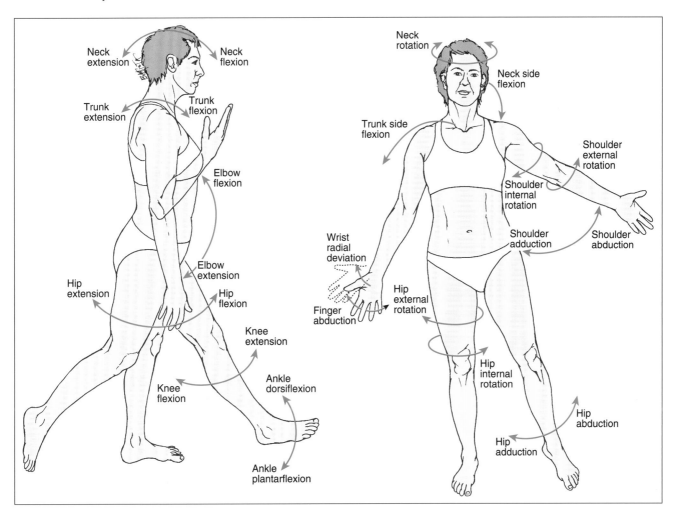

Figure 1-17 Osteokinematic movement terminology.

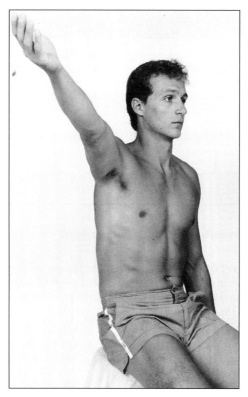

Figure 1-18 Shoulder elevation: plane of the scapula.

Lateral (upward) rotation of the scapula—movement of the inferior angle of the scapula away from the midline and movement of the glenoid cavity in a cranial or upward direction.

Circumduction: a combination of the movements of flexion, extension, abduction, and adduction.

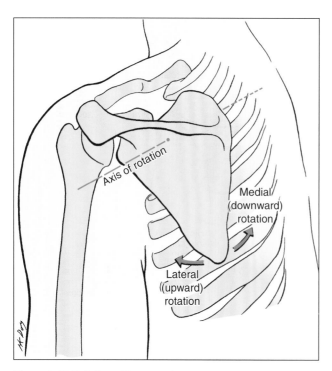

Figure 1-19 Rotation of the scapula.

Opposition of the thumb and little finger: the tips of the thumb and little finger come together.

Reposition of the thumb and little finger: the thumb and little finger return to anatomical position from a position of opposition.

Horizontal abduction (extension): occurs at the shoulder and hip joints. With the shoulder joint in 90° of either abduction or flexion, or the hip joint in 90° flexion, the arm or the thigh, respectively, is moved in a direction either away from the midline of the body or in a posterior direction.

Horizontal adduction (flexion): occurs at the shoulder and hip joints. With the shoulder joint in 90° of either abduction or flexion, or the hip joint in 90° flexion, the arm or the thigh, respectively, is moved in a direction either toward the midline of the body or in an anterior direction.

Tilt: describes movement of either the scapula or the pelvis.

Anterior tilt of the scapula—"the coracoid process moves in an anterior and caudal direction while the inferior angle moves in a posterior and cranial direction".[11 (p. 303)]

Posterior tilt of the scapula—the coracoid process moves in a posterior and cranial direction while the inferior angle of the scapula moves in an anterior and caudal direction.

Anterior pelvic tilt—the anterior superior iliac spines of the pelvis move in an anterior and caudal direction.

Posterior pelvic tilt—the anterior superior iliac spines of the pelvis move in a posterior and cranial direction.

Lateral pelvic tilt—movement of the ipsilateral iliac crest in the frontal plane either in a cranial direction (elevation or hiking of the pelvis) or in a caudal direction (pelvic drop).

Shoulder girdle elevation: movement of the scapula and lateral end of the clavicle in a cranial direction.

Shoulder girdle depression: movement of the scapula and lateral end of the clavicle in a caudal direction.

Hypermobility: an excessive amount of movement; joint ROM that is greater than the normal ROM expected at the joint.

Hypomobility: a reduced amount of movement; joint ROM that is less than the normal ROM expected at the joint.

Passive insufficiency of a muscle occurs when the length of a muscle prevents full ROM at the joint or joints that the muscle crosses over (Fig. 1-20).[12]

Movement Description: Arthrokinematics

The study of movement occurring within the joints, between the articular surfaces of the bones, is called *arthrokinematics*.[4] Arthrokinematic motion can be indirectly observed and determined when assessing active and passive joint ROM by knowing the shape of the articular surfaces and observing the direction of movement of the bone.

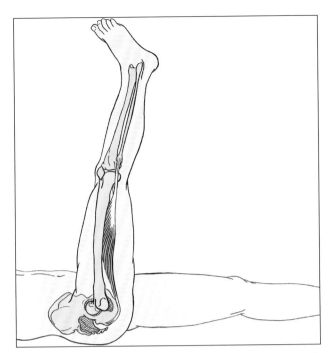

Figure 1-20 Passive insufficiency of the hamstring muscles. Hip flexion range of motion (ROM) is limited by the length of the hamstring muscles when the knee joint is held in extension.

Joints are classified on the basis of the general form of the joint (see Table 1-1). Regardless of the joint classification, the shape of all articular surfaces of synovial joints is, to varying degrees, either concave or convex, even for articulations classified as plane.[4] All joint surfaces are either concave or convex in all directions, as in the hip joint (see Fig. 1-4) (i.e., the acetabulum is concave and the head of the femur is convex), or sellar (i.e., saddle-shaped). The saddle-shaped surface has a convexity at right angles to a concave surface, as in the first carpometacarpal joint (i.e., formed by the distal surface of the trapezium and base of the first metacarpal) (see Fig. 1-8). At all joints, concave articular surfaces mate with corresponding convex surfaces.

When movement occurs at a joint, two types of articular motion—glide (i.e., slide) and roll—are present.[4] Both glide and roll occur together in varying proportions to allow normal joint motion. *Glide* is a translatory motion that occurs when a point on one joint surface contacts new points on the opposing surface. Glide at a joint is analogous to a car tire sliding over an icy surface when the brakes are applied. *Roll* occurs when new points on one joint surface contact new equidistant points on an opposing joint surface. Roll is analogous to a car tire rolling over the ground.

According to Kaltenborn,[13] decreased motion at a joint is due to decreased glide and roll, with glide being the more significant motion that is restricted. In the presence of decreased joint ROM due to decreased joint glide, an appropriate treatment plan to restore normal motion is determined based on the therapist's knowledge of the normal direction of glide at the joint for the limited joint movement.

The therapist determines the normal direction of glide at a joint for a specific movement by the following:

1. Knowing the shape of the moving articular surface (described at the beginning of each chapter).

2. Observing the direction of movement of the bone during the assessment of the PROM.

3. Applying the concave–convex rule.

   The concave–convex rule[13] states that:

   a. When a convex joint surface moves on a fixed concave surface, the convex joint surface glides in the opposite direction to the movement of the shaft of the bone (Fig. 1-21A).

      Example: during glenohumeral joint abduction ROM, the shaft of the humerus moves in a superior direction and the convex humeral articular surface moves in an inferior direction on the fixed concave surface of the scapular glenoid fossa. Restricted inferior glide of the convex humeral head would result in decreased glenohumeral joint abduction ROM.

   b. When a concave joint surface moves on a fixed convex surface, the concave joint surface glides in the same direction as the movement of the shaft of the bone (Fig. 1-21B).

      Example: during knee extension ROM, the shaft of the tibia moves in an anterior direction and the concave tibial articular surface moves in an anterior direction on the fixed convex femoral articular surface. Restricted anterior glide of the concave tibial articular surface would result in decreased knee extension ROM.

Arthrokinematics, specifically the glide that accompanies the bone movement for normal ROM at the extremity joints, is identified in subsequent chapters. The normal joint glide is introduced to facilitate integration of osteokinematic (i.e., bone movement) findings with arthrokinematics (i.e., the corresponding motion between the joint surfaces) when assessing and measuring ROM of the extremity joints. The techniques used to assess and restore joint glide are beyond the scope of this text.

Spin,[4] the third type of movement that occurs between articular surfaces is a rotary motion that occurs around an axis. During normal joint ROM, spin may occur alone or accompany roll and glide. Spin occurs alone during flexion and extension at the shoulder (Fig. 1-22A) and hip joints, and pronation and supination at the humeroradial joint (Fig. 1-22B). Spin occurs in conjunction with roll and glide during flexion and extension at the knee joint.

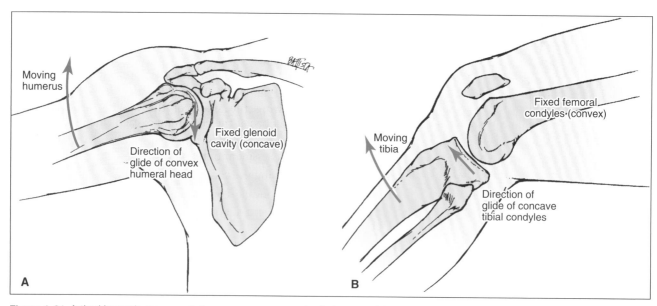

Figure 1-21 Arthrokinematic movement: the concave–convex rule. **A.** A convex joint surface glides on a fixed concave surface in the opposite direction to the movement of the shaft of the bone. **B.** A concave joint surface glides on a fixed convex surface in the same direction as the movement of the shaft of the bone.

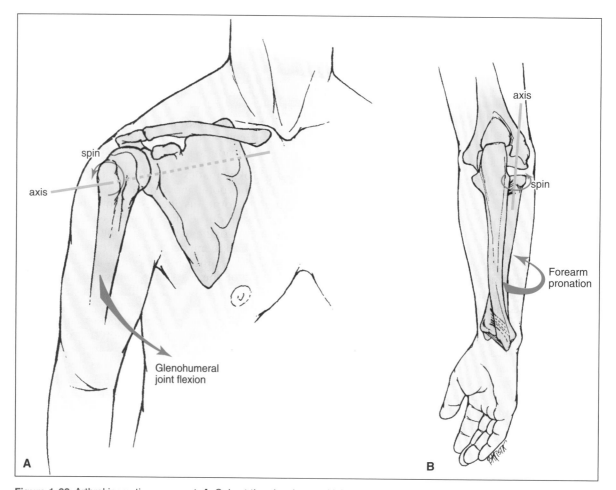

Figure 1-22 Arthrokinematic movement. **A.** Spin at the glenohumeral joint when the shoulder is flexed or extended. **B.** Spin at the humeroradial joint when the forearm is supinated or pronated.

ASSESSMENT AND MEASUREMENT OF JOINT RANGE OF MOTION

Contraindications and Precautions

AROM or PROM must not be assessed or measured if contraindications to these assessment procedures exist. In special instances, the assessment techniques may have to be performed with a modified approach to be employed safely.

AROM and PROM assessment techniques are contraindicated where muscle contraction (i.e., in the case of AROM) or motion of the part (i.e., in the case of either AROM or PROM) could disrupt the healing process or result in injury or deterioration of the patient's condition. A few examples are the following:

1. If motion to the part will cause further damage or interrupt the healing process immediately after injury or surgery.

2. If the therapist suspects a subluxation or dislocation or fracture.

3. If myositis ossificans or ectopic ossification is suspected or present, AROM and PROM should not be undertaken without first ensuring the patient is assessed by a professional who has expertise in the management of these conditions.[14]

After ensuring that no contraindications to AROM or PROM exist, the therapist must take extra care when assessing AROM and PROM if movement to the part might aggravate the patient's condition. A few examples are as follows:

1. In painful conditions.

2. In the presence of an inflammatory process in a joint or the region around a joint.

3. In patients taking medication for pain or muscle relaxants, because the patient may not be able to respond appropriately and movement may be performed too vigorously.

4. In the presence of marked osteoporosis or in conditions where bone fragility is a factor, perform PROM with extreme care or not at all.

5. In assessing a hypermobile joint.

6. In patients with hemophilia.

7. In the region of a hematoma, especially at the elbow, hip, or knee.

8. In assessing joints if bony ankylosis is suspected.

9. After an injury where there has been a disruption of soft tissue (i.e., tendon, muscle, ligament).

10. In the region of a recently healed fracture.

11. After prolonged immobilization of a part.

After ensuring no contraindications to AROM or PROM exist, the therapist must take extra care when performing AROM assessment where strenuous and resisted movement could aggravate or worsen the patient's condition. A few examples are as follows:

1. Following neurosurgery[15] or recent surgery of the abdomen, intervertebral disc, or eye[16]; in patients with intervertebral disc pathology[15] or herniation of the abdominal wall; or in patients with a history or risk of cardiovascular problems (e.g., aneurysm, fixed-rate pacemaker, arrhythmias, thrombophlebitis, recent embolus, marked obesity, hypertension, cardiopulmonary disease, angina pectoris, myocardial infarctions, and cerebrovascular disorders). Instruct these patients to avoid the *Valsalva maneuver* during the strength testing procedure.

   Kisner and Colby[15] described the sequence of events in the Valsalva maneuver, which consists of an expiratory effort against a closed glottis during a strenuous and prolonged effort. A deep breath is taken at the beginning of the effort and held by closing the glottis. The abdominal muscles contract, causing an increase in the intra-abdominal and intrathoracic pressures, and blood is forced from the heart, causing a temporary and abrupt rise in the arterial blood pressure. The abdominal muscle contraction may also put unsafe stress on the abdominal wall.

   To avoid the Valsalva maneuver, instruct the patient not to hold his or her breath during the assessment of AROM. Should this be difficult, instruct the patient to breathe out[17] or talk during the test.[15]

2. If fatigue may be detrimental to or exacerbate the patient's condition (e.g., extreme debility, malnutrition, malignancy, chronic obstructive pulmonary disease, cardiovascular disease, multiple sclerosis, poliomyelitis, postpoliomyelitis syndrome, myasthenia gravis, lower motor neuron disease, and intermittent claudication), strenuous testing should not be carried out. Signs of fatigue include complaints or observation of tiredness, pain, muscular spasm, a slow response to contraction, tremor, and a decreased ability to perform AROM.

3. In situations where overwork may be detrimental to the patient's condition (e.g., patients with certain neuromuscular diseases or systemic, metabolic, or inflammatory disease), care should be used to avoid fatigue or exhaustion. Overwork[15] is a phenomenon that causes a temporary or permanent loss of strength in already weakened muscle due to excessively vigorous activity or exercise relative to the patient's condition.

Assessment of AROM

Assessment of the AROM can provide the following patient information:

- Willingness to move
- Level of consciousness
- Ability to follow instructions
- Attention span
- Coordination
- Joint ROM
- Movements that cause or increase pain
- Muscle strength
- Ability to perform functional activities

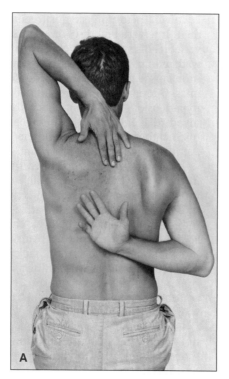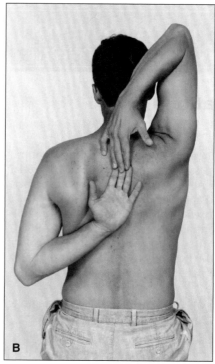

Figure 1-23 A and B. End positions: scan of active range of motion (AROM) of the upper extremities.

AROM may be decreased due to the following patient factors:

- Unwillingness to move
- Inability to follow instructions
- Restricted joint mobility
- Muscle weakness
- Pain

To perform a scan of the AROM available at the joints of the upper and lower limb, instruct the patient to perform activities that include movement at several joints simultaneously. Scans of the AROM for the upper and lower extremity joints are described and illustrated in this text.

Example: a scan of upper extremity joint AROM is illustrated in Figure 1-23A and B: instruct the patient to try and touch the fingertips of each hand together behind the back.

- As the hand reaches down the back, observe the AROM of scapular abduction and lateral (upward) rotation, shoulder elevation and external rotation, elbow flexion, forearm supination, wrist radial deviation, and finger extension.

- As the hand reaches up the back, observe the AROM of scapular adduction and medial (downward) rotation, shoulder extension and internal rotation, elbow flexion, forearm pronation, wrist radial deviation, and finger extension.

- Elbow extension is observed as the patient moves from position A to position B. If required, to scan wrist, finger, and thumb AROM, instruct the patient to make a fist, and then open the hand and spread the fingers as far apart as possible.

The results of the scan(s) are used to guide the need for subsequent assessment procedures.

For a more detailed assessment of the AROM, instruct the patient to perform all of the active movements that normally occur at the affected joint(s) and at the joints immediately proximal and distal to the affected joint(s). Observe the patient's ability to perform each active movement, if possible, bilaterally and symmetrically (Fig. 1-24A). Bilateral and symmetrical movement allows comparison of the AROM with the unaffected side, if available. When the patient actively moves through the range, emphasize the exactness of the movement to the patient so that substitute motion at other joints is avoided. The AROM can be measured using a universal goniometer (Fig. 1-24B) or OB "Myrin" goniometer to provide an objective measure of the patient's ability to perform functional activity.

In the presence of full joint movement (i.e., full PROM) and muscle weakness, the effect of gravity on the part being moved may affect the AROM. When the part is moved in a vertical plane against the force of gravity rather than in a horizontal plane when gravity is not a factor, the AROM may be less. Consider the patient's position and the effect of gravity on the movement to interpret the AROM assessment findings.

When manually assessing muscle strength, a grade is assigned to indicate the strength of a muscle or muscle group. The grade indicates the strength of a voluntary muscle contraction and the AROM possible relative to the existing PROM available at the joint. The muscle grade assigned to indicate muscle strength provides a general indication of the AROM from which to extrapolate the patient's functional capability.

Assessment of AROM is followed by an assessment of PROM and muscle strength.

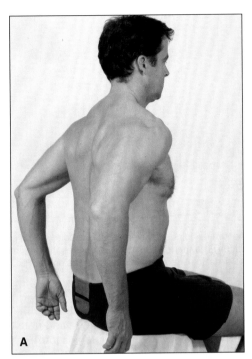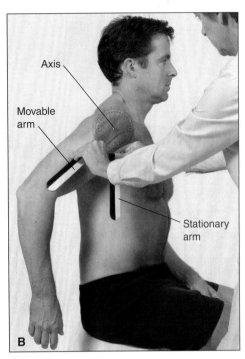

Figure 1-24 Assessment and measurement of active range of motion (AROM) using glenohumeral joint extension as an example. **A.** Observe and evaluate the AROM. **B.** Use an instrument such as a universal goniometer to measure the AROM.

Measurement of AROM

The measurement procedures for the universal goniometer and the OB "Myrin" goniometer are described in the section "Measurement of ROM," later in this chapter. The measurement of AROM may use the same or different positions to those used for PROM; for example, functional positions or activities may be used to measure AROM. When the patient actively moves through the range, emphasize the exactness of the movement to the patient so that substitute motion at other joints is avoided.

Assessment of PROM

Assessment of the PROM provides information about the following:

- Amount of movement possible at the joint
- Factors responsible for limiting movement
- Movements that cause or increase pain

PROM is usually slightly greater than AROM, owing to the slight elastic stretch of tissues and in some instances due to the decreased bulk of relaxed muscles. However, the PROM can also be greater than the AROM in the presence of muscle weakness.

The passive joint ROM must be assessed before assessing muscle strength because the full available PROM at the joint establishes the range the muscle(s) can be expected to move the limb through. Therefore, the full available PROM is defined as the full available ROM for the purpose of grading muscle strength.

To assess the PROM at a joint, for each joint movement, stabilize the proximal joint segment(s) and move the distal joint segment(s) through the full PROM (Fig. 1-25) and do the following:

- Visually estimate the PROM.
- Determine the quality of the movement throughout the PROM.
- Determine the end feel and factors that limit the PROM.
- Note the presence of pain.
- Determine whether a capsular or noncapsular pattern of movement is present.

If the PROM is either less than or greater than normal, measure and record the PROM using a goniometer.

The following concepts and terms are important to understanding joint motion restriction when assessing PROM.

Normal Limiting Factors and End Feels

The unique anatomical structure of a joint determines the direction and magnitude of its PROM. The factors that normally limit movement and determine the range of the PROM at a joint include:

- The stretching of soft tissues (i.e., muscles, fascia, and skin)
- The stretching of ligaments or the joint capsule
- The apposition of soft tissues
- Bone contacting bone

When assessing the PROM of a joint, observe whether the range is full, restricted, or excessive, and by feel determine which structure(s) limits the movement. The *end feel* is the sensation transmitted to the therapist's hand at the extreme end of the PROM that indicates the structures that limit the joint movement.[18] The end feel may be normal (physiological) or abnormal (pathological).[19]

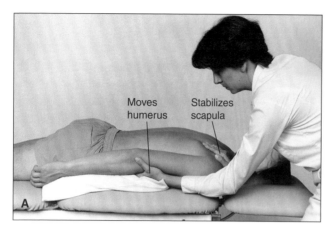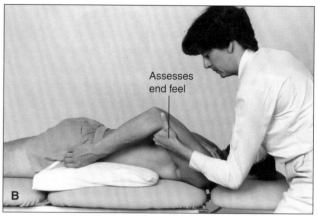

Figure 1-25 Assessment of passive range of motion (PROM) using glenohumeral joint extension as an example. **A.** The patient is comfortable, well supported, and relaxed with the joint in the anatomical position. The therapist manually stabilizes the proximal joint segment (e.g., scapula) and moves the distal joint segment (e.g., humerus). **B.** The distal joint segment is moved to the end of PROM and gentle overpressure is applied to determine the end feel.

A normal end feel exists when there is full PROM at the joint and the normal anatomy of the joint stops movement. An abnormal end feel exists when there is either a decreased or an increased passive joint ROM, or when there is a normal PROM but structures other than the normal anatomy stop joint movement. Normal and abnormal end feels are presented in Tables 1-3 and 1-4. The end feel(s) for joint movements are documented in subsequent chapters based on knowledge of the anatomy of the region, clinical experience, and available references. Although several different end feels may be possible for a particular joint motion, only one end feel will be present. When several different end feels are possible at a joint, this will be indicated using a "/" between each possible end feel. For example, the end feel for elbow flexion may be soft/firm/hard (i.e., soft, firm, or hard).

Method to Assess End Feel

Movement is isolated to the joint being assessed (Fig. 1-25A). With the patient relaxed, stabilize the proximal joint segment and move the distal joint segment to the end of its PROM for the test movement (Fig. 1-25B). Apply gentle overpressure at the end of the PROM and note the end feel.

When assessing the PROM at a joint, in addition to determining the end feel, visually estimate the available PROM for each movement at the joint and establish the presence or absence of pain.

Capsular and Noncapsular Patterns

If there is a decreased PROM, assess the *pattern of joint movement restriction*. The description of capsular and noncapsular patterns is derived from the work of Cyriax.[18]

Capsular Pattern

If a lesion of the joint capsule or a total joint reaction is present, a characteristic pattern of restriction in the PROM will occur: the capsular pattern. Only joints that are controlled by muscles exhibit capsular patterns. When painful stimuli from the region of the joint provoke involuntary muscle spasm, a restriction in motion at the joint in the capsular proportions results. Each joint capsule resists stretching in selective ways; therefore, in time, certain aspects of the capsule

TABLE 1-3 Normal (Physiological) End Feels[18–20]

End Feel General Terminology (Specific Terminology)	Description
Hard (bony)	A painless, abrupt, hard stop to movement when bone contacts bone; for example, passive elbow extension, the olecranon process contacts the olecranon fossa.
Soft (soft tissue apposition)	When two body surfaces come together a soft compression of tissue is felt; for example, in passive knee flexion, the soft tissue on the posterior aspects of the calf and thigh come together.
Firm (soft tissue stretch)	A firm or springy sensation that has some give when muscle is stretched; for example, passive ankle dorsiflexion performed with the knee in extension is stopped due to tension in the gastrocnemius muscle.
(capsular stretch)	A hard arrest to movement with some give when the joint capsule or ligaments are stretched. The feel is similar to stretching a piece of leather; for example, passive shoulder external rotation.

TABLE 1-4 Abnormal (Pathological) End Feels[18–20]

End Feel	Description
Hard	An abrupt hard stop to movement, when bone contacts bone, or a bony grating sensation, when rough articular surfaces move past one another; for example, in a joint that contains loose bodies, degenerative joint disease, dislocation, or a fracture.
Soft	A boggy sensation that indicates the presence of synovitis or soft tissue edema.
Firm	A springy sensation or a hard arrest to movement with some give, indicating muscular, capsular, or ligamentous shortening.
Springy block	A rebound is seen or felt and indicates the presence of an internal derangement; for example, the knee with a torn meniscus.
Empty	If considerable pain is present, there is no sensation felt before the extreme of passive ROM as the patient requests the movement be stopped, this indicates pathology such as an extra-articular abscess, a neoplasm, acute bursitis, joint inflammation, or a fracture.
Spasm	A hard sudden stop to passive movement that is often accompanied by pain, is indicative of an acute or subacute arthritis, the presence of a severe active lesion, or fracture. If pain is absent, a spasm end feel may indicate a lesion of the central nervous system with resultant increased muscular tonus.

become more contracted than others do. The capsular pattern manifests as a proportional limitation of joint motions that are characteristic to each joint; for example, the capsular pattern of the shoulder joint differs from the pattern of restriction at the hip joint. The capsular pattern at each joint is similar between individuals. Joints that rely primarily on ligaments for their stability do not exhibit capsular patterns, and the degree of pain elicited when the joint is strained at the extreme of movement indicates the severity of the total joint reaction or arthritis. The capsular pattern for each joint is provided in each chapter, with movements listed in order of restriction (most restricted to least restricted). However, be advised that research[21–23] indicates capsular patterns may not be relied upon as much as previously thought.

Noncapsular Pattern

A noncapsular pattern exists when there is limitation of movement at a joint but not in the capsular pattern of restriction. A noncapsular pattern indicates the absence of a total joint reaction. Ligamentous sprains or adhesions, internal derangement, or extra-articular lesions may result in a noncapsular pattern at the joint.

Ligamentous sprains or adhesions affect specific regions of the joint or capsule. Motion is restricted, and there is pain when the joint is moved in a direction that stretches the affected ligament. Other movements at the joint are usually full and pain-free.

Internal derangement occurs when loose fragments of cartilage or bone are present within a joint. When the loose fragment impinges between the joint surfaces, the movement is suddenly blocked and there may be localized pain. All other joint movements are full and pain-free. Internal derangements occur in joints such as the knee, jaw, and elbow.

Extra-articular lesions that affect nonarticular structures, such as muscle adhesions, muscle spasm, muscle strains, hematomas, and cysts, may limit joint ROM in one direction while a full and painless PROM is present in all other directions.

Measurement of ROM

Instrumentation

A goniometer is an apparatus used to measure joint angles.[7] The goniometer chosen to assess joint ROM depends on the degree of accuracy required in the measurement, the time, and resources available to the clinician, and the patient's comfort and well-being. Radiographs, digital images, photographs, photocopies, and the use of the electrogoniometer, flexometer, or plumb line may give objective, valid, and reliable measures of ROM but are not always practical or available in the clinical setting. When doing clinical research, the therapist should investigate alternative instruments that will offer a more stringent assessment of joint ROM.

In the clinical setting, the universal goniometer (Figs. 1-26 and 1-27) is the goniometer most frequently used to

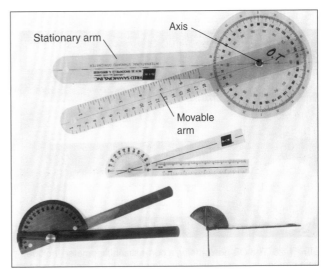

Figure 1-26 Various sizes of 180° and 360° universal goniometers.

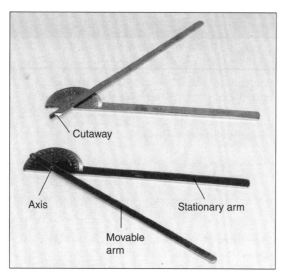

Figure 1-27 Universal goniometer with a 180° protractor. *Top*: range of motion (ROM) cannot be read as the cutaway portion of the movable arm is off the scale. *Bottom*: With the cutaway portion of the movable arm on the scale, the ROM can be read.

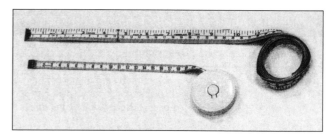

Figure 1-29 Tape measures used to measure joint range of motion (ROM).

measure ROM for the extremity joints. In this text, the universal goniometer is described and illustrated for the measurement of the ROM for the joints of the extremities and spine. The OB "Myrin" goniometer[24] (OB Rehab, Solna, Sweden) (Fig. 1-28), although less commonly used in the clinic, is a useful tool and is described and illustrated for the measurement of selected ROM at the forearm, hip, knee, and ankle.

The universal goniometer, tape measure (Fig. 1-29), standard inclinometer (Fig. 1-30), and the Cervical Range-of-Motion Instrument (CROM)[25] (Performance Attainment Associates, Roseville, MN) (Fig. 1-31) are the tools used to measure spinal AROM as presented in this text. AROM measurements of the temporomandibular joints (TMJs) are performed using a ruler or calipers. These instruments and the measurement procedures employed when using these instruments to measure spinal and TMJ AROM are described and illustrated in Chapter 9.

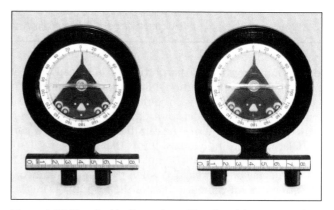

Figure 1-30 Standard inclinometers with adjustable contact points to facilitate placement on the surface of the body.

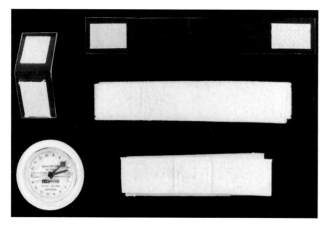

Figure 1-28 The OB goniometer, a compass/inclinometer, includes Velcro straps and plastic extension plates used to attach the goniometer to the body part being measured.

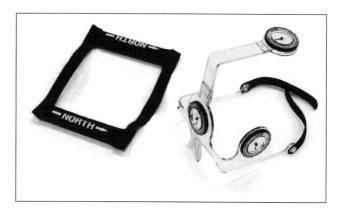

Figure 1-31 The Cervical Range-of-Motion Instrument (CROM) consists of two gravity inclinometers, a magnetic compass inclinometer, and a magnetic yoke.

Validity and Reliability

Validity

Validity is "the degree to which an instrument measures what it is supposed to measure".[26 (p. 171)] Validity indicates the accuracy of a measurement. A goniometer, inclinometer, or tape measure is used to provide measurements of the number of degrees or distance in centimeters, of movement or the position of a joint. Measurements must be accurate because the results, taken to be valid representations of actual joint angles, are used to plan treatment and determine treatment effectiveness, patient progress, and degree of disability.

Criterion-related validity is one means of assessing the accuracy of the instruments for assessing joint angles or positions. To establish this validity, the measures of the instrument being assessed are compared to the measures obtained with an instrument that is an accepted standard (criterion) for the measurement of joint angles, for example, a radiograph. When the supporting evidence from the accepted standard is collected at the same time as the measurement from the test instrument, concurrent validity is assessed. If a close relationship is found between the measures obtained with the instrument and the accepted standard, the instrument measures are valid.

Reliability

Reliability is "the extent to which the instrument yields the same measurement on repeated uses either by the same operator (intraobserver reliability) or by different operators (interobserver reliability)".[27 (p. 49)] Reliability indicates the consistency or repeatability of a measurement.

The therapist measures ROM and compares measurements taken over time to evaluate treatment effectiveness and patient progress. It is important for the therapist to know that joint position and ROM can be measured consistently (i.e., with minimal deviation due to measurement error). If this is possible, then in comparing ROM measurements, the similarity or divergence between the measures can be relied on to indicate when a true change has occurred that is not due to measurement error or lack of measurement consistency.

The universal goniometer and OB "Myrin" goniometer are described here, along with the validity and reliability of the universal goniometer. Validity and reliability of the tape measure/ruler, inclinometer, and the CROM is discussed in Chapter 9, along with the description and application of these instruments.

Universal Goniometer

The *universal goniometer* (see Figs. 1-26 and 1-27) is a 180° or 360° protractor with one axis that joins two arms. One arm is stationary, and the other arm is movable around the axis or fulcrum of the protractor. The size of universal goniometer used is determined by the size of the joint being assessed. Larger goniometers are usually used for measurement of joint range at large joints.

Validity and Reliability — Universal Goniometer

Radiographs, "the most accurate means of assessing joint motion,"[28 (p. 116)] and photographs are accepted standards used for comparison to determine the accuracy of the universal goniometer. When the supporting evidence from the radiographs or photographs is collected at the same time as the measurement from the universal goniometer, concurrent validity can be assessed.

There has been little study of the criterion-related validity of the universal goniometer. Using x-ray bone angle measurements compared to goniometric measurements of knee joint position,[29,30] high criterion-related validity has been found, along with disparate findings of goniometric accuracy in only a small part of the range, thought to be due to the increased complexity of movement in approaching terminal extension. Using a photographic reference standard to assess elbow joint positions, the "results indicate that relatively inexperienced raters should be able to use goniometers accurately to measure elbow position when given standardized methods to follow".[31 (p. 1666)]

Reliability of joint position and ROM using the universal goniometer depends on the joint being assessed but has generally been found to be good to excellent. Reliability study results indicate that:

1. The universal goniometer is more reliable than visual estimation of joint ROM.[32-37] The use of the goniometer becomes even more critical when the examiner is inexperienced.[36,38]

2. The reliability of goniometric measurement varies depending on the joint and motion assessed.[34,39-42]

3. Intratester reliability is better than intertester reliability; therefore, the same therapist should perform all measures when possible.[32,33,39,40,43-45] Different therapists should not be used interchangeably to obtain ROM measurements on the same patient unless the intertester reliability is known.[46]

4. The size of the goniometer selected to assess ROM at a joint does not affect measurement reliability.[47,48]

5. The findings are mixed on whether taking the average of repeated measures improves[33,44,49] or makes no difference to[41,42,47,50] the reliability of goniometric measures.

6. Research[50-56] regarding the reliability of goniometric measurement in the presence of spasticity appears inconclusive.

Joint ROM can be measured reliably using a universal goniometer when preferably the same therapist performs the repeated measures using a "rigid standardized measurement protocol",[43 (p. 57)] in the absence of spasticity. Miller[28] provides a method for clinicians to determine the intratester and intertester reliability within their clinical facility. Knowing the measurement error factor allows therapists to better determine patient progress.

Joint ROM Assessment and Measurement Procedure

Expose the Area

Explain to the patient the need to expose the area to be assessed. Adequately expose the area and drape the patient as required.

Explanation and Instruction

Briefly explain the ROM assessment and measurement procedure to the patient. Explain and demonstrate the movement to be performed, and/or passively move the patient's uninvolved limb through the ROM.

Assessment of the Normal ROM

Initially assess and record the ROM of the uninvolved limb to determine the patient's normal ROM and normal end feels and to demonstrate the movement to the patient before performing the movement on the involved side. If there is bilateral limb involvement, use your clinical knowledge and experience to judge the patient's normal PROM, keeping in mind that PROM is usually slightly greater than the AROM.

Use the tables of normal AROM values provided by the American Academy of Orthopaedic Surgeons[57] and the suggested normal AROM values derived from an evaluation of the research literature by Berryman Reese and Bandy,[58] as a guide to normal AROM. These "normal" AROM values are presented in table form at the beginning of each chapter.

"Normal" ranges can be misleading because joint ROM can vary between individuals depending on gender, age, occupation, and health status.[59] Therefore, "normal" ranges should be used only as a guide when assessing and treating patients. More importantly, determine the essential functional ROM required by the patient to perform activities of daily living (ADL) and the patient's ability to meet these requirements.

Assessment and Measurement Procedure

Patient Position. Ensure the patient is:

- Comfortable.
- Well supported.

Position the patient so that the:

- Joint to be assessed is in the anatomical position.
- Proximal joint segment can be stabilized to allow only the desired motion.
- Movement can occur through the full ROM unrestricted.
- Goniometer can be properly placed to measure the ROM.

If the patient's position varies from the standard assessment position outlined in this text, make a special note on the ROM assessment form.

Substitute Movements. When assessing and measuring AROM and PROM, ensure that only the desired movement occurs at the joint being assessed. Substitute movements may take the form of additional movements at the joint being assessed or at other joints, thus giving the appearance of having a greater joint ROM than is actually present. An example of substitute movements used when performing a functional activity is illustrated in Figure 1-32.

When assessing and measuring AROM and PROM, try to eliminate substitute movements. For AROM, this may be accomplished through adequate explanation and instruction to the patient regarding the movement to be performed and the substitute movement(s) to be avoided. In addition, substitute motion(s) may be avoided for AROM and PROM by the following:

- Using proper patient positioning
- Adequately stabilizing the proximal joint segment as required
- Acquiring substantial practice in assessing AROM and PROM.

To assess joint ROM accurately, the therapist must know and recognize the possible substitute movements. If the presence of substitute movements results in inaccurate AROM or PROM assessment and measurement, the treatment plan may be inappropriate.

Stabilization. Stabilize the proximal joint segment to limit movement to the joint being assessed or measured and prevent substitute movement for lack of joint range by making use of the following:

1. The patient's body weight.
   Examples:
   - To measure shoulder elevation through flexion PROM, position the patient supine on a firm plinth

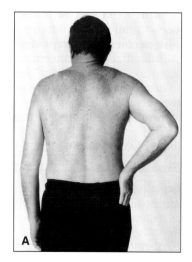
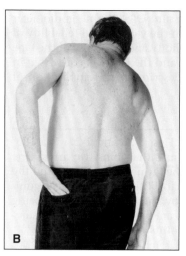

Figure 1-32 A. Patient reaches into a back pocket using normal right upper extremity. **B.** Substitute motions at the left shoulder girdle and trunk compensate for restricted left shoulder joint range of motion (ROM) as the patient attempts to reach into a back pocket.

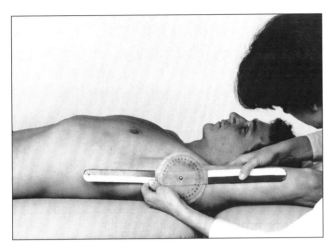

Figure 1-33 The weight of the trunk on the plinth serves to stabilize the scapula as the therapist measures the passive range of motion (PROM) of shoulder elevation through flexion.

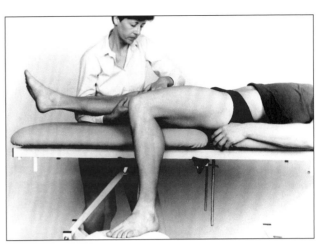

Figure 1-35 The position of the patient's nontest leg stabilizes the pelvis when testing hip abduction passive range of motion (PROM).

so that the weight of the trunk stabilizes the shoulder girdle (Fig. 1-33).

- To assess hip internal rotation PROM, position the patient supine on a firm plinth so that the weight of the body stabilizes the pelvic girdle (see Fig. 1-34).

2. The patient's position.
   Example:
   - To assess hip abduction ROM (Fig. 1-35), position the patient supine on a firm plinth with the contralateral leg over the opposite side of the plinth and the foot resting on a stool. This leg position prevents the tilting or shifting of the pelvis toward the test side, which would give the appearance of a greater hip abduction PROM than actually exists.

3. External forces in the form of external pressure applied directly by the therapist and devices such as belts or sandbags. Ensure that manual contacts or devices avoid tender or painful areas, for example, in some viral diseases (i.e., poliomyelitis), muscle bellies may be tender.
   Examples:
   - Manually stabilize the pelvis to assess hip extension PROM (Fig. 1-36) and employ a belt to stabilize

the pelvis when both hands are needed to place the goniometer to measure hip extension PROM (Fig. 1-37).
- Manually stabilize the tibia and fibula to assess ankle (i.e., talocrural) joint dorsiflexion and plantarflexion PROM (Fig. 1-38).

Assessment of Passive ROM and End Feel. With the patient relaxed, positioned comfortably on a firm surface, and the joint in anatomical position:

- Stabilize the proximal joint segment (see Fig. 1-39A)
- Move the distal joint segment to the end of the PROM for the test movement (see Fig. 1-39B) and apply slight (i.e., gentle) overpressure at the end of the PROM
- Visually estimate the PROM
- Note the end feel, presence of pain
- Return the limb to the start position
- Following the assessment of the PROM for all movements at a joint, determine the presence of a capsular or noncapsular pattern of movement.

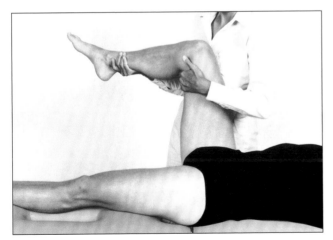

Figure 1-34 The weight of the trunk and position of the pelvis on a firm surface serves to stabilize the pelvis as the therapist assesses hip internal rotation passive range of motion (PROM) and end feel.

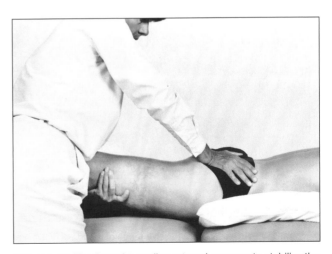

Figure 1-36 The therapist applies external pressure to stabilize the pelvis to assess hip extension passive range of motion (PROM).

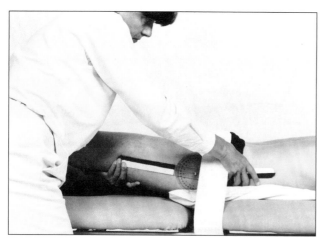

Figure 1-37 A belt may be used to stabilize the pelvis to measure hip joint extension passive range of motion (PROM).

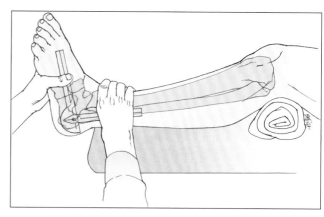

Figure 1-38 The therapist manually stabilizes the tibia and fibula proximal to the ankle joint to measure ankle dorsiflexion and plantarflexion passive range of motion (PROM).

Measurement. It is not necessary to measure the joint ROM when the involved joint has a full AROM and PROM. Record the full ROM as full, normal (N), or within normal limits (WNL).

Neutral Zero Method[57]

The neutral zero method is the most common method used to assess and measure joint ROM. All joint motions are measured from a defined zero position, either the anatomical position (see Figs. 1-14 to 1-16) or a position specified as zero. Any movement on either side of zero is positive and moves toward 180°.

Universal Goniometer—Measurement Procedure

- *Goniometer placement*: The preferred placement of the goniometer is lateral to the joint, just off the surface of the limb (see Fig. 1-40), but it may also be placed over the joint (see Fig. 1-41) using only light contact between the goniometer and the skin. If joint swelling is present, placing the goniometer over the joint may give erroneous results when assessing joint ROM as the degree of swelling changes.

- *Axis*: The axis of the goniometer is placed over the axis of movement of the joint. A specific bony prominence or anatomical landmark can be used to represent the axis of motion, even though this may not represent the exact location of the axis of movement throughout the entire ROM.

- *Stationary arm*: The stationary arm of the goniometer normally lies parallel to the longitudinal axis of the fixed proximal joint segment and/or points toward a distant bony prominence on the proximal segment.

- *Movable arm*: The movable arm of the goniometer normally lies parallel to the longitudinal axis of the moving distal joint segment and/or points toward a distant bony prominence on the distal segment.

If careful attention is paid to the correct positioning of both goniometer arms and the positions are maintained as the joint moves through the ROM, the goniometer axis will be aligned approximately with the axis of motion.[59]

The goniometer is first aligned to measure the defined zero position for the ROM at a joint (see Figs. 1-40A and 1-41A). If it is not possible to attain the defined zero position, the joint is positioned as close as possible to the zero position, and the distance the movable arm is positioned away from the 0° start position on the protractor is recorded as the start position.

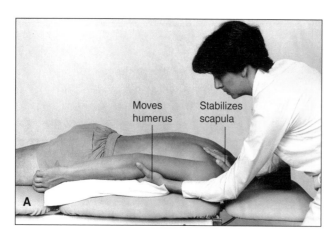

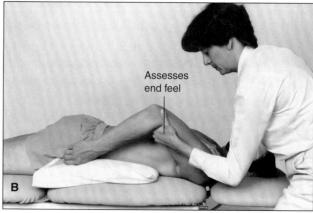

Figure 1-39 Assessment of passive range of motion (PROM) using glenohumeral joint extension as an example. **A.** The patient is comfortable, well supported, and relaxed with the joint in the anatomical position. The therapist manually stabilizes the proximal joint segment (e.g., scapula) and moves the distal joint segment (e.g., humerus). **B.** The distal joint segment is moved to the end of joint PROM and gentle overpressure is applied to determine the end feel.

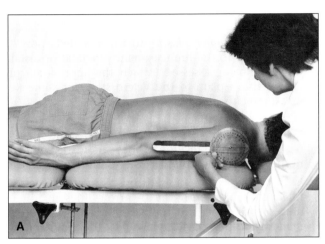

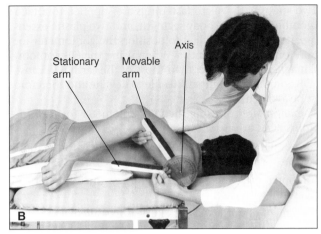

Figure 1-40 Measurement of passive range of motion (PROM) using glenohumeral joint extension as an example. **A.** Start position: the universal goniometer is aligned with the joint in anatomical position (0°). **B.** End position: measurement of shoulder extension PROM (60°).

To Measure AROM. To measure the AROM, have the patient move actively through the full AROM and either move the movable arm of the goniometer along with the limb through the entire range of movement to the end of the AROM or realign the goniometer at the end of the AROM (see Fig. 1-24B).

To Measure PROM. One of the following two techniques is used to measure the PROM at a joint:

1. Have the patient actively move through the joint ROM, and realign the goniometer at the end of the AROM. Have the patient relax, and passively move the goniometer and the limb segment through the final few degrees of the PROM.

2. Passively move the movable arm of the goniometer and the limb segment through the entire range of movement to the end of the PROM.

Using either technique, the distance the movable arm moves away from the 0° start position on the protractor is recorded as the joint ROM. When using a goniometer with a 180° protractor (see Fig. 1-27), ensure that the goniometer is positioned such that the cutaway portion of the moving arm remains on the protractor so that the ROM can be read at the end of the assessed joint ROM.

To avoid parallax when reading a goniometer, look directly onto the scale and view the scale with both eyes open or by closing one eye. Be consistent and use the same methodology on subsequent readings.

Proficiency in assessing and measuring joint ROM is gained through PRACTICE. It is important to practice the techniques on as many persons as possible to become familiar with the variation between individuals.

OB "Myrin" Goniometer

The OB "Myrin" goniometer (see Fig. 1-28), a compass inclinometer, consists of a fluid-filled rotatable container mounted on a plate.[24] The container has the following:

- A compass needle that reacts to earth's magnetic field and measures movements in the horizontal plane.

- An inclination needle that is influenced by the force of gravity and measures movements in the frontal and sagittal planes.

- A scale on the container floor is marked in 2° increments.

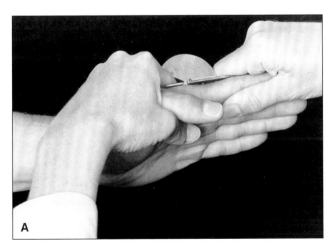

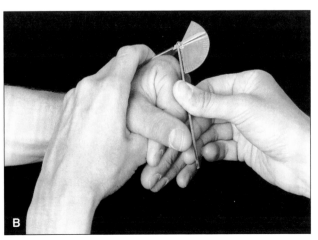

Figure 1-41 **A.** Start position (0°) for metacarpophalangeal (MCP) joint flexion with the universal goniometer placed over the dorsum of the MCP joint. **B.** End position: MCP flexion PROM (90°) with the goniometer aligned over the joint.

Two straps with Velcro fastenings are supplied to attach the goniometer to the body segment, and two plastic extension plates are also supplied to position the goniometer for certain joint measurements.[24] When using the OB goniometer, magnetic fields other than those of the earth will cause the OB goniometer compass needle to deviate and therefore must be avoided.

The *advantages* of using the OB goniometer for measuring joint ROM are as follows:

- It is not necessary to align the inclinometer with the joint axis.
- Rotational movements using a compass inclinometer are measured with ease.
- Assessment of trunk and neck ROM is measured with ease.
- There is little change in the alignment of the goniometer throughout the ROM.
- PROM is more easily assessed using the OB goniometer, as the therapist does not have to hold the goniometer and can stabilize the proximal joint segment with one hand and passively move the distal segment with the other.

The *disadvantages* of the OB goniometer are as follows:

- It is expensive and bulky compared to the universal goniometer.
- It cannot be used to measure the small joints of the hand and foot.
- Magnetic fields other than those of the earth will cause the compass needle to deviate and must be avoided.

OB "Myrin" Goniometer—Measurement Procedure

- *Velcro strap and/or plastic extension plate*: Apply the Velcro strap to the limb segment proximal or distal to the joint being assessed. Attach the appropriate plastic extension plate to the Velcro strap for some ROM measurements.

- *OB Goniometer*: Attach the goniometer container to the Velcro strap or the plastic extension plate. The goniometer is positioned in relation to bony landmarks and placed in the same location on successive measurements.[60]

- With the patient in the start position, rotate the fluid-filled container until the 0° arrow lines up directly underneath either the inclination needle, if the movement occurs in a vertical plane (i.e., the frontal or sagittal planes) (Fig. 1-42A), or the compass needle, if the movement occurs in the horizontal plane[24] (Fig. 1-43).

- Ensure that the needle is free to swing during the measurement.[24] Do not deviate the goniometer during the measurement by touching the strap or goniometer dial or by applying hand pressure to change the contour of the soft tissue mass near the OB goniometer.

- At the end of the AROM or PROM, the number of degrees the inclination needle (Fig. 1-42B) or the compass needle (Fig. 1-44) moves away from the 0° arrow on the compass dial is recorded as the joint ROM.

- The OB goniometer is especially useful for measuring forearm supination and pronation, tibial rotation, and hamstring and gastrocnemius muscle length. The ROM measurements of these movements are described and illustrated in this text as examples of how to apply the OB goniometer.

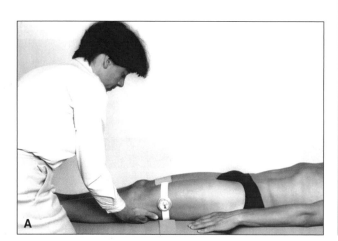
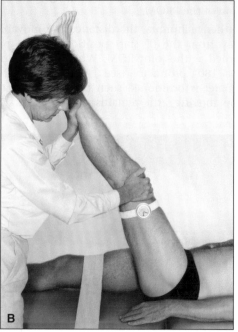

Figure 1-42 A. Start position: length of hamstrings utilizing the OB goniometer. **B.** End position: OB goniometer measurement of hip flexion angle, which indirectly represents the hamstrings length.

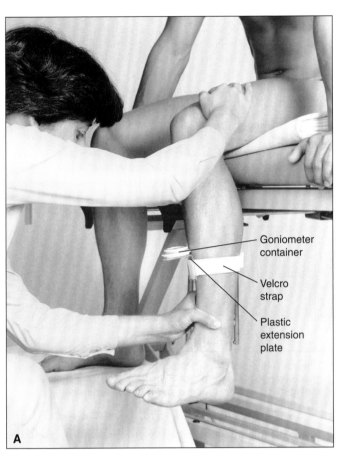

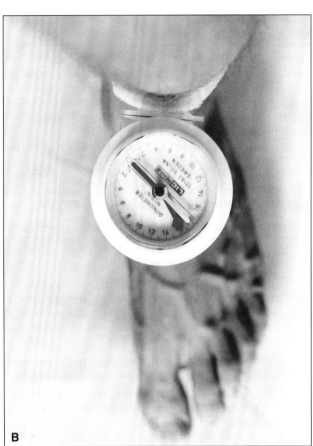

Goniometer
container

Velcro
strap

Plastic
extension
plate

A

B

Figure 1-43 **A and B.** Start position for total tibial rotation: tibial internal rotation.

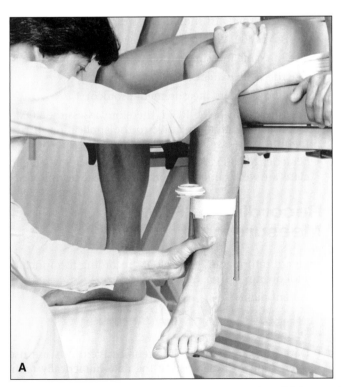

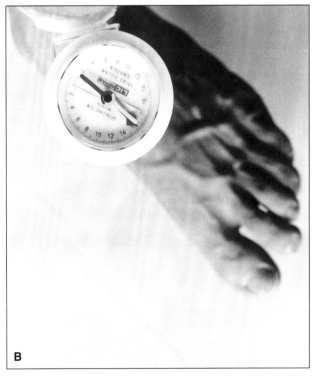

A

B

Figure 1-44 **A and B.** End position for total tibial rotation: tibial external rotation.

Assessing and Measuring Joint ROM with a Two- or Multi-Joint Muscle in the Region

If during the assessment of joint ROM the movement will lengthen or stretch a two- or multi-joint muscle, move the nontest joint crossed by the muscle into position so that the two-joint or multi-joint muscle is placed on slack. This prevents the muscle from becoming passively insufficient and restricting the assessed joint ROM.

Example: When the hip is flexed to assess hip flexion ROM (Fig. 1-45), the knee is positioned in flexion to place the two-joint hamstring muscles on slack and prevent restriction of the hip flexion ROM due to passive insufficiency of the hamstrings as illustrated in Figure 1-46.

Sources of Error in Measuring Joint ROM

Read the goniometer scale carefully to avoid erroneous ROM measurements. Sources of error to be avoided when measuring joint ROM are[61] the following:

- Reading the wrong side of the scale on the goniometer (e.g., when the goniometer pointer is positioned midway between 40° and 50°, reading the value of 55° rather than 45°).

- A tendency to read values that end in a particular digit, such as zero (i.e., "_0°").

- Having expectations of what the reading "should be" and allowing this to influence the recorded result. For example, the patient has been attending treatment for 2 weeks and the therapist expects and sees an improvement in the ROM that is not actually present.

- A change in the patient's motivation to perform.

- Taking successive ROM measurements at different times of the day.

- Measurement procedure error: Make sure sources of error do not occur or are minimized so that ROM measurements

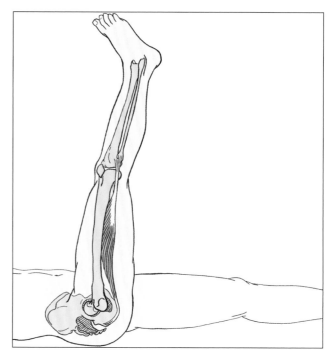

Figure 1-46 Passive insufficiency of the hamstring muscles. Hip flexion range of motion (ROM) is limited by the length of the hamstring muscles when the knee joint is held in extension.

are reliable and the patient's progress will be accurately monitored.

For reliable ROM measurements, the following are essential:

- The same therapist should assess the ROM.
- Assess the ROM at the same time each day.
- Use the same measuring tool.
- Use the same patient position.
- Follow a standard measurement protocol.[59]
- Treatment may affect ROM; therefore, assess the ROM in a consistent manner relative to the application of treatment techniques.
- "Practice Makes Perfect": reliability improves when clinicians are well trained and practiced in the techniques.

Recording of ROM Measurement

Standard information on an ROM recording form includes the following:

- Patient name
- Age
- Diagnosis
- Date of examination: Different conventions are used internationally when listing the date numerically (either day/month/year or month/day/year); to ensure clear communication when recording dates, write the month in full or abbreviated form, as shown in Figures 1-47 and 1-48
- Assessing therapist's name, signature, and credentials

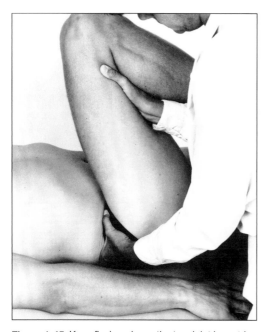

Figure 1-45 Knee flexion places the two-joint hamstring muscles on slack so that hip flexion range of motion (ROM) is not restricted by the length of the hamstrings.

RANGE OF MOTION MEASUREMENT

Patient's Name   *Jane Donner*   Age   *31*

Diagnosis   *# Ⓡ distal humeral shaft, depressed # Ⓡ tibial plateau*   Date of Onset   *July 10/20*

Therapist Name   *Tom Becker*   AROM or PROM   *PROM*

Signature   *T Becker BPT, MA*   Measurement Instrument

Recording:

1. The Neutral Zero Method defined by the American Academy of Orthopaedic Surgeons[1] is used for measurement and recording.
2. Average ranges defined by the American Academy of Orthopaedic Surgeons[1] are provided in parentheses.

3. The columns designated with asterisks (*) are used for indicating limitation of range of motion and referencing for summarization.
4. Space is left at the end of each section to record hypermobile ranges and comments regarding positioning of the patient or body part, edema, pain, and/or end feel.

Left Side					Right Side		
*	Oct 8/20	*	**Date of Measurement**	*	Oct 8/20	*	
			Shoulder Complex				
	0-180°		Elevation through flexion (0–180°)	*	0-160°		
	N		Elevation through abduction (0–180°)		N		
			Shoulder Glenhumeral Joint				
			Extension (0–60°)				
			Horizontal abduction (0–45°)				
			Horizontal adduction (0–135°)				
			Internal rotation (0–70°)				
	↓		External rotation (0–90°)		↓		
			Hypermobility:				
			Comments: *end feel: Ⓡ Shoulder flexion firm*				
			Elbow and Forearm				
	0-150°		Flexion (0–150°)	*	10-120°		
	N		Supination (0–80°)		N		
	↓		Pronation (0–80°)		↓		
			Hypermobility: Ⓛ elbow hyperextension 5°				
			Comments: *end feels: Ⓡ elbow extension firm; flexion firm*				
			Knee				
	0-135°		Flexion (0–135°)	*	0-75°		
	NT		Tibial rotation		NT		
			Hypermobility:				
			Comments: *end feel: Ⓡ knee flexion firm*				

Figure 1-47 Example of recording range of motion (ROM) using a numeric recording form.

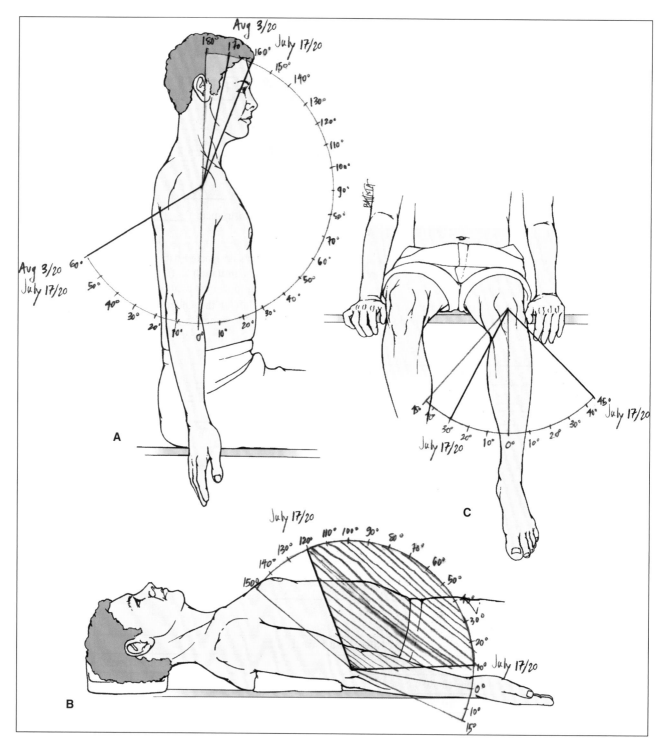

Figure 1-48 Examples of recording range of motion (ROM) using a pictorial recording form: **(A)** right shoulder flexion and extension, **(B)** left hip internal and external rotation, and **(C)** right elbow flexion and extension/hyperextension. The use of shading to show the available elbow flexion ROM is illustrated in **C**.

- Type of ROM being recorded, that is, AROM or PROM
- Type of goniometer or instrument used to measure the ROM.

Numerical or pictorial charts are used to record ROM. See Figure 1-47 and Appendix A for examples of a numerical recording form; Figure 1-48 gives examples of selected joint motion recordings from a pictorial recording form.

If the AROM and PROM are full, the joint ROM does not have to be measured with a goniometer or tape measure and the ROM may be recorded as full, normal (N), within normal limits (WNL), or numerically.

If the ROM is less than or greater than the normal ROM, the existing ROM is indicated on a pictorial chart or the number of degrees of motion is recorded on a numerical chart.

Every space on the ROM recording form should include an entry.[8] If the measurement was not performed, not tested (NT) should be entered and a line may be drawn from the first such entry to the end of several adjacent entries so that NT does not have to be recorded in every space.[8]

Any changes from the standard method of assessing joint ROM as presented in this text should be noted on the assessment form.

The ranges of motion are recorded on the *numerical chart* as follows (Fig. 1-47).

- When it is possible to begin the movement at the 0° start position, the ROM is recorded by writing the number of degrees the joint has moved away from 0°—for example, right shoulder elevation through flexion (i.e., shoulder flexion) 160° or 0°–160°, right knee flexion 75° or 0°–75°, right knee extension 0°.

- When it is not possible to begin the movement from the 0° start position, the ROM is recorded by writing the number of degrees the joint is away from 0° at the beginning of the ROM, followed by the number of degrees the joint is away from 0° at the end of the ROM—for example, the patient cannot achieve 0° right elbow extension due to a contracture (abnormal shortening) of the elbow flexor muscles; the end feel is firm. More specifically, the right elbow cannot be extended beyond 10° of elbow flexion and can be flexed to 120°. The ROM would be recorded as right elbow flexion 10°–120°.

- For a joint that is in a fixed position or ankylosed, this is recorded on the chart along with the fixed position of the joint.

On *pictorial charts* (Fig. 1-48), the therapist extends lines from the joint axis on the diagram to the appropriate number of degrees marked on the arc of movement at the start and end positions for the movement. The area between the two lines may be shaded in to provide a visual image of the ROM (see Fig. 1-48C). The date is recorded at the end of each line drawn to a degree marking on the arc of movement.

Figure 1-48 provides examples of ranges of motion recorded using a pictorial chart for the following:

- Right shoulder elevation through flexion (i.e., shoulder flexion) 160° or 0°–160° and right shoulder extension 60° or 0°–60° as assessed on July 17, 2020. The patient was reassessed on August 3, 2020, and the ROM for right shoulder elevation through flexion increased to 170° or 0°–170°, and there was no change in the ROM for right shoulder extension.

- The July 17, 2020 assessment of left hip external rotation of 30° or 0°–30° and left hip internal rotation of 45° or 0°–45°.

- Right elbow flexion 10°–120° assessed on July 17, 2020.

The *SFTR Method*[62] is a less commonly used method of recording joint ROM and is included here for completeness. The letters S, F, and T represent the plane of motion (sagittal, frontal, and transverse, respectively; see Fig. 1-13) of the joint ROM assessed; the R represents rotational motions. To record ROM, the letter identifying the plane of motion or rotational motion is noted. The letter is followed by three numbers that represent the start position, 0° with normal movement, and the ROM present on either side of the start position. The start position is recorded as the middle number. The ROM present on either side of the start position is recorded before and after the start position using the conventions indicated below.[62] If a joint is ankylosed, only two numbers are recorded, 0° and the joint position to either the right or left of 0° using the conventions.

Conventions and examples of recording ROM using the SFTR Method are as follows:

- Motion occurring in the S (i.e., sagittal plane) is extension and flexion. The number to the left of the start position represents extension ROM, and the number to the right represents flexion ROM.

Example: Shoulder left S: 60°–0°–180° right S: 60°–0°–80°.

Interpretation: Left shoulder ROM is WNL, with 60° extension and 180° shoulder elevation through flexion. Right shoulder extension is 60° and shoulder elevation through flexion 80°.

Example: Elbow left S: 0°–0°–150° right S: 0°–10°–120°.

Interpretation: The ROM recorded indicates motion in the sagittal plane. Left elbow ROM is WNL with a start position of 0°, 0° extension, and 150° flexion. Right elbow extension and flexion has a start position of 10°, elbow flexion is 10° to 120°, or right elbow flexion is 120°.

Example: Knee right S: 0°–15°.

Interpretation: The use of only two numbers indicates that the knee joint is ankylosed. The S indicates the ankylosed position is in the sagittal plane; therefore, the joint is in either an extended or flexed position. The number is to the right of the 0 and by convention represents flexion. Thus, the knee is ankylosed in 15° flexion.

Motion occurring in the F (i.e., frontal plane) is abduction and adduction. The number to the left of the start position represents abduction, eversion, or left spinal lateral flexion ROM, and the number to the right of the start position represents adduction, inversion, or right spinal lateral flexion ROM.

Example: Hip right F: 45°–0°–30°.

Interpretation: Right hip abduction is 45°, and adduction is 30°.

- Motion occurring in the T (i.e., transverse plane) is horizontal abduction and horizontal adduction, and retraction and protraction. The number to the left of the start position represents horizontal abduction or retraction ROM, and the number to the right of the start position represents horizontal adduction or protraction ROM.

Example: Shoulder left T(F90): 35°–0°–90°.

Interpretation: The (F90) following the T indicates frontal plane 90°, meaning the motions of horizontal abduction and adduction were performed with the left shoulder in a start position of 90° abduction. Left shoulder horizontal abduction is 35°, and horizontal adduction is 90°.

- An R indicates rotational motion. The number left of the start position represents external rotation, forearm supination, or spinal rotation to the left. The number right of the start position represents internal rotation, forearm pronation, or spinal rotation to the right.

Example: Hip right R(S90): 45°–0°–30°.

Interpretation: The (S90) after the R indicates that hip rotation was measured with the hip in the sagittal plane 90° (i.e., with the hip flexed 90°). Right hip external rotation ROM is 45°, and internal rotation is 30°.

Progress Guideline

If upper or lower extremity ROM is measured by the same therapist, a 3° or 4° increase in the ROM indicates improvement.[42] If different therapists measure the ROM, an increase of more than 5° for the upper extremity and 6° for the lower extremity would be needed to indicate progress.[42]

ASSESSMENT AND MEASUREMENT OF MUSCLE LENGTH

To assess and measure the length of a muscle, passively stretch (i.e., lengthen) the muscle across the joint(s) crossed by the muscle. When the muscle is on full stretch, the end feel will be firm, and the patient will report a pulling sensation or discomfort in the region of the muscle. Use a universal goniometer, inclinometer (e.g., OB goniometer), or tape measure to measure the PROM possible at the last joint moved to place the muscle on full stretch, or note any observed limitation in joint PROM due to muscle tightness. The PROM measurement indirectly represents the length of the shortened muscle. Retesting the joint PROM with the nontest joint(s) crossed by the muscle placed into position so that the two- or multi-joint muscle is on slack, will normally result in an increased PROM at the joint. Procedures used to assess and measure specific muscle length are described and illustrated for each joint complex in Chapters 3 through 9.

One-Joint Muscle

To assess and measure the length of a muscle that crosses one joint, the joint crossed by the muscle is positioned so that the muscle is lengthened across the joint. The position of the joint is measured, and this represents an indirect measure of the muscle length. The end feel will be firm.

Example: To assess and measure the length of the one-joint hip adductor muscles, stabilize the ipsilateral pelvis, and passively abduct the hip to the limit of range to place the hip adductors on stretch. If the hip adductor muscles limit the motion (Fig. 1-49A), the end feel will be firm. To measure the length of the hip adductor muscles, use a universal goniometer and measure the hip abduction PROM (Fig. 1-49B). This measurement serves as an indirect measurement of hip adductor muscle length.

Two-Joint Muscle

To assess and measure the length of a two-joint muscle, position one of the joints crossed by the muscle so as to lengthen the muscle across the joint. Then move the second joint crossed by the muscle, through a PROM until the muscle is placed on full stretch and prevents further joint motion. If the muscle is shortened, the end feel will be firm, the patient should feel a pulling sensation or discomfort over the stretched muscle. Assess and measure the final position of the second joint; the joint position represents an indirect measure of the muscle length.

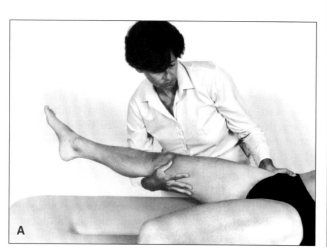

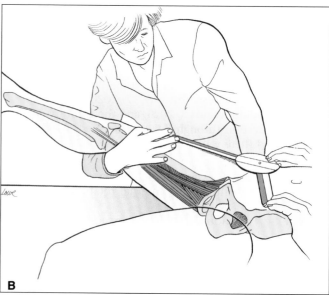

Figure 1-49 **A.** Hip abduction places the one-joint hip adductor muscles on stretch. **B.** Goniometer measurement: length of the hip adductors as the muscles limit hip abduction passive range of motion (PROM).

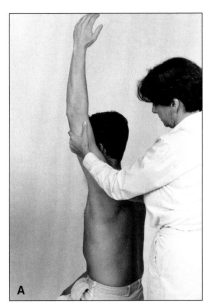
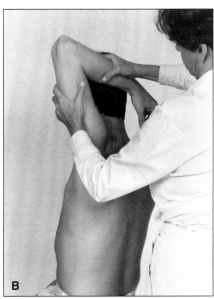
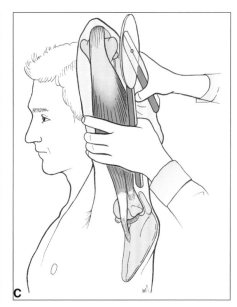

Figure 1-50 **A.** Start position: length of triceps, the muscle is stretched across the shoulder joint. **B.** The elbow is flexed to place triceps on full stretch. **C.** Goniometer measurement: length of the triceps as the muscle limits elbow flexion range of motion (ROM).

Example: To assess and measure the length of the two-joint triceps muscle, place the shoulder in full elevation to stretch the triceps across the shoulder joint, and stabilize the humerus (Fig. 1-50A). Then flex the elbow to place triceps on full stretch (Fig. 1-50B). If the triceps muscle limits the motion, the end feel will be firm. The elbow flexion PROM measured using a universal goniometer (Fig. 1-50C) indirectly represents the triceps muscle length.

Multi-Joint Muscle

To assess and measure the length of a multi-joint muscle, successively position all but one of the joints crossed by the muscle so that the muscle is lengthened across the joints. Then move the one remaining joint crossed by the muscle through a PROM, until the muscle is on full stretch and prevents further motion at the joint. Assess and measure the final position of the joint; the joint position represents an indirect measure of the muscle length.

Example: To assess and measure the length of the multi-joint finger flexor muscles, stabilize the humerus and forearm, successively place the elbow and fingers in full extension to stretch the muscles across these joints (Fig. 1-51A). Extend the wrist to place the flexors on full stretch (Fig. 1-51B and C). The end feel will be firm if the finger flexors limit wrist extension PROM. The end position of wrist extension PROM can be measured using a universal goniometer to indirectly represent the muscle length of the finger flexors.

PRACTICE MAKES PERFECT

Proficiency in assessing and measuring joint ROM and muscle length is gained through **PRACTICE**. It is important to practice the assessment and measurement techniques

on as many persons as possible to become familiar with the variation between individuals.

 Practice Makes Perfect

To aide you in practicing the Joint ROM and Muscle Length Assessment and Measurement skills covered in this textbook, or for a handy review, use the Practice Makes Perfect—Summary & Evaluation Forms found at http://thepoint.lww.com/ClarksonJM2e.

These Summary & Evaluation Forms list the criteria for each joint ROM and muscle length assessment and measurement technique in a chart/checklist format. These Forms serve as a valuable tool to promote proficiency in the clinical assessment and measurement techniques, allow for evaluation of student proficiency, and serve as a handy summary review of the techniques.

Practice Makes Perfect icons 🔵 and Form numbers appear next to clinical assessment and measurement techniques throughout Chapters 3 through 9 of the textbook to cross-reference the corresponding online Summary & Evaluation Forms.

FUNCTIONAL APPLICATION OF ASSESSMENT OF JOINT RANGE OF MOTION

Evaluation of functional activities, through task analysis and observation of the patient's performance in activities, can guide the therapist in proceeding with a detailed assessment

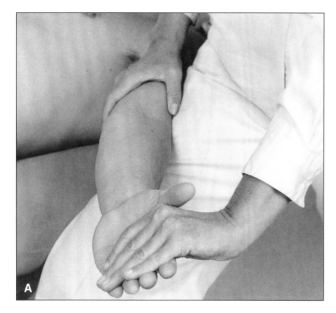

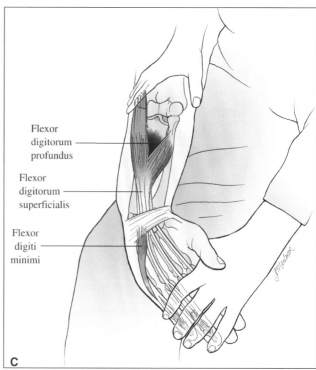

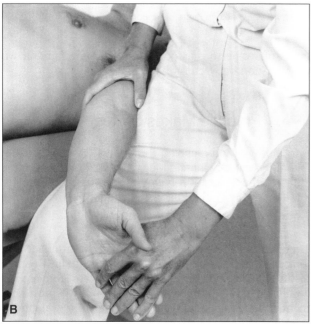

Figure 1-51 A. Start position: length of multi-joint finger flexors (i.e., flexor digitorum superficialis, flexor digitorum profundus, and flexor digiti minimi). Elbow and finger joint extension places the muscles on stretch across these joints. **B.** The wrist is extended to place the finger flexors on full stretch. **C.** The therapist observes the passive range of motion (PROM) and assesses a firm end feel at the limit of wrist extension PROM.

and provide objective and meaningful treatment goals. The therapist may ask the patient about his or her ability to perform activities. It is essential the therapist observes the patient performing the functional activities.[63] The patient is observed performing some functional activities, such as, walking, standing, dressing, sitting, and moving into different recumbent positions during the initial assessment.

Assessment of joint ROM is not performed in isolation of function. On completion of the evaluation of ROM, the therapist must consider the impact of deficit on the patient's daily life. Knowledge of functional anatomy of the musculoskeletal system is required to integrate the assessment findings into meaningful and practical treatment options. The knowledge of functional anatomy assists the therapist in gaining insight into the effect of joint ROM limitations in the patient's daily life.

The final section of each chapter is devoted to the functional application of assessment. The specific function of

the joint complex is described. The functional ROM at the joint is documented. Emphasis is placed on the ranges required for performance of daily activities. These ranges serve as guidelines, as the ranges required for a task may differ based on environmental factors, and the manner in which the task is completed.

The influence of environmental factors is illustrated when one sits in an arm chair versus an armless chair, to pull on a sock. In Figure 1-52A, the patient flexes the hip and knee in the sagittal plane to bring the foot close to pull on a sock. Without the restriction of chair arms (see Fig. 1-52B), the task is completed with quite different hip ROM requirements, that is, hip flexion, abduction, and external rotation.

The importance of observing the patient performing the functional activity is illustrated in the following example. Reaching for a wallet in one's back pocket and completing the activity in a normal manner is illustrated in Figure 1-53A. In Figure 1-53B, the patient presents

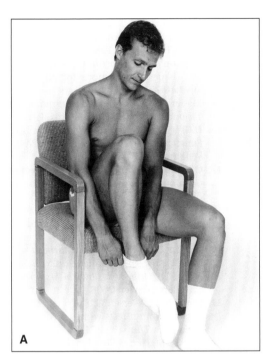
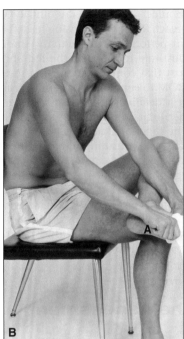

Figure 1-52 Environmental factors, such as style of chair **(A)** with or **(B)** without arms influences hip ROM requirements as one pulls on a sock.

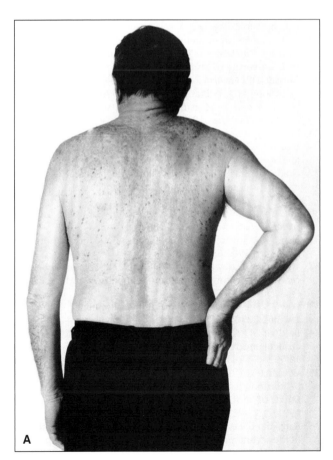
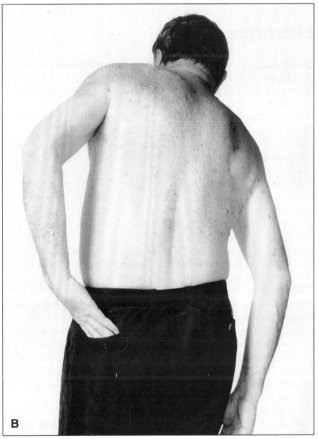

Figure 1-53 Reaching for a wallet in a back pocket completed with **(A)** normal ROM and **(B)** restricted shoulder glenohumeral joint ROM.

with restricted left shoulder glenohumeral joint ROM and reports being able to reach for his wallet using his left hand. Observing the patient performing this activity, the therapist takes note of substitute motions at the left shoulder girdle, trunk, and wrist that compensate for the restricted left shoulder joint PROM to enable the patient to reach for his wallet. Based on a detailed assessment that includes evaluation of shoulder joint ROM and observation of the patient performing the functional activity, the therapist is able to provide objective and meaningful goals and means of treatment.

Through knowledge of the ROM required in daily activities, the therapist can elicit relevant information from the assessments. The therapist correlates the assessment findings with the patient's ability to perform daily activities and, in conjunction with other physical assessment measures, plans an appropriate treatment plan to restore or maintain function.

Outline of the Assessment Process

"An Outline of the Assessment Process," located on the inside back cover of this text, serves as an overview of the assessment process and a review of some of the main points presented in this chapter.

References

1. Basmajian JV. *Surface Anatomy: An Instructional Manual*. Baltimore, MD: Williams & Wilkins; 1983.
2. Neumann DA. *Kinesiology of the Musculoskeletal System: Foundations for Rehabilitation*. St. Louis, MO: Mosby Elsevier; 2010.
3. Hollis M. *Safer Lifting for Patient Care*. 2nd ed. Oxford, England: Blackwell Scientific Publications; 1985.
4. MacConaill MA, Basmajian JV. *Muscles and Movements: A Basis for Human Kinesiology*. 2nd ed. New York, NY: Robert E. Krieger; 1977.
5. Kapandji IA. *The Physiology of the Joints. Vol. 1. The Upper Limb*. 6th ed. New York, NY: Churchill Livingstone; 2007.
6. Standring S, ed. *Gray's Anatomy: The Anatomical Basis of Clinical Practice*. 39th ed. London, UK: Elsevier Churchill Livingstone; 2005.
7. Stedman TL. *Stedman's Medical Dictionary for the Health Professions and Nursing*. 6th ed. Philadelphia, PA: Lippincott Williams & Wilkins; 2008.
8. Duesterhaus Minor MA, Duesterhaus Minor S. *Patient Evaluation Methods for the Health Professional*. Reston, VA: Reston Publishing; 1985.
9. Soderberg GL. *Kinesiology: Application to Pathological Motion*. 2nd ed. Baltimore, MD: Williams & Wilkins; 1997.
10. Perry J. Shoulder function for the activities of daily living. In: Matsen FA, Fu FH, Hawkins RJ, eds. *The Shoulder: A Balance of Mobility and Stability*. Rosemont, IL: American Academy of Orthopaedic Surgeons; 1993.
11. Kendall FP, McCreary EK, Provance PG, et al. *Muscles Testing and Function with Posture and Pain*. 5th ed. Baltimore, MD: Lippincott Williams & Wilkins; 2005.
12. Gowitzke BA, Milner M. *Understanding the Scientific Bases of Human Movement*. 2nd ed. Baltimore, MD: Williams & Wilkins; 1980.
13. Kaltenborn FM. *Mobilization of the Extremity Joints. Examination and Basic Treatment Techniques*. 3rd ed. Oslo, Norway: Olaf Norlis Bokhandel; 1985.
14. Lundon K, Hampson D. Acquired ectopic ossification of soft tissues: implications for physical therapy. *Can J Rehabil*. 1997;10:231-246.
15. Kisner C, Colby LA. *Therapeutic Exercise: Foundations and Techniques*. 5th ed. Philadelphia, PA: FA Davis; 2007.
16. Hall CM, Brody LT. *Therapeutic Exercise: Moving Toward Function*. 2nd ed. Philadelphia, PA: Lippincott Williams & Wilkins; 2005.
17. O' Connor P, Sforzo GA, Frye P. Effect of breathing instruction on blood pressure responses during isometric exercise. *Phys Ther*. 1989;69:55-59.
18. Cyriax J. *Textbook of Orthopaedic Medicine: Vol 1. Diagnosis of Soft Tissue Lesions*. 8th ed. London, UK: Bailliere Tindall; 1982.
19. Norkin CC, White DJ. *Measurement of Joint Motion: A Guide to Goniometry*. 4th ed. Philadelphia, PA: FA Davis; 2009.
20. Magee DJ. *Orthopedic Physical Assessment*. 5th ed. St. Louis, MO: Saunders Elsevier; 2008.
21. Hayes KW, Petersen C, Falconer J. An examination of Cyriax's passive motion tests with patients having osteoarthritis of the knee. *Phys Ther*. 1994;74:697-707.
22. Klassbo M, Harms-Ringdahl K. Examination of passive ROM and capsular patterns in the hip. *Physiother Res Int*. 2003;8:1-12.
23. Mitsch J, Casey J, McKinnis R, Kegerreis S, Stikeleather J. Investigation of a consistent pattern of motion restriction in patients with adhesive capsulitis. *J Man Manip Ther*. 2004;12:153-159.
24. *Instruction Manual: OB Goniometer "Myrin."* Available from OB Rehab, Solna, Sweden.
25. Performance Attainment Associates. *CROM Procedure Manual: Procedure for Measuring Neck Motion with the CROM*. St. Paul, MN: University of Minnesota; 1988.
26. Currier DP. *Elements of Research in Physical Therapy*. 3rd ed. Baltimore, MD: Williams & Wilkins; 1990.
27. Sim J, Arnell P. Measurement validity in physical therapy research. *Phys Ther*. 1993;73:48-56.
28. Miller PJ. Assessment of joint motion. In: Rothstein JM, ed. *Measurement in Physical Therapy*. New York, NY: Churchill Livingstone; 1985.
29. Gogia PP, Braatz JH, Rose SJ, Norton BJ. Reliability and validity of goniometric measurements at the knee. *Phys Ther*. 1987;67:192-195.
30. Enwemeka CS. Radiographic verification of knee goniometry. *Scand J Rehabil Med*. 1986;18:47-49.
31. Fish DR, Wingate L. Sources of goniometric error at the elbow. *Phys Ther*. 1985;65:1666-1670.
32. Youdas JW, Carey JR, Garrett TR. Reliability of measurements of cervical spine range of motion—comparison of three methods. *Phys Ther*. 1991;71:23-29.
33. Low J. The reliability of joint measurement. *Physiotherapy*. 1976;62:227-229.
34. Baldwin J, Cunningham K. Goniometry under attack: a clinical study involving physiotherapists. *Physiother Can*. 1974;26:74-76.
35. Watkins MA, Riddle DL, Lamb RL, Personius WJ. Reliability of goniometric measurements and visual estimates of knee range of motion obtained in a clinical setting. *Phys Ther*. 1991;71:15-22.
36. Banskota B, Lewis J, Hossain M, Irvine A, Jones MW. Estimation of the accuracy of joint mobility assessment in a group of health professionals. *Eur J Orthop Surg Traumatol*. 2008;18:287-289.
37. Lavernia C, D'Apuzzo M, Rossi MD, Lee D. Accuracy of knee range of motion assessment after total knee arthroplasty. *J Arthroplasty*. 2008;23(6 suppl 1):85-91.

38. Rachkidi R, Ghanem I, Kalouche I, et al. Is visual estimation of passive range of motion in the pediatric lower limb valid and reliable. *BMC Musculoskelet Disord.* 2009;10:126-135.

39. Bovens AMPM, van Baak MA, Vrencken JGPM, et al. Variability and reliability of joint measurements. *Am J Sports Med.* 1990;18:58-63.

40. Pandya S, Florence JM, King WM, et al. Reliability of goniometric measurements in patients with Duchenne muscular dystrophy. *Phys Ther.* 1985;65:1339-1342.

41. Elveru RA, Rothstein JM, Lamb RL. Goniometric reliability in a clinical setting: subtalar and ankle joint measurements. *Phys Ther.* 1988;68:672-677.

42. Boone DC, Azen SP, Lin C-M, et al. Reliability of goniometric measurements. *Phys Ther.* 1978;58:1355-1360.

43. Dijkstra PU, deBont LGM, van der Weele LTh, Boering G. Joint mobility measurements: reliability of a standardized method. *Cranio.* 1994;12:52-57.

44. Youdas JW, Bogard CL, Suman VJ. Reliability of goniometric measurements and visual estimates of ankle joint active range of motion obtained in a clinical setting. *Arch Phys Med Rehabil.* 1993;74:1113-1118.

45. Horger MM. The reliability of goniometric measurements of active and passive wrist motions. *Am J Occup Ther.* 1990;44:342-348.

46. Hellebrant FA, Duvall EN, Moore ML. The measurement of joint motion: Part III, reliability of goniometry. *Phys Ther Rev.* 1949;29:302-307.

47. Rothstein JM, Miller PJ, Roettger RF. Goniometric reliability in a clinical setting: elbow and knee measurements. *Phys Ther.* 1983;63:1611-1615.

48. Riddle DL, Rothstein JM, Lamb RL. Goniometric reliability in a clinical setting: shoulder measurements. *Phys Ther.* 1987;67:668-673.

49. Watkins B, Darrah J, Pain K. Reliability of passive ankle dorsiflexion measurements in children: comparison of universal and biplane goniometers. *Pediatr Phys Ther.* 1995;7:3-8.

50. Kilgour G, McNair P, Stott NS. Intrarater reliability of lower limb sagittal range-of-motion measures in children with spastic diplegia. *Dev Med Child Neurol.* 2003;45:385-390.

51. Stuberg WA, Fuchs RH, Miedaner JA. Reliability of goniometric measurements of children with cerebral palsy. *Dev Med Child Neurol.* 1988;30:657-666.

52. Ashton B, Pickles B, Roll JW. Reliability of goniometric measurements of hip motion in spastic cerebral palsy. *Dev Med Child Neurol.* 1978;20:87-94.

53. Harris SR, Smith LH, Krukowski L. Goniometric reliability for a child with spastic quadriplegia. *J Pediatr Orthop.* 1985;5:348-351.

54. Mutlu A, Livanelioglu A, Gunel MK. Reliability of goniometric measurements in children with spastic cerebral palsy. *Med Sci Monit.* 2007;13(7):CR323-CR329.

55. McWhirk LB, Glanzman AM. Within-session inter-rater reliability of goniometric measures in patients with spastic cerebral palsy. *Pediatr Phys Ther.* 2006;18(4):262-265.

56. ten Berge SR, Habertsma JPK, Maathius PGM, Verheij NP, Dijkstra PU, Maathuis KGB. Reliability of popliteal angle measurement: a study in cerebral palsy patients and healthy controls. *J Pediatr Orthop.* 2007;27(6):648-652.

57. American Academy of Orthopaedic Surgeons. *Joint Motion: Method of Measuring and Recording.* Chicago, IL: AAOS; 1965.

58. Berryman Reese N, Bandy WD. *Joint Range of Motion and Muscle Length Testing.* 2nd ed. St. Louis, MO: Saunders Elsevier; 2010.

59. Moore ML. Clinical assessment of joint motion. In: Basmajian JV, ed. *Therapeutic Exercise.* 4th ed. Baltimore, MD: Williams & Wilkins; 1984.

60. Ekstrand J, Wiktorsson M, Oberg B, Gillquist J. Lower extremity goniometric measurements: a study to determine their reliability. *Arch Phys Med Rehabil.* 1982;63:171-175.

61. Stratford P, Agostino V, Brazeau C, Gowitzke BA. Reliability of joint angle measurement: a discussion of methodology issues. *Physiother Can.* 1984;36:5-9.

62. Gerhardt JJ, Cocchiarella L, Randall LD. *The Practical Guide to Range of Motion Assessment.* Chicago, IL: American Medical Association; 2002.

63. Smith LK. Functional tests. *Phys Ther Rev.* 1954;34:19-21.

EXERCISES AND QUESTIONS

See the Answer Guide in Appendix E for suggested answers to the following exercises and questions.

1. JOINT MOVEMENTS

Define the following movements and identify the opposite movement. Starting from anatomical position, demonstrate each movement and the opposite movement at one joint. Identify the plane and axis of each movement.

   i.   Flexion
   ii. Abduction
   iii. Internal rotation
   iv. Lateral flexion
   v.   Horizontal adduction

2. OSTEOKINEMATICS AND ARTHROKINEMATICS

A. Define the terms *osteokinematics* and *arthrokinematics*.
B. Explain how a therapist applies osteokinematics and arthrokinematics when assessing restricted knee flexion PROM.

3. CONTRAINDICATIONS AND PRECAUTIONS FOR ROM ASSESSMENT

A. When are AROM and PROM assessment techniques contraindicated?
B. Case: Mrs. Smith, a frail 76 year-old, was involved in a car accident and suffered a fracture of the midshaft of her left humerus. She is just out of cast and is referred for physical therapy. On her initial visit, Mrs. Smith appears to be slightly intoxicated and protects her left upper extremity. Would the therapist assess Mrs. Smith's ROM? Explain.

4. THE RATIONALE FOR THE ASSESSMENT OF AROM AND PROM

A. Case: Mr. Fitzgerald, a 30 year-old teacher, suffered a fracture of his right distal femur. The femoral fracture is now well united. The therapist assesses the AROM of Mr. Fitzgerald's lower extremities with the patient high sitting (i.e., sitting on a plinth with his feet off the ground). The therapist assesses and measures all AROM of the lower extremities and finds all AROM to be normal bilaterally except for the following right knee and ankle AROM:

AROM	Left	Right
Knee flexion	135°	60° (R knee pain)
Knee extension	0°	20° flexion
Ankle dorsiflexion	20°	0°

   i.   When measuring joint ROM using the neutral zero method, identify the defined zero positions for measuring knee and ankle ROM.
   ii. Assume the high sitting position and demonstrate the following:
        a. Mr. Fitzgerald's left knee AROM

           Identify any two- or multi-joint muscle(s) in the region that could restrict knee AROM with Mr. Fitzgerald in the high sitting position. Explain why the muscle(s) would restrict the ROM. Identify an alternate start position that could be used for the assessment of Mr. Fitzgerald's left knee AROM that would eliminate any two- or multi-joint muscle(s) identified above from restricting knee ROM.
        b. Mr. Fitzgerald's right knee AROM
   iii. What information can the therapist gather from an assessment of Mr. Fitzgerald's AROM?

iv. From the AROM assessment, can the therapist determine the reason for Mr. Fitzgerald's decreased right knee and ankle AROM? Explain.

v. Explain why the therapist would go on to assess Mr. Fitzgerald's PROM.

B. The therapist assesses Mr. Fitzgerald's PROM and finds all PROM of the lower extremities to be normal bilaterally except for the following right knee and ankle PROM:

PROM	Left	Right
Knee flexion	135° soft end feel	60° empty end feel (pain R knee)
Knee extension	0° firm end feel	0° firm end feel
Ankle dorsiflexion	20° firm end feel	5° firm end feel (pulling sensation over calf muscles)

Comparing only the AROM and PROM findings, what could the therapist conclude regarding Mr. Fitzgerald's right knee and ankle?

5. ASSESSMENT AND MEASUREMENT OF AROM AND PROM USING THE UNIVERSAL GONIOMETER

The following exercises are designed to facilitate learning of the AROM and PROM assessment and measurement process. The assessment and measurement of elbow flexion and extension/hyperextension serve as an example of the process as described and illustrated on pages 100 and 101.

Working in a group of three persons:

- One person, having normal elbow joints (i.e., no history of pathology/injury), serves as the patient.
- The second person is the therapist, who carries out the assessment and measurement of AROM and PROM.
- The third person assists the therapist by reading the instructions below and the description of the assessment and measurement of elbow flexion–extension/hyperextension on pages 100 and 101 to guide the therapist through the assessment and measurement process.

Before beginning the assessment and measurement of AROM and/or PROM, the therapist:

- Tells the patient about the assessment and measurement process and may demonstrate the movement(s) to be performed to the patient.
- Explains the need to expose the area to be assessed and drapes the patient as required.

A. _Demonstrate assessment of AROM_ for elbow flexion and extension/hyperextension.

i. Whenever possible, observe the AROM by having the patient perform the movements bilaterally and symmetrically. Ask the patient to communicate any pain or other symptoms during the performance of the test movements.

Start position. The patient is sitting on a chair or stool with the arms hanging by the side with the shoulder, elbow, and forearm in anatomical position.

Stabilization. The patient is instructed to sit up straight, keep the upper arms in at his or her sides, and move only the forearms and hands.

End positions. Flexion—The patient is instructed, "Bend your elbows to bring the palms of your hands towards your shoulders as far as you can." Extension/Hyperextension—The patient is instructed, "Straighten your elbows as far as you can." The therapist may also demonstrate these movements to the patient.

The therapist observes the AROM to determine:

- The patient's willingness to move and ability to follow directions, perform well-coordinated movement, and move the part through the full AROM.
- Movement(s) that cause or increase pain.

ii. All three persons in the group can perform the following exercise.

- Assume the start position for the assessment of elbow flexion AROM as described above.
- Next, position your elbow in 90° flexion and assume this is as far as you can actively flex your elbow.
- Without allowing further elbow flexion, try to give the appearance that your elbow flexion is greater than 90° ROM.

a) What substitute movement(s) did you use to give the appearance of a greater AROM than was actually possible?

b) Substitute movement(s) should be avoided when performing the assessment and measurement of AROM. How can this be accomplished?

c) Assume the supine position and repeat the above exercise. Did the change in position affect the substitute movement(s) possible when performing elbow flexion AROM? Explain.

B. *Demonstrate measurement of AROM* for elbow flexion and extension/hyperextension using the universal goniometer.

Start position. The patient is sitting on a chair or stool with the arms hanging by the side in anatomical position. The goniometer is aligned at the start position of 0°.

Goniometer alignment. The goniometer alignment for AROM is the same as that for the measurement of PROM as described and illustrated on pages 100 and 101. The anatomical landmarks required for the alignment of the goniometer are described and illustrated on page 99.

Stabilization. The patient is instructed to sit up straight, keep the upper arms in at his or her sides, and move only the forearms and hands.

End positions. Flexion—The patient is instructed, "Bend your elbows to bring the palms of your hands towards your shoulders as far as you can." Extension/hyperextension—The patient is instructed, "Straighten your elbows as far as you can." The therapist may also demonstrate the above movements to the patient.

As the patient moves through the AROM, the goniometer is either moved through the range along with the limb to the end of the AROM or realigned at the end of the movement. The ROM, in degrees, is read from the goniometer at the end of the AROM and recorded.

C. *Demonstrate assessment of PROM* for elbow flexion and extension/hyperextension.

• Assess the PROM carefully and slowly.

• Ask the patient to communicate any pain or other symptoms during the test movements.

• Reassure the patient that you will stop the movement at any time if there is pain.

The patient must be relaxed during the assessment of PROM, but it is often difficult for the patient to relax. Tell the patient, "Relax, and let me do all the work to move your arm." If the patient continues to have difficulty relaxing, support the forearm and hand and instruct the patient to, "Let your arm drop into my hand so that I can feel the whole weight of your arm." When performing passive elbow flexion, instruct the patient, "Relax while I bring your hand toward your shoulder." When performing passive elbow extension/hyperextension, instruct the patient to, "Relax while I straighten your elbow."

Refer to pages 100 and 101 and follow the description and illustrations to demonstrate the assessment of PROM. The therapist:

• Observes the amount of movement possible at the joint.

• Determines the quality of movement throughout the PROM.

• Notes the presence or absence of pain.

• Assesses and records the end feels.

D. *Demonstrate measurement of PROM* for elbow flexion and extension/hyperextension using the universal goniometer. Refer to pages 100 and 101 and follow the description and illustrations to demonstrate and record the measurement of PROM.

E. When carrying out the assessment/measurement procedures, did the therapist:

• Ensure the patient was comfortable and well supported?

• Communicate well with the patient?

• Assume an appropriate position and stance, and appear comfortable (see Fig. 1-1)?

• Adequately stabilize the humerus (i.e., proximal joint segment)?

After completion of the above exercises, change roles and repeat the exercises.

6. VALIDITY AND RELIABILITY—UNIVERSAL GONIOMETER

A. Define the terms *validity* and *reliability*.

B. Explain how the therapist would best obtain reliable joint ROM measurements using the universal goniometer.

7. ASSESSMENT AND MEASUREMENT OF MUSCLE LENGTH

Work in a group of three as described in Exercise 5 above. Before beginning an assessment and measurement of muscle length, the therapist:

- Tells the patient about the assessment and measurement process and demonstrates the movement(s) to be performed.
- Explains the need to expose the area to be assessed and drapes the patient as required.

Refer to pages 189 and 190 and follow the description and illustrations to demonstrate the assessment and measurement of muscle length using the hamstrings as an example. The person serving as the patient should have normal back and hip joints (i.e., no history of pathology or injury in these regions).

8. USING THE OB "MYRIN" GONIOMETER TO MEASURE JOINT ROM

A. Briefly describe the OB "Myrin" goniometer, a compass/inclinometer, and explain how it is applied to measure joint ROM.

B. Identify the advantages and disadvantages of using the OB "Myrin" goniometer compared to the universal goniometer to measure joint ROM.

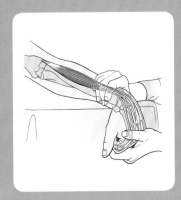

Relating Assessment to Treatment

2

Chapter Rationale

- Although the guidelines for diagnosis and treatment protocols are beyond the scope of this text, this chapter links the techniques used to assess active range of motion (AROM), passive range of motion (PROM), and muscle length with the techniques used for treatment.

- Through illustration and description, the reader is provided with an overview of the similarities and differences between clinical assessments presented in this textbook and complementary treatments.

- Knowing the similarities between assessment and treatment, and using the knowledge and skills for assessing AROM, PROM, and muscle length, the reader will be able to utilize similar techniques for treatments using active or passive movement.

- Understanding the link between assessment and treatment is essential for the reader to be able to integrate patient assessment and treatment in the clinical setting.

Optional learning approach: Should the reader prefer to learn the assessment techniques presented in this text prior to considering how assessment and treatment techniques are related, then this chapter would be considered the final chapter of this text.

SIMILAR ASSESSMENT AND TREATMENT METHODS

Similar assessments and treatments are categorized according to the type of movement used (i.e., active or passive movement, as set out in Table 2-1).

KEY STEPS WHEN APPLYING ASSESSMENTS AND TREATMENTS

The key steps used when applying assessments and treatments are listed in order in the first column of Table 2-1. These steps are set out in detail for assessment in Chapter 1 and are summarized here and in Table 2-1 to compare with those for treatment.

Purpose

The therapist performs an assessment to evaluate how an injury or disease affects the patient's status. Treatment, if appropriate, is then used to eliminate or lessen the effects of an injury or disease. Assessment is repeated as required to evaluate the outcome of treatment.

Common Technique

Technique is the same when using active or passive movement for similar assessment and treatment.

Explanation and Instruction

Before carrying out an assessment or treatment, explain the assessment or treatment to the patient and obtain the patient's informed consent. When applying a specific assessment or treatment for the first time, explain and/or demonstrate the movement to be performed and/or ask the patient to relax and passively move the patient's limb through the movement.

Expose Region

For assessment and treatment, expose the area to be assessed or treated and drape the patient as required.

Start Position

For assessment and treatment, ensure the patient is in a safe, comfortable position and is adequately supported. When positioning the patient, the effect of gravity on the movement may be relevant.

Stabilization

For assessment and treatment, provide adequate stabilization to ensure only the required movement occurs. For assessment and treatment, perform either of the following:

(a) The proximal joint segment or site of attachment of the origin of the muscle(s) is(are) stabilized.

(b) The distal joint segment or site of insertion of the muscle(s) is(are) stabilized.

Movement

For assessment and treatment, either of the following should be performed:

TABLE 2-1 Comparing of Assessment and Treatment

Key Steps	Active Movement		Passive Movement			
	Assessment	Treatment	Assessment	Treatment	Assessment	Treatment
	Active ROM (AROM)	*Active Exercise*	*Passive ROM (PROM)*	*Relaxed Passive Movement*	*Muscle Length*	*Prolonged Passive Stretch*
PURPOSE	Assessment of: • AROM • Muscle strength (grades 0–3) • Ability to perform ADL	Treatment to maintain/ increase: • Joint ROM • Muscle strength • Ability to perform ADL	Assessment of: • Joint PROM • End feel	Treatment to maintain/ increase: • Joint ROM	Assessment of: • Muscle length	Treatment to maintain/ increase: • Muscle length

COMMON TECHNIQUE

Key Steps						
Explanation/ Instruction	←———————— Verbal (clear, concise), demonstration and/or passive movement ————————→					
Expose Area	←———————————— Expose area and drape as required ————————————→					
Start Position	• Safe, comfortable, adequate support • Consider effect of gravity		• Safe, comfortable, adequate support, relaxed			
Stabilization*	• Proximal joint segment(s) • Muscle origin(s)		• Proximal joint segment(s)		• Muscle origin(s)	
Movement*	• Distal joint segment(s)		• Distal joint segment(s)		• Joint(s) crossed by muscle(s)	
Assistance	n/a		• Assistance applied at distal end of distal joint segment(s)		• Assistance applied at distal end of segment(s) muscle(s) inserts into	
End Position	• End of full or available AROM		• End of full available PROM		• Muscle(s) on full stretch	
Substitute Movement	←———————————— Ensure no substitute movement ————————————→					
PURPOSE-SPECIFIC PROCEDURE	• Estimate and/or measure AROM • Determine the presence of muscle contraction and the AROM when moving without (i.e., for grades of 0 to 2) and/or against the force of gravity (i.e., for grades of 2+, 3– or 3).	• Active movement performed according to exercise prescription	• Observe and/ or measure joint PROM • Note end feel	• Passive movement performed according to treatment prescription	• Visually observe and/ or measure joint position at maximum stretch of muscle • Note end feel	• Joint held at position of maximal muscle stretch for prescribed length of time
CHARTING	• Joint AROM • MMT grade	• Describe exercise prescribed • Note any change in patient's condition	• Joint PROM • End feel	• Describe treatment prescribed • Note any change in patient's con-dition	• Joint position • End feel	• Describe position and duration of stretch • Note any change in pa-tient's condition

NOTE: The area shaded in orange highlights COMMON TECHNIQUE that is the same for similar assessment and treatment.

*For ease of explanation and understanding, the proximal joint segment or site of attachment of the muscle origin is stabilized and the distal joint segment or site of attachment of the muscle insertion is described as the moving segment.

ADL, activities of daily living.

(a) The distal joint segment or site of attachment of the insertion of the muscle(s) is(are) moved.

(b) The proximal joint segment or site of origin of the muscle(s) is(are) moved.

Assistance

For passive movements used in assessment and treatment, assistance is normally applied at the distal end of either the distal joint segment or the segment into which the muscle(s) is(are) inserted.

End Position

For assessment and treatment, either instruct the patient to move the body segment(s) (for active movement) or passively move the limb segment(s) (for passive movement) through either a selected part of or the full ROM possible. For prolonged passive stretch, the therapist passively moves the body segment(s) to the point in the ROM that provides maximal stretch of the muscle(s).

Substitute Movement

For assessment and treatment, ensure there are no substitute movements that may exaggerate the actual joint ROM and/or muscle strength or interfere with the patient's capacity to perform an exercise. To avoid unwanted movements, explain/demonstrate to the patient how the movement is to be performed and the substitute movements to be avoided. Pay attention to positioning and stabilizing the patient. Experience and careful observation enable the therapist to prevent substitute movements and detect any that may occur.

Purpose-Specific Procedure

After applying the "common technique," specific procedure is used to provide outcomes that meet the specific purpose of the assessment or treatment technique. Purpose-specific assessment procedures include observing and/or measuring the AROM or PROM, and noting the end feel for PROM, or grading muscle strength for AROM. Purpose-specific treatment procedures normally follow a specific treatment prescription that may include changing the number of times a movement is performed, changing the length of time a position is held, and/or changing the magnitude of the resistance used.

Charting

For assessment, deviations from standardized testing procedure and the findings are noted in the chart. For treatment, details of the exercise or treatment prescription used and any change in the patient's condition are noted in the chart.

EXAMPLES OF SIMILAR ASSESSMENT AND TREATMENT METHODS

Specific joint movements and muscles are used as examples to illustrate similar assessments and treatments using active, passive, or resisted movement.

In the examples, note that for assessment and treatment, which use a similar type of movement, the "common technique" is the same, but the "purpose," "purpose-specific procedure," and "charting" are different.

In Table 2-1 and in these examples, for ease of explanation and understanding, the proximal joint segment or site of attachment of the origin of the muscle is stabilized, and the distal joint segment or site of attachment of the insertion of the muscle is described as the moving segment.

Knee Extension*: Active Range of Motion (AROM) Assessment and Treatment Using Active Exercise

Assessment AROM	Treatment Active Exercise
PURPOSE To assess AROM and quadriceps muscle strength and determine the ability to perform ADL.	**PURPOSE** To maintain or increase AROM, quadriceps muscle strength, and the ability to perform ADL.

COMMON TECHNIQUE

Explanation/Instruction. The therapist explains, demonstrates, and/or passively moves the limb through knee extension. The therapist instructs the patient to straighten the knee as far as possible.

Expose Region. The patient wears shorts.

Start Position. The patient is sitting, grasps the edge of the plinth, and has the nontest foot supported on a stool (Fig. 2-1).

Stabilization. The patient is instructed to maintain the thigh in the start position or the therapist may stabilize the thigh.

Movement. The patient performs knee extension.

End Position. The knee is extended as far as possible through the ROM (Fig. 2-2). The hamstrings may restrict knee extension in this position.

Substitute Movement. The patient leans back to posteriorly tilt the pelvis and extend the hip joint.

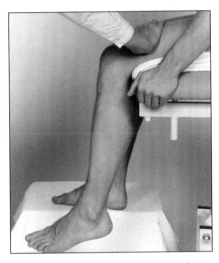

Figure 2-1 Start position knee extension: AROM assessment and active exercise.

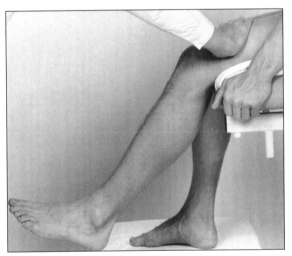

Figure 2-2 End position: AROM assessment and active exercise. The therapist may stabilize the femur and/or palpate for contraction of the knee extensors.

PURPOSE-SPECIFIC PROCEDURE

AROM is visually assessed or measured using the universal goniometer. Following the assessment of PROM, the therapist grades the strength of the knee extensors using AROM.

PURPOSE-SPECIFIC PROCEDURE

Knee extension is performed actively by the patient a predetermined number of times according to the exercise prescription.

CHARTING

Knee extension AROM is recorded in degrees and/or the knee extensors are assigned a grade for strength.

CHARTING

The prescribed exercise is described, and any change in the patient's condition is noted.

Note: Movement performed with gravity eliminated could also be used to illustrate the similarity between AROM assessment and active exercise.

*To show an example of movement performed against gravity.

Hip Flexion: Passive Range of Motion (PROM) Assessment and Treatment Using Relaxed Passive Movement

Assessment **PROM**	Treatment **Relaxed Passive Movement**
PURPOSE To assess hip flexion PROM and determine an end feel.	**PURPOSE** To maintain or increase hip flexion ROM.

COMMON TECHNIQUE

Explanation/Instruction. The therapist explains, demonstrates, and/or passively moves the limb through hip flexion. The therapist instructs the patient to relax as the movement is performed.

Expose Region. The patient wears shorts and is draped as required.

Start Position. The patient is supine. The hip and knee on the test side are in the neutral position. The other hip is extended on the plinth (Fig. 2-3).

Stabilization. The therapist stabilizes the pelvis. The trunk is stabilized through body positioning.

Movement. The therapist raises the lower extremity off the plinth and moves the femur anteriorly to flex the hip.

End Position. The femur is moved to the limit of hip flexion (Fig. 2-4).

Substitute Movement. Posterior pelvic tilt and flexion of the lumbar spine.

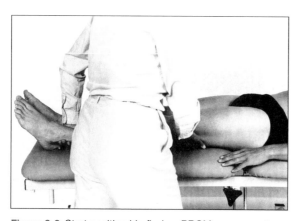

Figure 2-3 Start position hip flexion: PROM assessment and relaxed passive movement.

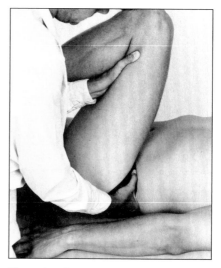

Figure 2-4 End position hip flexion: PROM assessment and relaxed passive movement.

PURPOSE-SPECIFIC PROCEDURE

The therapist applies slight overpressure at the end of the PROM to identify the end feel. The therapist observes and measures the joint PROM.

CHARTING

The end feel and number of degrees of hip flexion PROM are recorded.

PURPOSE-SPECIFIC PROCEDURE

The hip is passively moved into flexion a predetermined number of times according to the treatment prescription.

CHARTING

The prescribed treatment is described, and any change in the patient's condition is noted.

Long Finger Extensors: Muscle Length Assessment and Treatment Using Prolonged Passive Stretch

Assessment Muscle Length	Treatment Prolonged Passive Stretch
PURPOSE To assess the length of the long finger extensor muscles.	**PURPOSE** To maintain or increase the length of the long finger extensor muscles.

COMMON TECHNIQUE

Explanation/Instruction. The therapist explains, demonstrates, and/or passively positions the patient in the stretch position. The therapist instructs the patient to relax as the movement is performed and held.

Expose Region. The patient wears short-sleeved shirt.

Start Position. The patient is sitting. The elbow is extended, the forearm is pronated, and the fingers are flexed (Fig. 2-5).

Stabilization. The therapist stabilizes the radius and ulna.

Movement. The therapist flexes the wrist.

End Position. The wrist is flexed to the limit of motion so that the long finger extensors are fully stretched (Figs. 2-6 and 2-7).

Substitute Movement. Finger extension.

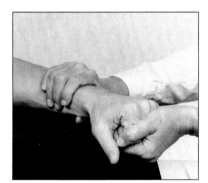

Figure 2-5 Start position long finger extensors: muscle length assessment and prolonged passive stretch.

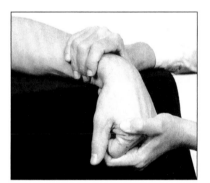

Figure 2-6 End position long finger extensors on stretch: muscle length assessment and prolonged passive stretch.

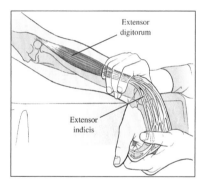

Figure 2-7 Long finger extensors on stretch.

PURPOSE-SPECIFIC PROCEDURE

With the long finger extensors on full stretch, the angle of wrist flexion is observed and/or measured, and the therapist identifies the end feel.

CHARTING

The long finger extensors may be described as being shortened, and the angle of wrist flexion may be recorded. The end feel is noted.

PURPOSE-SPECIFIC PROCEDURE

The position of maximum wrist flexion is maintained so that the long finger extensors are placed on full stretch for a prescribed length of time, and the therapist identifies the end feel.

CHARTING

The stretch position and the length of time the stretch is applied to the long finger extensors are recorded. Any change in the patient's condition is noted.

EXERCISES AND QUESTIONS

See the Answer Guide in Appendix E for suggested answers to the following exercises and questions.

1. LIST THE KEY STEPS USED TO APPLY THE SIMILAR ASSESSMENTS AND TREATMENTS THAT USE ACTIVE AND PASSIVE MOVEMENTS.

2. DESCRIBE THE FUNDAMENTAL DIFFERENCE BETWEEN ASSESSMENT AND TREATMENT.

3. IDENTIFY THE KEY STEPS THAT ARE THE SAME AND THE KEY STEPS THAT ARE DIFFERENT WHEN APPLYING SIMILAR ASSESSMENTS AND TREATMENTS.

4. IDENTIFY THE TREATMENTS THAT ARE SIMILAR TO THE FOLLOWING ASSESSMENTS:

A. Active ROM (AROM): _____

B. Passive ROM (PROM): _____

C. Muscle length: _____

5. ASSESSMENT FINDING: SHORTENED HIP ADDUCTORS

A. Identify the assessment a therapist used to assess this muscle length deficiency.

B. Identify the treatment that is similar to the assessment identified in 5.A. and would be used to treat the shortened muscle.

C. Demonstrate the general procedure for the treatment identified in 5.B. that would be used to lengthen the hip adductors.

6. ASSESSMENT FINDING: HIP MUSCLE PARALYSIS, DECREASED HIP FLEXION PROM WITH SOFT END FEEL

A. Identify the assessment the therapist used to assess this PROM deficiency.

B. Identify the treatment that is similar to the assessment identified in 6.A. and would be used to maintain hip flexion ROM.

C. Demonstrate the general procedure for the treatment identified in 6.B. that would be used to maintain the hip flexion PROM.

7. ASSESSMENT FINDING: DECREASED ELBOW FLEXION AROM

A. Identify the assessment the therapist used to assess this AROM deficiency.

B. Identify the treatment that is similar to the assessment identified in 7.A. and would be used to maintain or increase elbow flexion AROM.

C. Demonstrate the general procedure for the treatment identified in 7.B. that would be used to maintain or increase the elbow flexion AROM.

SECTION II

Regional Evaluation Techniques

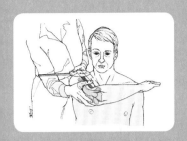

Shoulder Complex 3

ARTICULATIONS AND MOVEMENTS

The *shoulder complex* is a related group of articulations. This group of articulations (Fig. 3-1) includes the sternoclavicular, acromioclavicular, scapulothoracic, and glenohumeral joints. The shoulder complex can be subdivided into two main components:

a. The *shoulder girdle*, which includes the sternoclavicular, acromioclavicular, and scapulothoracic joints

b. The shoulder joint, that is, the *glenohumeral joint.*

The Shoulder Girdle

The shoulder girdle is connected directly to the trunk via the *sternoclavicular joint.* The medial end of the clavicle forms the lateral sternoclavicular joint surface, and the lateral aspect of the manubrium sternum and adjacent superior surface of the first costal cartilage make up the medial joint surface. An articular disc lies between the articular surfaces. Categorized as a saddle joint, the clavicular surface of

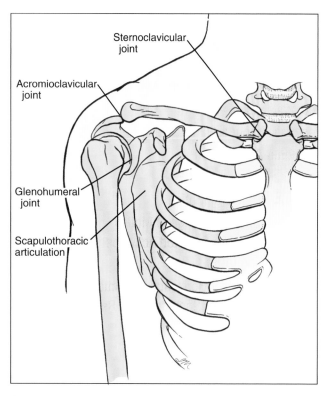

Figure 3-1 Shoulder complex articulations.

the joint is convex vertically and concave horizontally, and articulates with the reciprocal surfaces on the medial aspect of the joint.[1]

Movements at the sternoclavicular joint include elevation, depression, protraction, retraction, and rotation of the clavicle. During elevation and depression, the lateral end of the clavicle moves superiorly and inferiorly, respectively, in the frontal plane around a sagittal axis. The lateral end of the clavicle moves in an anterior direction with protraction and in a posterior direction with retraction. Protraction and retraction movements of the clavicle occur in a horizontal plane about a vertical axis. Rotation of the clavicle takes place in a sagittal plane around a frontal axis (i.e., an axis that passes along the long axis of the clavicle). Mobility at the sternoclavicular joint is requisite for the clavicular and scapular motion essential to the normal performance of shoulder elevation (i.e., movement of the arm above shoulder level to a vertical position alongside the head).

The *acromioclavicular joint*, linking the clavicle and scapula, is classified as a plane joint formed by the relatively flat articular surfaces of the lateral end of the clavicle and the acromion process of the scapula. In some instances, the joint surfaces are partially separated by an articular disc.[1] At the acromioclavicular joint, limited gliding motions between the clavicle and scapula during shoulder girdle movement allow scapular motion independent of clavicular motion, and alignment of the scapula against the chest wall.[2]

A physiological or functional joint, the *scapulothoracic joint* consists of flexible soft tissues (i.e., subscapularis and serratus anterior) sandwiched between the scapula and the chest wall that allow the scapula to move over the thorax. Scapular motions are accompanied by movement of the clavicle via the acromioclavicular joint.

Scapular motions include elevation, depression, retraction, protraction, lateral (upward) rotation, and medial (downward) rotation. Movement of the scapula in a cranial direction is called elevation and is accompanied by elevation of the clavicle. The scapula and clavicle move in a caudal direction with scapular depression. Scapular retraction and protraction occur in the horizontal plane around a vertical axis as the medial border of the scapula moves either toward (retraction) or away from (protraction) the vertebral column. Scapular retraction and protraction are accompanied by retraction and protraction of the clavicle, respectively. The scapula also rotates laterally and medially, with reference to the movement of the inferior angle, so that the glenoid cavity moves in either an upward (cranial) or a downward (caudal) direction, respectively (Fig. 3-2).

In the clinical setting, motion at the sternoclavicular joint and scapula is not easily measured, and it is not possible to measure motion at the acromioclavicular joint. Therefore,

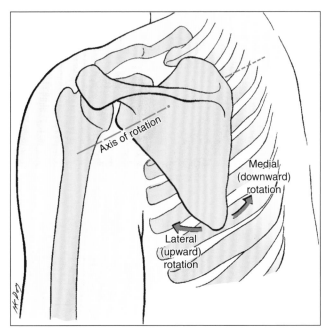

Figure 3-2 Scapular axis of rotation.

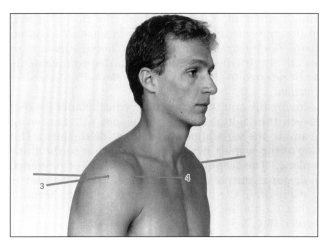

Figure 3-4 Glenohumeral axes: *(3)* flexion–extension; *(4)* abduction–adduction.

scapular and clavicular motions are normally assessed by visual observation of active movement and through passive movement.

The Glenohumeral Joint

The *glenohumeral or shoulder joint* is a ball-and-socket joint formed medially by the concave surface of the scapular glenoid cavity and laterally by the convex surface of the head of the humerus. The axes around which glenohumeral joint motions occur are illustrated in

Figures 3-3 and 3-4. In Figure 3-4, from the anatomical position, the glenohumeral joint may be flexed and extended in the sagittal plane with movement occurring around a frontal axis. The movements of shoulder abduction and adduction occur in the frontal plane around a sagittal axis. In Figure 3-3, the shoulder is positioned in 90° abduction for the purpose of illustrating the vertical axis around which the movements of shoulder horizontal adduction and abduction occur in the transverse plane. With the shoulder in 90° abduction, shoulder internal and external rotation takes place in a sagittal plane about the longitudinal axis of the humerus (Fig. 3-3). However, with the arm at the side in anatomical position, internal and external rotation takes place in a horizontal plane about the longitudinal axis of the humerus.

The Shoulder Complex

Normal function in performing activities of daily living (ADL) depends on the integrated movement patterns of the joints of the shoulder girdle and the shoulder (glenohumeral) joint. Shoulder (glenohumeral joint) movements are accompanied at varying points in the range of motion (ROM) by scapular, clavicular, and trunk motions. The movements at the scapulothoracic, acromioclavicular, sternoclavicular, and spinal articulations extend the ROM capabilities of the glenohumeral joint. Shoulder elevation is an example of movement that requires the integrated movement patterns of all the joints of the shoulder complex.

Shoulder elevation is the term used to describe movement of the arm above shoulder level (i.e., 90°) to a vertical position alongside the head (i.e., 180°). The vertical position may be arrived at by moving the arm

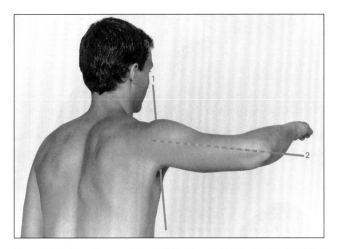

Figure 3-3 Glenohumeral axes: *(1)* horizontal abduction–adduction; *(2)* internal–external rotation.

through either the sagittal plane or the frontal plane, and the movements are referred to as *shoulder elevation through flexion* or *shoulder elevation through abduction,* respectively. In the clinical setting, these movements may be referred to simply as *shoulder flexion* and *shoulder abduction.*

Moving the arm through other vertical planes located between the sagittal and frontal planes will also bring the arm to the vertical position alongside the head. The plane of the scapula lies 30° to 45° anterior to the frontal plane.[3] The scapular plane is the plane of reference for diagonal movements of shoulder elevation and is the plane often used when the arm is raised to perform overhead activities. This midplane elevation is called *scaption*[4] (Fig. 3-5).

Figures 3-6A and 3-7A illustrate the integrated movement patterns of the joints of the shoulder complex during the normal performance of two ADL, combing one's hair and reaching into a back pocket. Figures 3-6B and 3-7B illustrate the changes that occur in the integrated movement patterns when motion is restricted at one of the joints of the shoulder complex, in this case the glenohumeral joint. Observe how increased movement (i.e., substitute motion) of the scapula and trunk is used to compensate for the loss of motion at the glenohumeral joint. The completion of the two ADL would not be possible without employing the substitute motions.

The joints and movements of the shoulder complex are summarized in Tables 3-1 to 3-3.

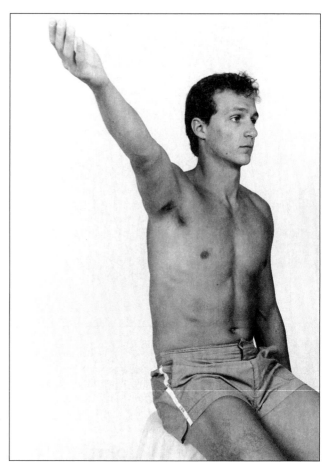

Figure 3-5 Elevation: plane of the scapula.

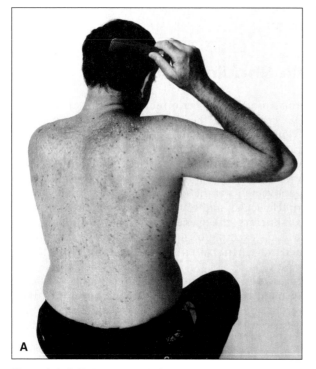

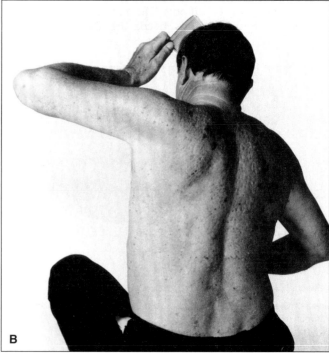

Figure 3-6 **A.** Patient combs hair using normal right upper extremity. **B.** Patient attempts to comb hair using left upper extremity with restricted glenohumeral joint movement. Substitute motions are observed at the left shoulder girdle and more distant joints.

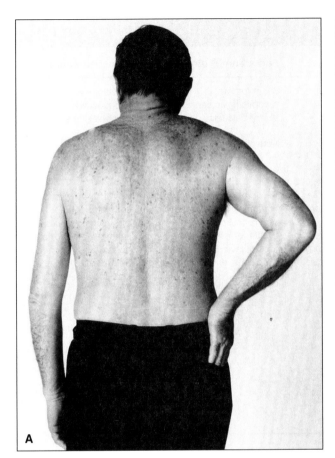
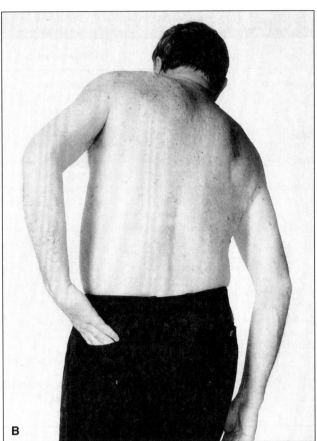

Figure 3-7 **A.** Patient reaches into back pocket using normal right upper extremity. **B.** Patient attempts to reach into back pocket using left upper extremity with restricted glenohumeral joint movement. Substitute motions are observed at the left shoulder girdle and more distant joints.

TABLE 3-1 Joint Structure: Scapular Movements

	Elevation	Depression	Abduction (Protraction)	Adduction (Retraction)
Articulation[1,5]	Scapulothoracic Acromioclavicular Sternoclavicular	Scapulothoracic Acromioclavicular Sternoclavicular	Scapulothoracic Acromioclavicular Sternoclavicular	Scapulothoracic Acromioclavicular Sternoclavicular
Plane	Frontal	Frontal	Horizontal	Horizontal
Axis	Sagittal	Sagittal	Vertical	Vertical
Normal limiting factors[5-9,*] (See Fig. 3-8A and B)	Tension in the costo-clavicular ligament, inferior sternoclavicu-lar joint capsule, lower fibers of trapezius, pectoralis minor, and subclavius	Tension in the interclavicular ligament, sternoclavicular ligament, articular disk, upper fibers of trapezius, and levator scapulae; bony contact between the clavicle and the superior aspect of the 1st rib	Tension in the trapezoid ligament, posterior ster-noclavicular ligament, posterior lamina of the costoclavicular ligament, trapezius, and rhomboids	Tension in the conoid ligament, anterior lamina of the costoclavicular ligament, anterior ster-noclavicular ligament, pectoralis minor, and serratus anterior
Normal end feel[6,10]	Firm	Firm/hard	Firm	Firm
Normal AROM[5,†]	10–12 cm (total range for elevation–depression)		10–12 cm (total range for abduction–adduction)	

	Medial Rotation (Downward Rotation)	Lateral Rotation (Upward Rotation)
Articulation[1,5]	Scapulothoracic Acromioclavicular Sternoclavicular	Scapulothoracic Acromioclavicular Sternoclavicular
Plane	Frontal	Frontal
Axis	Sagittal	Sagittal
Normal limiting factors[5-9,*] (See Fig. 3-8A and B)	Tension in the conoid ligament and serratus anterior	Tension in the trapezoid liga-ment, the rhomboid muscles and the levator scapulae
Normal end feel[6,10]	Firm	Firm
Normal AROM[5]	45°–60° (total range for medial-lateral rotation)	

Note: Medial and lateral rotations of the scapula are associated with extension and/or adduction, and flexion and/or abduction of the shoulder, respectively.

*There is a paucity of definitive research that identifies the normal limiting factors (NLF) of joint motion. The NLF and end feels listed here are based on knowledge of anatomy, clinical experience, and available references.

†AROM, active range of motion.

TABLE 3-2 Joint Structure: Glenohumeral Joint Movements

	Extension	Internal Rotation	External Rotation	Horizontal Abduction	Horizontal Adduction
Articulation[1,5]	Glenohumeral	Glenohumeral	Glenohumeral	Glenohumeral	Glenohumeral
Plane	Sagittal	Horizontal	Horizontal	Horizontal	Horizontal
Axis	Frontal	Longitudinal	Longitudinal	Vertical	Vertical
Normal limiting factors[5–9,*] (See Fig. 3-8B)	Tension in the anterior band of the coracohumeral ligament, anterior joint capsule, and clavicular fibers of pectoralis major	Tension in the posterior joint capsule, infraspinatus, and teres minor	Tension in all bands of the glenohumeral ligament, coracohumeral ligament, the anterior joint capsule, subscapularis, pectoralis major, teres major, and latissimus dorsi	Tension in the anterior joint capsule, the glenohumeral ligament, and pectoralis major	Tension in the posterior joint capsule. Soft tissue apposition
Normal end feel[6,10]	Firm	Firm	Firm	Firm	Firm/soft
Normal AROM[11] **(AROM[12])**	0°–60° (0°–60°)	0°–70° (0°–70°)	0°–90° (0°–90°)	0°–45° (–)	0°–135° (–)

*There is a paucity of definitive research that identifies the normal limiting factors (NLF) of joint motion. The NLF and end feels listed here are based on knowledge of anatomy, clinical experience, and available references.

TABLE 3-3 Joint Structure: Shoulder Complex Movements

	Elevation Through Flexion	Elevation Through Abduction
Articulation[1,5]	Glenohumeral Acromioclavicular Sternoclavicular Scapulothoracic	Glenohumeral Acromioclavicular Sternoclavicular Scapulothoracic Subdeltoid[1]
Plane	Sagittal	Frontal
Axis	Frontal	Sagittal
Normal limiting factors[5–9,*] (See Fig. 3-8B)	Tension in the posterior band of the coracohumeral ligament, posterior joint capsule, shoulder extensors, and external rotators; scapular movement limited by tension in rhomboids, levator scapulae, and the trapezoid ligament	Tension in the middle and inferior bands of the glenohumeral ligament, inferior joint capsule, shoulder adductors; greater tuberosity of the humerus contacting the upper portion of the glenoid and glenoid labrum or the lateral surface of the acromion; scapular movement limited by tension in rhomboids, levator scapulae, and the trapezoid ligament
Normal end feel[6,10]	Firm	Firm/hard
Normal AROM[1,5,11] **(AROM[12])**	0°–180° (0°–165°) 0°–60°, glenohumeral 60°–180°, glenohumeral, scapular movement, and trunk movement	0°–180° (0°–165°) 0°–30°, glenohumeral 30°–180°, glenohumeral, scapular movement, and trunk movement
Capsular pattern[10,13]	Glenohumeral: external rotation, abduction (only through 90°–120° range), internal rotation Sternoclavicular/acromioclavicular: pain at extreme range of motion notably horizontal adduction and full elevation	

*There is a paucity of definitive research that identifies the normal limiting factors (NLF) of joint motion. The NLF and end feels listed here are based on knowledge of anatomy, clinical experience, and available references.

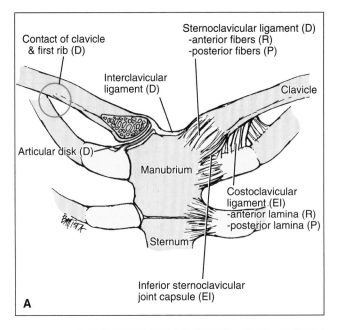

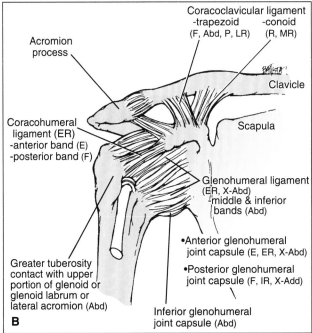

Figure 3-8 **Normal Limiting Factors. A.** Anterior view of sternoclavicular joints showing noncontractile structures that normally limit motion. **B.** Anterior view of the shoulder showing noncontractile structures that normally limit motion.*

*Motion limited by structure is identified in brackets, using the following abbreviations for (1) Scapular movements, (2) Glenohumeral joint movements, and (3) Shoulder complex movements:

(1) Scapular movements:
El, elevation;   P, protraction;
D, depression;   R, retraction;
MR, medial (downward) rotation;   LR, lateral (upward) rotation.

(2) Glenohumeral joint movements:
E, extension;   X-Add, horizontal adduction;
IR, internal rotation;   X-Abd, horizontal abduction.
ER, external rotation;

(3) Shoulder complex movements:
F, elevation through flexion;   Abd, elevation through abduction.

Muscles normally limiting motion are not illustrated.

ANATOMICAL LANDMARKS (FIGS. 3-9 THROUGH 3-14)

Anatomical landmarks are described and illustrated below. Anatomical landmarks, numbered 2 through 7 and 9 through 14, are used to assess scapular ROM and to align the goniometer axis and arms to measure ROM at the shoulder complex.

Structure	Location
1. Inion	Dome-shaped process that marks the center of the superior nuchal line.
2. Vertebral border of the scapula	Approximately 5–6 cm lateral to the thoracic spinous processes covering ribs 2–7.
3. Inferior angle of the scapula	At the inferior aspect of the vertebral border of the scapula.
4. Spine of the scapula	The bony ridge running obliquely across the upper four-fifths of the scapula.
5. Acromion process	Lateral aspect of the spine of the scapula at the tip of the shoulder.
6. Clavicle	Prominent S-shaped bone on the anterosuperior aspect of the thorax.
7. Coracoid process	Approximately 2 cm distal to the junction of the middle and lateral thirds of the clavicle in the delto-pectoral triangle. Press firmly upward and laterally, deep to the anterior fibers of the deltoid.
8. Brachial pulse	Palpate pulse on the medial, proximal aspect of the upper arm posterior to the coracobrachialis.
9. Lateral epicondyle of the humerus	Lateral projection at the distal end of the humerus.
10. Olecranon process of the ulna	Posterior aspect of the elbow at the proximal end of the shaft of the ulna.
11. T12 spinous process	The most distal thoracic spinous process slightly above the level of the olecranon process of the ulna when the body is in the anatomical position.
12. Sternum	Flat bone surface along the midline of the anterior aspect of the thorax.
13. Styloid process of ulna	Bony projection on the posteromedial aspect of the forearm at the distal end of the ulna (see Figs. 4-4 through 4-6).
14. Fourth rib	Palpate the 2nd rib immediately lateral to the sternal angle (i.e., the slightly raised bony junction between the manubrium and sternum). From the 2nd rib, palpate the intercostal spaces down to the 4th rib.

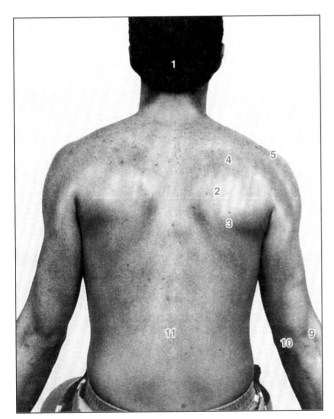

Figure 3-9 Posterior aspect of the shoulder complex.

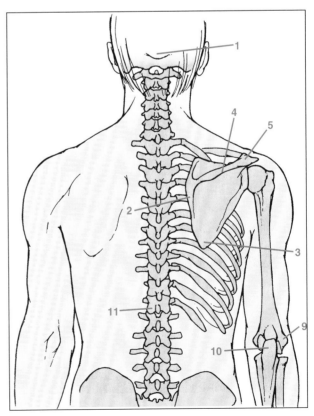

Figure 3-10 Bony anatomy, posterior aspect of the shoulder complex.

CHAPTER 3

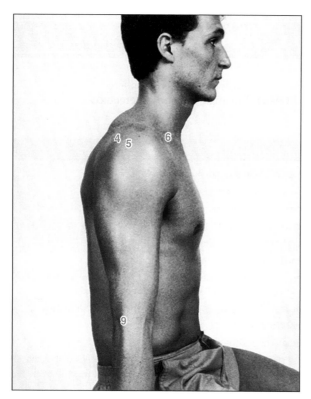

Figure 3-11 Lateral aspect of the shoulder complex.

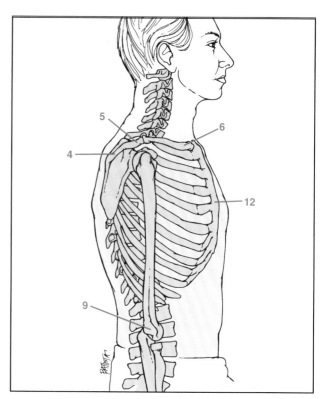

Figure 3-12 Bony anatomy, lateral aspect of the shoulder complex.

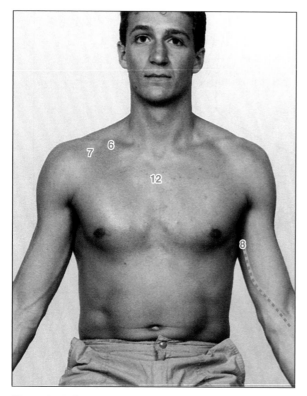

Figure 3-13 Anterior aspect of the shoulder complex.

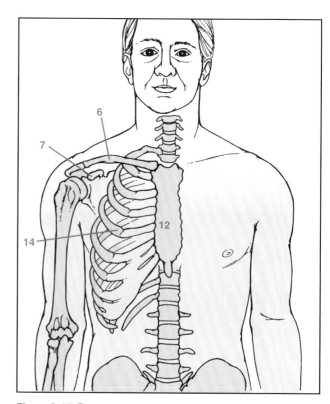

Figure 3-14 Bony anatomy, anterior aspect of the shoulder complex.

RANGE OF MOTION ASSESSMENT AND MEASUREMENT

 Practice Makes Perfect

To aid you in practicing the skills covered in this section, or for a handy review, use the Summary & Evaluation Forms found at

http://thepoint.lww.com/ClarksonJM2e.

Normal function of the shoulder complex depends on the integrated movement patterns of all joints that are a part of the shoulder complex. Therefore, a complete evaluation of ROM of the shoulder complex must include evaluation of scapular and glenohumeral joint active and passive ROM. Evaluation of scapular, glenohumeral, and integrated shoulder complex movement is presented.

General Scan: Upper Extremity Active Range of Motion

Scan the **active range of motion** (AROM) of the upper extremity joints, starting with the patient in the sitting or standing position with the arms at the sides (Fig. 3-15).

Instruct the patient to place the left hand behind the neck and reach down the spine as far as possible (Fig. 3-16A). Observe the ROM of scapular abduction and lateral (upward) rotation, shoulder elevation and external rotation, elbow flexion, forearm supination, wrist radial deviation, and finger extension.

Instruct the patient to place the right hand on the low back (Fig. 3-16A) and reach up the spine as far as possible. Observe the ROM of scapular adduction and medial (downward) rotation, shoulder extension and internal rotation, elbow flexion, forearm pronation, wrist radial deviation, and finger extension.

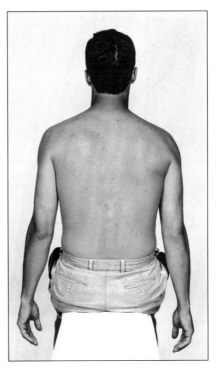

Figure 3-15 Start position: scan of AROM of the upper extremities.

The vertebral levels reached at the levels of the tips of the middle fingers as the patient reaches behind the neck or up the back may be used as a general measure of AROM of the upper extremity joints.

Instruct the patient to return to the start position and repeat the movements on the contralateral sides (see Fig. 3-16B).

As observed in Figure 3-16, there is often an appreciable difference in the ROM between sides that can be considered normal.

Figure 3-17 illustrates a general scan of the upper extremity AROM in the presence of normal right and decreased left glenohumeral joint ROM. As the patient attempts to perform the test movements, substitute movements at the left shoulder girdle and more distant joints are used to compensate for the restricted left shoulder joint ROM.

CHAPTER 3

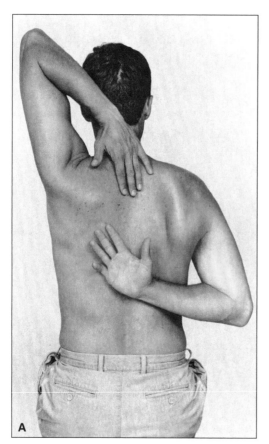
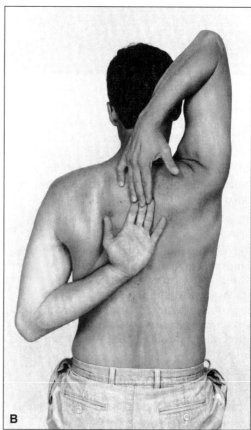

Figure 3-16 A and B. End positions: scan of AROM of the upper extremities.

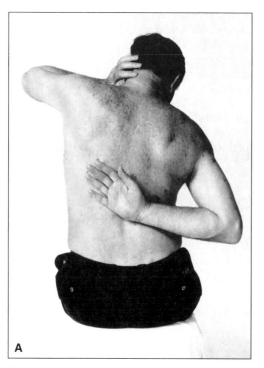
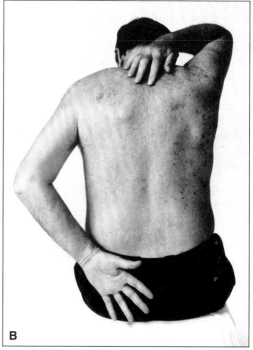

Figure 3-17 A and B. End positions: scan of AROM of the upper extremities with decreased left glenohumeral joint mobility. Substitute motions are observed at the left shoulder girdle and more distant joints.

Scapular Movements

Normal ROM at the sternoclavicular and acromioclavicular joints (i.e., clavicular motion) is required for normal scapular motion. In the clinical setting, motion at the sternoclavicular joint and scapula is not easily measured, and it is not possible to measure motion at the acromioclavicular joint.

Scapular movement (see Table 3-1) is assessed by visual observation of the AROM and the evaluation of passive movement. The ROM is estimated as either "full" or "restricted." In the presence of decreased scapular ROM, the motion at the sternoclavicular and acromioclavicular joints is assessed; however, these assessment techniques are beyond the scope of this text.

AROM Assessment

Start Position. The patient is sitting and assumes a relaxed, anatomical posture (Fig. 3-18). In this posture, the scapula normally lies between the 2nd and 7th ribs and the vertebral border lies approximately 5 to 6 cm lateral to the spine. The therapist stands behind the patient to observe the scapular movements.

Scapular Elevation

Movement. The patient moves the shoulders toward the ears in an upward or cranial direction (Fig. 3-19).

Scapular Depression

Movement. The patient moves the shoulders toward the waist in a downward or caudal direction (Fig. 3-20).

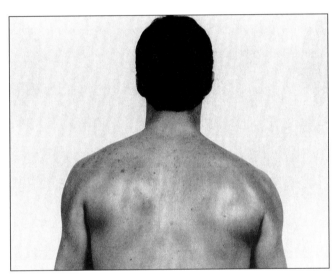

Figure 3-18 Start position for all active scapular movements.

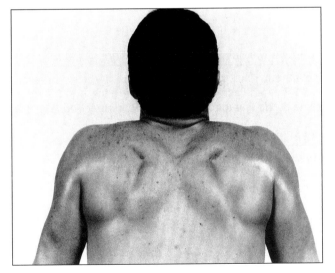

Figure 3-19 Active movement: scapular elevation.

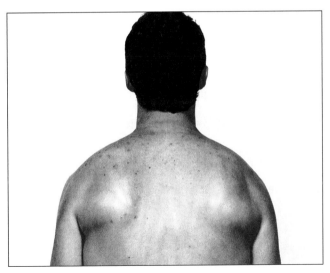

Figure 3-20 Active movement: scapular depression.

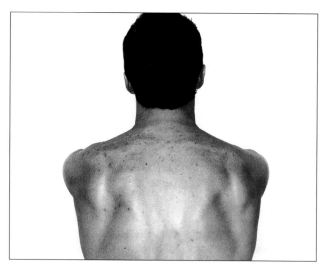

Figure 3-21 Active movement: scapular abduction.

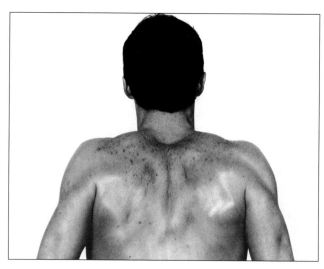

Figure 3-22 Active movement: scapular adduction.

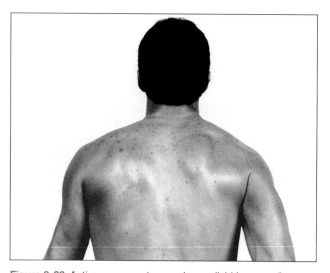

Figure 3-23 Active movement: scapular medial (downward) rotation.

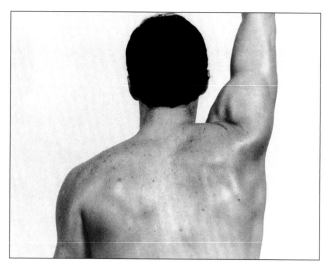

Figure 3-24 Active movement: scapular lateral (upward) rotation.

Scapular Abduction

Movement. From the start position, the patient flexes the arms to 90°, and scapular abduction is observed as the patient reaches forward (Fig. 3-21). The vertebral borders of the scapulae move away from the vertebral column.

Scapular Adduction

Movement. The patient moves the scapulae horizontally toward the vertebral column (Fig. 3-22).

Scapular Medial (Downward) Rotation

Movement. The patient extends and adducts the arm to place the hand across the small of the back, and the inferior angle of the scapula moves in a medial direction (Fig. 3-23).

Scapular Lateral (Upward) Rotation

Movement. The patient elevates the arm through flexion or abduction (Fig. 3-24). During elevation, the inferior angle of the scapula moves in a lateral direction.

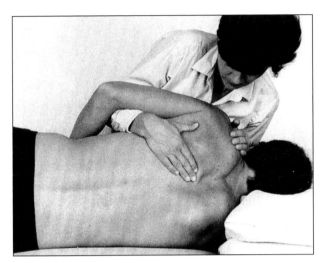

Figure 3-25 Passive movement: scapular elevation.

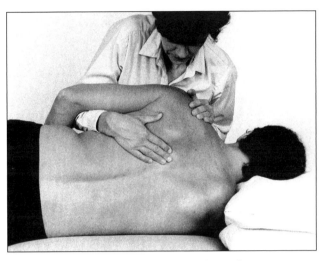

Figure 3-26 Passive movement: scapular depression.

PROM Assessment

Forms 3-1 to 3-4

Start Position. The patient is in a side-lying position with the hips and knees flexed, the head relaxed and supported on a pillow. This position remains unchanged for all scapular movements.

Stabilization. The weight of the trunk stabilizes the thorax.

Scapular Elevation

Procedure. The therapist cups the inferior angle of the scapula with one hand and elevates the scapula, while controlling the direction of movement with the other hand (Fig. 3-25).

End Feel. Firm

Joint Glides. *Scapular elevation*—the scapula glides in a cranial direction on the thorax. *Sternoclavicular joint:* elevation of the clavicle—the convex medial end of the clavicle glides inferiorly on the fixed concave surface of the manubrium. *Acromioclavicular joint*—gliding.

Scapular Depression

Procedure. The therapist places one hand on the top of the shoulder girdle to depress the scapula. The therapist's other hand cups the inferior angle of the scapula to control the direction of movement (Fig. 3-26).

End Feel. Firm/hard

Joint Glides. *Scapular depression*—the scapula glides in a caudal direction on the thorax. *Sternoclavicular joint:* depression of the clavicle—the convex medial end of the clavicle glides superiorly on the fixed concave surface of the manubrium. *Acromioclavicular joint*—gliding.

CHAPTER 3

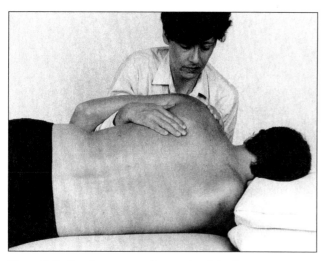

Figure 3-27 Passive movement: scapular abduction.

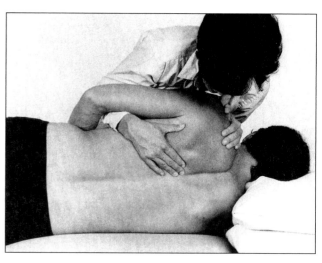

Figure 3-28 Passive movement: scapular adduction.

Scapular Abduction

Procedure. The therapist grasps the vertebral border and inferior angle of the scapula using the thumb and index finger of one hand and abducts the scapula. The therapist's other hand is placed on top of the shoulder girdle to assist in abduction (Fig. 3-27).

End Feel. Firm

Joint Glides. *Scapular abduction*—the scapula glides laterally on the thorax. *Sternoclavicular joint*: protraction of the clavicle—the concave medial end of the clavicle glides anteriorly on the fixed convex surface of the manubrium. *Acromioclavicular joint*—gliding.

Scapular Adduction

Procedure. The therapist grasps the axillary border and inferior angle of the scapula using the thumb and index finger of one hand and adducts the scapula. The therapist's other hand is placed on top of the shoulder girdle to assist in adduction (Fig. 3-28).

End Feel. Firm

Joint Glides. *Scapular adduction*—the scapula glides medially on the thorax. *Sternoclavicular joint*: retraction of the clavicle—the concave medial end of the clavicle glides posteriorly on the fixed convex surface of the manubrium. *Acromioclavicular joint*—gliding.

Shoulder Complex—Movements

Shoulder elevation depends on full ROM at the sternoclavicular, acromioclavicular, scapular, and glenohumeral joints (Tables 3-2 and 3-3). In the presence of decreased shoulder elevation ROM, the therapist must identify which joint(s) of the shoulder complex lack full ROM to effectively plan treatment to restore full ROM. The PROM at the shoulder girdle (i.e., scapular and clavicular motion) is evaluated independent of the PROM at the glenohumeral joint. To isolate the glenohumeral joint PROM, the therapist must stabilize the scapula and clavicle. To ensure adequate stabilization when measuring glenohumeral joint PROM, a second therapist may assist to align the goniometer. To assess and measure movements that require motion at all articulations of the shoulder complex, the trunk is stabilized.

Shoulder Elevation Through Flexion (Glenohumeral Joint, Scapular and Clavicular Motion)

AROM Assessment

Substitute Movement. Trunk extension and shoulder abduction.

PROM Assessment

Form 3-5

Start Position. The patient is in a crook-lying (Fig. 3-29) or a sitting position. The arm is at the side with the palm facing medially.

Stabilization. The weight of the trunk. The therapist stabilizes the thorax.

Therapist's Distal Hand Placement. The therapist grasps the distal humerus.

End Position. The therapist moves the humerus anteriorly and upward to the limit of motion for shoulder elevation through flexion (Fig. 3-30). The elbow is maintained in extension to prevent restriction of shoulder flexion ROM due to passive insufficiency of the two-joint triceps muscle.[14]

End Feel. Firm

Joint Glides/Spin. Shoulder elevation through flexion:

Scapular lateral (upward) rotation—the inferior angle of the scapula rotates in a lateral direction on the thorax.

Sternoclavicular joint: (a) elevation of the clavicle—the convex medial end of the clavicle glides inferiorly on the fixed concave surface of the manubrium, and (b) posterior rotation of the clavicle—the clavicle spins on the fixed surfaces of the manubrium.

Acromioclavicular joint—gliding.

Glenohumeral joint flexion—the convex humeral head spins (i.e., rotates around a fixed point) on the fixed concave glenoid cavity.

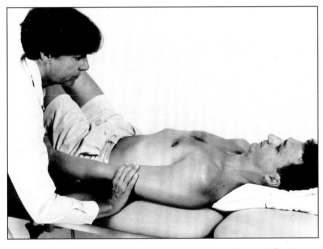

Figure 3-29 Start position for shoulder elevation through flexion.

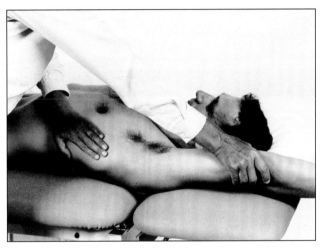

Figure 3-30 Firm end feel at limit of shoulder elevation through flexion.

Measurement: Universal Goniometer

Start Position. The patient is in a crook-lying position (Fig. 3-31) or sitting. The arm is at the side, with the palm facing medially.

Stabilization. The weight of the trunk. The scapula is left free to move.

Goniometer Axis. The axis is placed at the lateral aspect of the center of the humeral head. In anatomical position, the center of the humeral head is located about 2.5 cm inferior to the lateral aspect of the acromion process (see Figs. 3-31 and 3-36).

Stationary Arm. Parallel to the lateral midline of the trunk.

Movable Arm. Parallel to the longitudinal axis of the humerus.

End Position. The humerus is moved in an anterior and upward direction to the limit of motion **(shoulder elevation 180°).** This movement represents scapular, clavicular, and glenohumeral motion (Fig. 3-32).

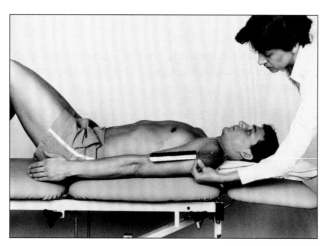

Figure 3-31 Start position for shoulder elevation through flexion: supine.

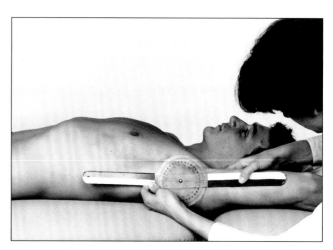

Figure 3-32 Shoulder elevation through flexion.

Glenohumeral Joint (Shoulder) Flexion

AROM Assessment

The patient cannot perform isolated glenohumeral joint flexion ROM without the scapula being stabilized.

PROM Assessment

Start Position. The patient is in a crook-lying or a sitting position. The arm is at the side with the palm facing medially.

Stabilization. The therapist places one hand on the axillary border of the scapula to stabilize the scapula.

Therapist's Distal Hand Placement. The therapist grasps the distal humerus.

End Position. While stabilizing the scapula, the therapist moves the humerus anteriorly and upward to the

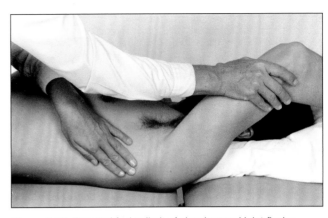

Figure 3-33 Firm end feel at limit of glenohumeral joint flexion.

limit of motion to assess glenohumeral joint motion (Fig. 3-33).

End Feel. Firm.

Joint Spin. *Glenohumeral joint flexion*—the convex humeral head spins on the fixed concave glenoid cavity.

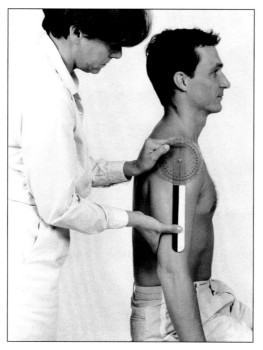

Figure 3-34 Start position for shoulder elevation through flexion: sitting.

Measurement: Universal Goniometer

Start Position. The patient is in sitting (Fig. 3-34) or crook-lying position. The arm is at the side, with the palm facing medially.

Stabilization. The therapist stabilizes the scapula.

Goniometer Axis. The axis is placed at the lateral aspect of the center of the humeral head about 2.5 cm inferior to the lateral aspect of the acromion process when in anatomical position (see Figs. 3-34 and 3-36).

Stationary Arm. Parallel to the lateral midline of the trunk.

Movable Arm. Parallel to the longitudinal axis of the humerus.

End Position. The humerus is moved in an anterior and upward direction to the limit of motion **(glenohumeral joint flexion 120°)**[8] (Figs. 3-35 and 3-36).

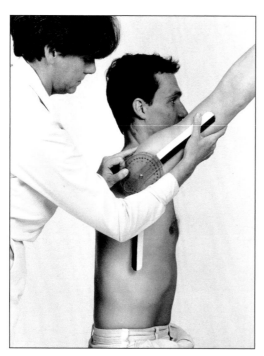

Figure 3-35 Goniometer alignment: shoulder elevation through flexion, glenohumeral joint flexion, and extension.

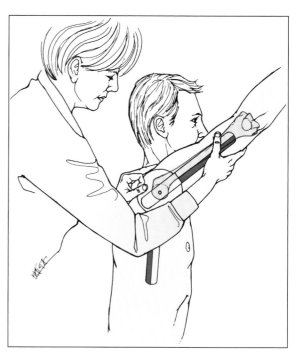

Figure 3-36 Glenohumeral joint flexion ROM.

Shoulder Extension

AROM Assessment

Substitute Movement. Scapular anterior tilting, scapular elevation, and shoulder abduction. In sitting, the patient may flex and ipsilaterally rotate the trunk.

PROM Assessment

Form 3-7

Start Position. The patient is prone (Fig. 3-37) or sitting. The arm is at the side, with the palm facing medially.

Stabilization. The therapist stabilizes the scapula to isolate and assess glenohumeral joint motion.

Therapist's Distal Hand Placement. The therapist grasps the distal humerus.

End Position. The therapist moves the humerus posteriorly until the scapula begins to move (Fig. 3-38). The elbow is flexed to prevent restriction of shoulder extension ROM due to passive insufficiency of the two-joint biceps brachii muscle.[14]

End Feel. Firm.

Joint Spin. *Glenohumeral joint extension*—the convex humeral head spins on the fixed concave glenoid cavity.

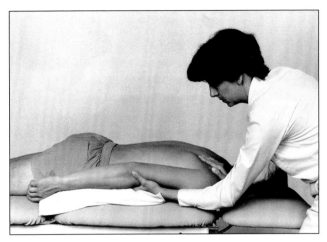

Figure 3-37 Start position for glenohumeral joint extension.

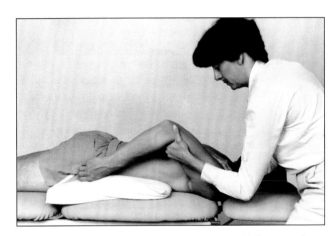

Figure 3-38 Firm end feel at limit of glenohumeral joint extension.

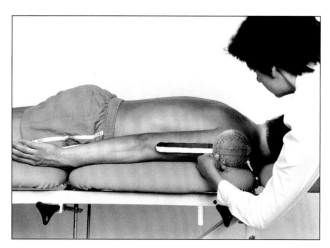

Figure 3-39 Start position for shoulder extension.

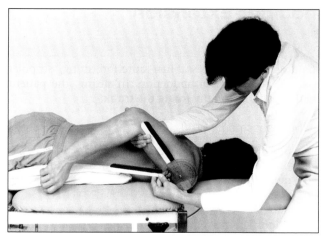

Figure 3-40 Shoulder extension: prone.

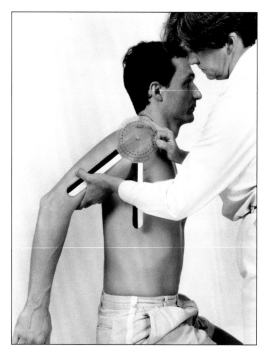

Figure 3-41 Shoulder extension: sitting.

Measurement: Universal Goniometer

Start Position. The patient is prone (Fig. 3-39) or sitting. The arm is at the side, with the palm facing medially.

Stabilization. The therapist's forearm may be used to stabilize the scapula.

Goniometer Axis. The axis is placed at the lateral aspect of the center of the humeral head about 2.5 cm inferior to the lateral aspect of the acromion process when in anatomical position (see Figs. 3-36 and 3-39).

Stationary Arm. Parallel to the lateral midline of the trunk.

Movable Arm. Parallel to the longitudinal axis of the humerus, pointing toward the lateral epicondyle of the humerus.

End Position. The humerus is moved posteriorly to the limit of motion (**shoulder extension 60°**) (Figs. 3-40 and 3-41).

Shoulder Elevation Through Abduction (Glenohumeral Joint, Scapular, and Clavicular Motion)

AROM Assessment

Substitute Movement. Contralateral trunk lateral flexion, scapular elevation, and shoulder flexion.

PROM Assessment

Form 3-8

The humerus is externally rotated when performing shoulder elevation through abduction to allow the greater tuberosity of the humerus to clear the acromion process. Prior to testing elevation through abduction, ensure the patient is capable of full shoulder external rotation.

Start Position. The patient is supine (Fig. 3-42) or sitting. The arm is at the side with the shoulder in external rotation. Ensure the patient sits in an upright posture, as the slouched sitting posture has been shown[15] to result in decreased shoulder abduction ROM.

Stabilization. The therapist stabilizes the trunk.

Therapist's Distal Hand Placement. The therapist grasps the distal humerus.

End Position. The therapist moves the humerus laterally and upward to the limit of motion for elevation through abduction (Fig. 3-43).

End Feel. Firm.

Joint Glides. Shoulder elevation through abduction:

Scapular lateral (upward) rotation—the inferior angle of the scapula rotates in a lateral direction on the thorax.

Sternoclavicular joint: (1) elevation of the clavicle—the convex medial end of the clavicle glides inferiorly on the fixed concave surface of the manubrium, and (2) posterior rotation of the clavicle—the clavicle spins on the fixed surface of the manubrium.

Acromioclavicular joint—gliding.

Glenohumeral joint abduction—the convex humeral head glides inferiorly on the fixed concave glenoid cavity.

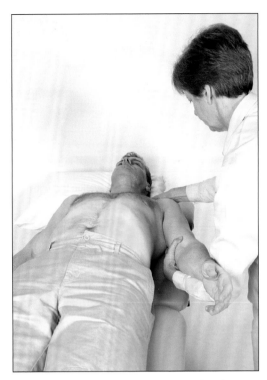

Figure 3-42 Start position for shoulder elevation through abduction.

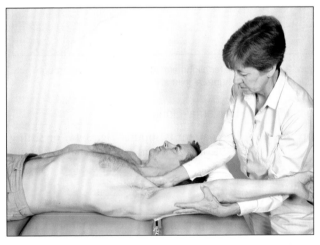

Figure 3-43 Firm end feel at limit of shoulder elevation through abduction.

CHAPTER 3

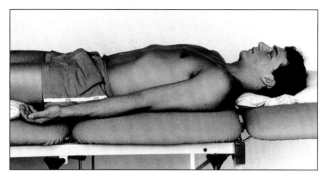

Figure 3-44 Start position for shoulder elevation through abduction.

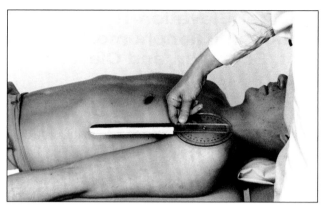

Figure 3-45 Goniometer placement for shoulder elevation through abduction.

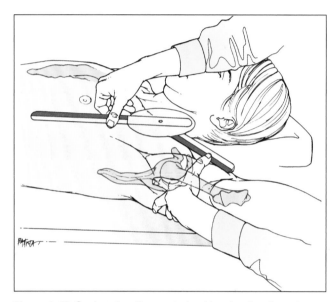

Figure 3-46 Goniometer alignment: shoulder elevation through abduction and glenohumeral joint abduction.

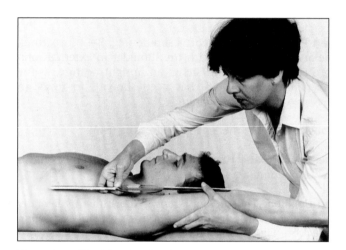

Figure 3-47 Shoulder elevation through abduction.

Measurement: Universal Goniometer

Start Position. The patient is supine (Fig. 3-44) or sitting. The arm is at the side in adduction and external rotation.

Stabilization. The weight of the trunk.

Goniometer Axis. The axis is placed at the midpoint of the anterior or posterior aspect of the glenohumeral joint, about 1.3 cm inferior and lateral to the coracoid process (Figs. 3-45 and 3-46).

Stationary Arm. Parallel to the sternum.

Movable Arm. Parallel to the longitudinal axis of the humerus.

End Position. The humerus is moved laterally and upward to the limit of motion **(shoulder elevation 180°)** (Fig. 3-47). This movement represents scapular and glenohumeral movement. The posterior aspect may be preferred for measurement of shoulder elevation through abduction range in women because the breast may interfere with the goniometer placement anteriorly (Fig. 3-48).

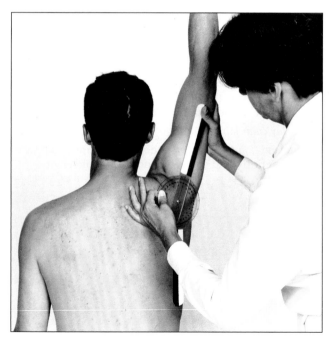

Figure 3-48 Shoulder elevation through abduction: sitting.

Glenohumeral Joint (Shoulder) Abduction

AROM Assessment

The patient cannot perform isolated glenohumeral joint abduction ROM without the scapula being stabilized.

PROM Assessment

Form 3-9

Start Position. The patient is supine (Fig. 3-49) or sitting. The arm is at the side with the elbow flexed to 90°.

Stabilization. The therapist stabilizes the scapula and clavicle.

Therapist's Distal Hand Placement. The therapist grasps the distal humerus.

End Position. The therapist moves the humerus laterally and upward to the limit of motion of glenohumeral joint abduction (Fig. 3-50).

End Feel. Firm or hard

Joint Glide. *Glenohumeral joint abduction*—the convex humeral head glides inferiorly on the fixed concave glenoid cavity.

Measurement: Universal Goniometer (not shown)

Start Position. The patient is supine or sitting. The arm is at the side with the elbow flexed to 90° (see Fig. 3-49).

Goniometer Placement. The goniometer is placed the same as for shoulder elevation through abduction (see Figs. 3-45 and 3-46).

Stabilization. The therapist stabilizes the scapula and clavicle to isolate and measure glenohumeral joint abduction.

End Position. The humerus is moved laterally and upward to the limit of motion (**glenohumeral joint abduction 90° to 120°**)[8] to measure glenohumeral joint abduction.

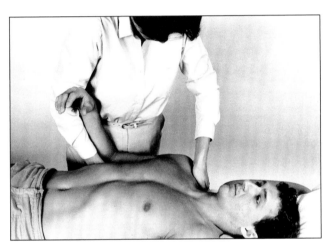

Figure 3-49 Start position for glenohumeral joint abduction.

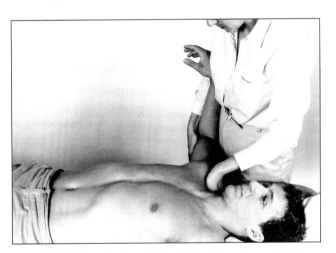

Figure 3-50 Firm or hard end feel at limit of glenohumeral joint abduction.

CHAPTER 3

Shoulder Horizontal Abduction and Adduction

AROM Assessment

Substitute Movement. Scapular retraction (horizontal abduction), scapular protraction (horizontal adduction), and trunk rotation.

PROM Assessment

Forms
3-10, 3-11

Start Position. The patient is sitting. The shoulder is in 90° of abduction and neutral rotation. The elbow is flexed, and the forearm is in midposition (Fig. 3-51).

Stabilization. The therapist stabilizes the trunk and scapula to isolate and assess glenohumeral joint motion.

Therapist's Distal Hand Placement. The therapist supports the arm in abduction and grasps the distal humerus.

End Position. The therapist moves the humerus posteriorly to the limit of motion for horizontal abduction (Fig. 3-52) and anteriorly to the limit of motion for horizontal adduction (Fig. 3-53).

End Feels. *Horizontal abduction—firm; horizontal adduction—firm/soft.*

Joint Glides. *Glenohumeral joint horizontal abduction—the convex humeral head glides anteriorly on the fixed concave glenoid cavity. Glenohumeral joint horizontal adduction—the convex humeral head glides posteriorly on the fixed concave glenoid cavity.*

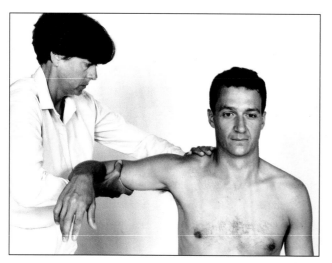

Figure 3-51 Start position for shoulder horizontal abduction and horizontal adduction.

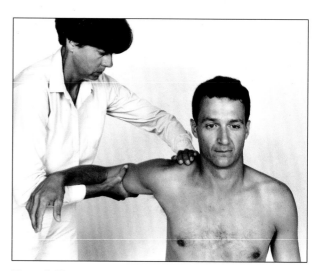

Figure 3-52 Firm end feel at limit of shoulder horizontal abduction.

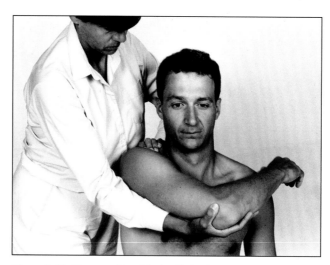

Figure 3-53 Firm or soft end feel at limit of shoulder horizontal adduction.

Measurement: Universal Goniometer

Start Position. The patient is sitting. The shoulder is in 90° of abduction and neutral rotation. The elbow is flexed, and the forearm is in midposition (Fig. 3-54). An alternate start position has the shoulder in 90° of flexion, the elbow is flexed, and the forearm is in midposition (Fig. 3-58). The start position of the shoulder should be recorded.

Stabilization. The therapist stabilizes the trunk and scapula.

Goniometer Axis. The axis is placed on top of the acromion process (Figs. 3-54 and 3-56).

Stationary Arm. Perpendicular to the trunk.

Movable Arm. Parallel to the longitudinal axis of the humerus.

End Position. The therapist supports the arm in abduction. The therapist moves the humerus anteriorly across the chest to the limit of motion (**shoulder horizontal adduction 135°**) (Figs. 3-55 and 3-56) and posteriorly to the limit of motion (**shoulder horizontal abduction 45°**) (Fig. 3-57).

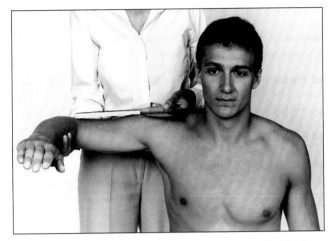

Figure 3-54 Start position for horizontal abduction and adduction.

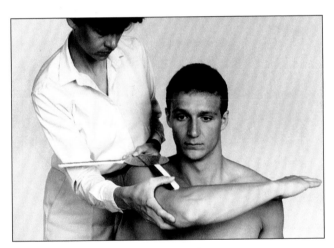

Figure 3-55 Shoulder horizontal adduction.

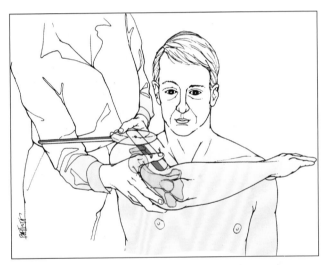

Figure 3-56 Goniometer alignment: shoulder horizontal adduction.

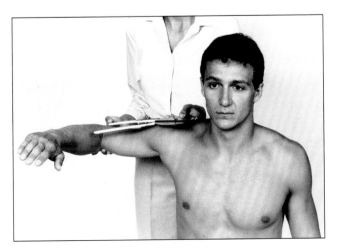

Figure 3-57 Shoulder horizontal abduction.

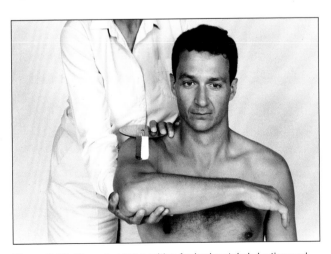

Figure 3-58 Alternate start position for horizontal abduction and adduction.

Shoulder Internal Rotation

AROM Assessment

Substitute Movement. In *prone* with the shoulder in 90° abduction: scapular elevation, shoulder abduction, and elbow extension. In *supine* with the shoulder in 90° abduction: scapular elevation, protraction, and anterior tilt, shoulder abduction, and elbow extension. In *sitting* with the arm at the side: scapular elevation, shoulder abduction, and trunk rotation.

PROM Assessment

Form 3-12

Start Position. The patient is prone or supine. In prone, the shoulder is in 90° of abduction, the elbow is flexed to 90°, and the forearm is in midposition (Fig. 3-59). A towel is placed under the humerus to achieve the abducted position. This start position is contraindicated if the patient has a history of posterior dislocation of the glenohumeral joint.

Stabilization. The therapist stabilizes the scapula and maintains the position of the humerus, without restricting movement. In prone, the plinth limits scapular protraction and anterior tilt. When assessing internal rotation ROM in supine with the shoulder in 90° of abduction, Boon and Smith[16] recommend the therapist place one hand over the clavicle and coracoid process to stabilize the scapula for more reliable and reproducible results.

Therapist's Distal Hand Placement. The therapist grasps the distal radius and ulna.

End Position. The therapist moves the palm of the hand toward the ceiling to the limit of internal rotation (Fig. 3-60)—that is, when scapular movement first occurs.

End Feel. Firm.

Joint Glide. *Glenohumeral joint internal rotation*—with the shoulder in the anatomical position, the convex humeral head glides posteriorly on the fixed concave glenoid cavity.

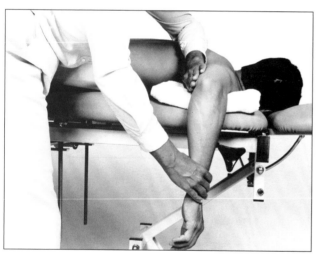

Figure 3-59 Start position for shoulder internal rotation.

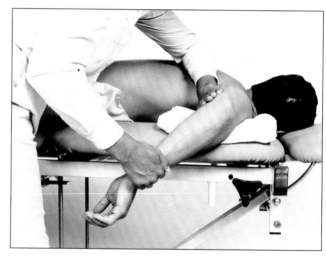

Figure 3-60 Firm end feel at limit of shoulder internal rotation.

Measurement: Universal Goniometer

Start Position. The patient is prone or supine. The shoulder is in 90° of abduction, the elbow is flexed to 90°, and the forearm is in midposition (Fig. 3-61). A towel is placed under the humerus to achieve the abducted position. This start position is contraindicated if the patient has a history of posterior dislocation of the glenohumeral joint.

Goniometer Axis. The axis is placed on the olecranon process of the ulna (Figs. 3-62 and 3-63).

Stationary Arm. Perpendicular to the floor.

Movable Arm. Parallel to the longitudinal axis of the ulna, pointing toward the ulnar styloid process.

End Position. The palm of the hand is moved toward the ceiling to the limit of motion **(shoulder internal rotation 70°)** (Figs. 3-63 and 3-64).

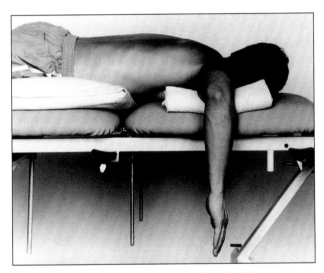

Figure 3-61 Start position for shoulder internal rotation.

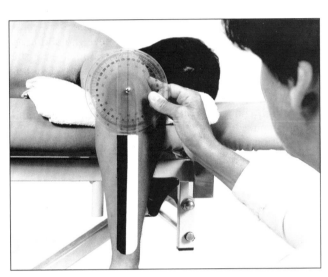

Figure 3-62 Goniometer placement for shoulder internal rotation.

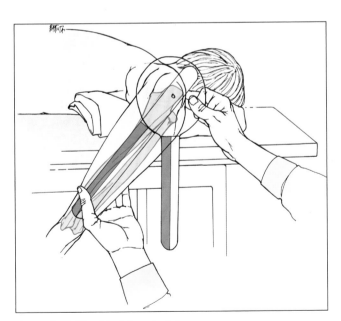

Figure 3-63 Shoulder internal rotation.

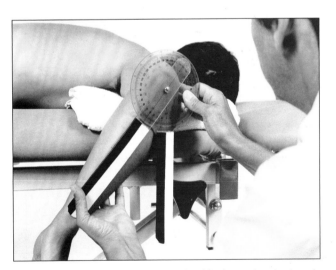

Figure 3-64 Goniometer alignment: shoulder internal and external rotation.

Shoulder External Rotation

AROM Assessment

Substitute Movement. In supine with the shoulder in 90° abduction: elbow extension, scapular depression, and shoulder adduction. In sitting with the arm at the side: scapular depression, shoulder adduction, and trunk rotation.

PROM Assessment

Start Position. The patient is supine. The shoulder is in 90° of abduction, the elbow is flexed to 90°, and the forearm is in midposition (Fig. 3-65). A towel is placed under the humerus to achieve the abducted position. This start position is contraindicated if the patient has a history of anterior dislocation of the glenohumeral joint.

Form 3-13

Stabilization. The weight of the trunk. The therapist stabilizes the scapula.

Therapist's Distal Hand Placement. The therapist grasps the distal radius and ulna.

End Position. The therapist moves the dorsum of the hand toward the floor to the limit of external rotation (Fig. 3-66);—that is, when scapular movement first occurs.

End Feel. Firm.

Joint Glide. *Glenohumeral joint external rotation*—with the shoulder in the anatomical position, the convex humeral head glides anteriorly on the fixed concave glenoid cavity.

Measurement: Universal Goniometer

The measurement process is similar to that for internal rotation with the following exceptions.

Start Position. The patient is supine (Fig. 3-67). This start position is contraindicated if the patient has a history of anterior dislocation of the glenohumeral joint.

End Position. The dorsum of the hand moves toward the floor to the limit of motion (**shoulder external rotation 90°**) (Fig. 3-68).

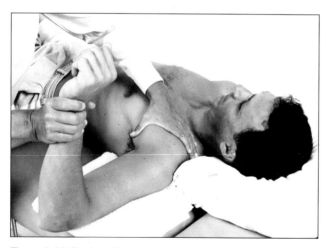

Figure 3-65 Start position for shoulder external rotation.

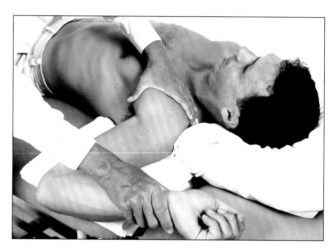

Figure 3-66 Firm end feel at limit of shoulder external rotation.

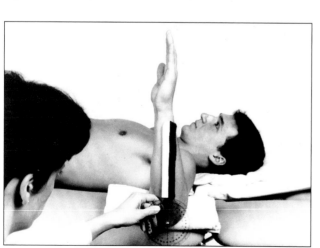

Figure 3-67 Start position for shoulder external rotation.

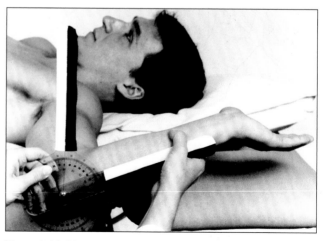

Figure 3-68 Shoulder external rotation.

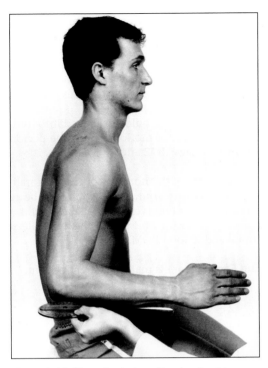

Figure 3-69 Alternate start position for shoulder internal rotation.

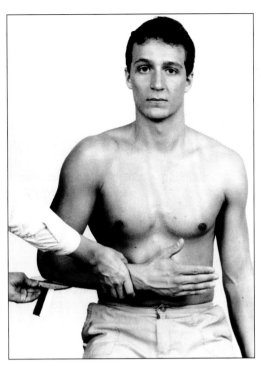

Figure 3-70 Shoulder internal rotation.

Alternate Assessment and Measurement: Internal/External Rotation

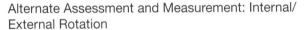

If the patient cannot achieve 90° of shoulder abduction, the end feel can be assessed (not shown) and the measurement can be taken while the patient is sitting. The starting position should be documented.

Start Position. The patient is sitting. To measure shoulder internal rotation, the shoulder is abducted to about 15°, the elbow is flexed to 90°, and the forearm is in midposition (Fig. 3-69). To measure external rotation (not shown), the arm is at the side in adduction, the elbow is flexed to 90°, and the forearm is in midposition.

Goniometer Axis. The axis is placed under the olecranon process.

Stationary Arm. Perpendicular to the trunk.

Movable Arm. Parallel to the longitudinal axis of the ulna.

End Positions. The palm of the hand is moved toward the abdomen to the limit of shoulder internal rotation (Fig. 3-70). The therapist moves the hand away from the abdomen to the limit of external rotation (not shown).

MUSCLE LENGTH ASSESSMENT
AND MEASUREMENT

 Practice Makes Perfect

To aid you in practicing the skills covered in this section, or for a handy review, use the Summary & Evaluation Forms found at

http://thepoint.lww.com/ClarksonJM2e.

Pectoralis Major

Form 3-14

This muscle length assessment technique is contraindicated if the patient has a history of anterior dislocation of the glenohumeral joint.

Start Position. The patient is supine with the shoulder in external rotation and 90° elevation through a plane midway between forward flexion and abduction. The elbow is in 90° flexion (Fig. 3-71).

Stabilization. The therapist stabilizes the trunk.

End Position. The shoulder is moved into horizontal abduction to the limit of motion, to put the pectoralis major on full stretch (Figs. 3-72 and 3-73).

Assessment. With shortness of the pectoralis major muscle, shoulder horizontal abduction will be restricted. The therapist either observes the available PROM or uses a goniometer to measure and record the available shoulder horizontal abduction PROM.

End Feel. Pectoralis major on stretch—firm.

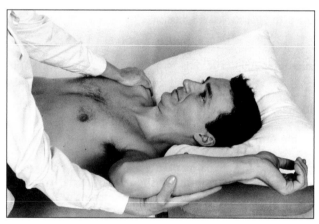

Figure 3-71 Start position: length of pectoralis major.

Origin[1]	Insertion[1]
Pectoralis Major	
a. Clavicular head: anterior border of the sternal half of the clavicle	Lateral lip of the intertubercular groove of the humerus
b. Sternal head: ipsilateral half of the anterior surface of the sternum; cartilage of the first 6 or 7 ribs; sternal end of the 6th rib; aponeurosis of the external abdominal oblique	

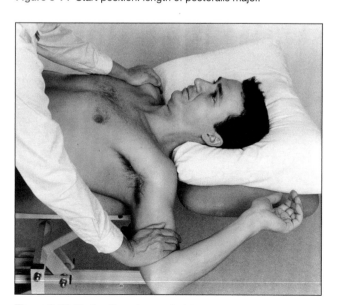

Figure 3-72 Pectoralis major on stretch.

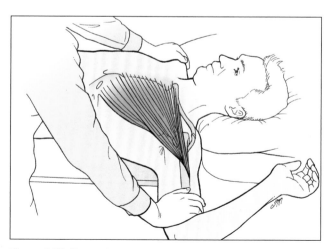

Figure 3-73 Pectoralis major.

Pectoralis Minor[17]

Form
3-15

This muscle length assessment technique is contraindicated if the patient has a history of posterior dislocation of the glenohumeral joint.

Start Position. The patient is supine with the scapula over the side of the plinth, with the shoulder in external rotation and about 80° flexion. The elbow is flexed (Fig. 3-74).

Stabilization. The weight of the trunk.

End Position. The therapist applies force through the long axis of the shaft of the humerus to move the shoulder girdle in a cranial and dorsal direction to put the pectoralis minor on full stretch (Figs. 3-75 and 3-76).

End Feel. Pectoralis minor on stretch—firm.

Measurement (not shown).[18] A second therapist palpates and places a mark at the inferomedial edge of the coracoid process and another mark at the inferior edge of the 4th rib adjacent to the sternum. A tape measure with 0.10 cm divisions is used as a reliable method to measure the distance between the two marks placed on the chest. The patient is instructed to exhale fully during the measurement. The distance measured represents the length of the pectoralis minor muscle on stretch.

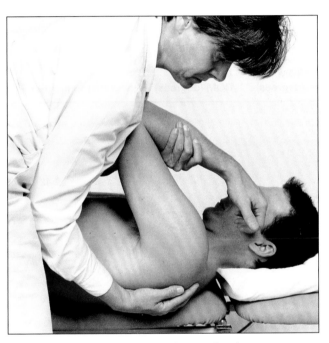

Figure 3-74 Start position: length of pectoralis minor.

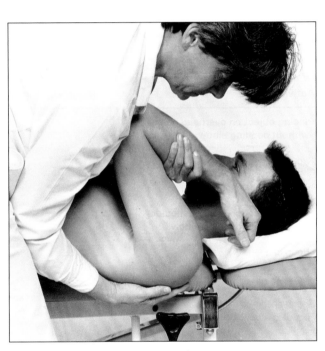

Figure 3-75 Pectoralis minor on stretch.

Origin[1]	Insertion[1]
Pectoralis Minor	
Outer surfaces of ribs 2–4 or 3–5 near the costal cartilages; fascia over corresponding external intercostals.	Medial border and upper surface of the coracoid process of the scapula.

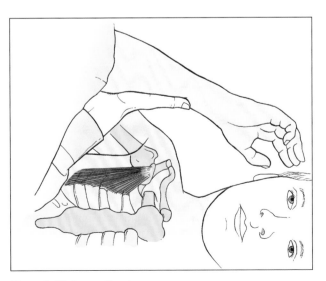

Figure 3-76 Pectoralis minor.

FUNCTIONAL APPLICATION

Joint Function

The function of the shoulder complex is to position or move the arm in space for the purpose of hand function. The shoulder complex is the most mobile joint complex in the body, providing an ROM that exceeds that of any other joint. Because of this mobility, stability is sacrificed.[8,19–23]

Functional Range of Motion

The glenohumeral joint may be flexed and extended, abducted and adducted, internally and externally rotated, and horizontally abducted and horizontally adducted. In the performance of functional activities, the glenohumeral movements are accompanied at varying points in the ROM by scapular, clavicular, and trunk motion. These motions extend the functional range capabilities of the shoulder joint, and without their contribution, movement of the upper limbs would be severely restricted.[20,22,23]

The ranges of motion required at the shoulder for selected activities of daily living (ADL) are presented in Tables 3-4

TABLE 3-4 Shoulder Range of Motion (ROM)* Required for Selected Activities of Daily Living (ADL)[24,25]

Activity	Flexion ROM (degrees)	Extension ROM (degrees)	Abduction ROM (degrees)	Adduction/ Horizontal Adduction† ROM (degrees)	Internal Rotation ROM (degrees)	External Rotation ROM (degrees)
Placing object on overhead shelf, without bending elbow:						
Soup can[24]	121					38
1 gallon container (8–10 lbs)[24]	120					42
Placing object on shelf at shoulder level, without bending elbow:						
Soup can[24]	105					34
1-gallon container (8–10 lbs)[24]	106					39
Reach shelf above head, without bending elbow[24]	119					30
Changing overhead bulb[25]	110		105			
Washing back of opposite shoulder[24]	95			−/116†		
Placing hand behind head with elbow straight out at side[24]			127			61
Combing hair[24]	108			−/86†		
Washing hair[25]	118		112			
Washing middle of back/unhooking bra[24]		47			99	
Washing back[25]		68		61/−		
Reaching small of back to tuck in shirt with hand[24]		46			88	

*Mean values from original sources[24,25] rounded to the nearest degree. Namdari and colleagues[24] reported ROM values for dominant and nondominant arms and found these did not differ significantly in the majority of cases, or were clinically insignificant. Therefore, only the dominant arm ROM mean values are reported.

†Horizontal adduction measured from a start position of 90° shoulder abduction.

TABLE 3-5 **Shoulder Horizontal Adduction/Abduction and Other Shoulder ROM* Required for Selected Functional Activities**[26]

Activity	Horizontal Adduction ROM (degrees)[†]	Other Shoulder ROM (degrees)	
Washing axilla	104 ± 12	flexion	52 ± 14
Eating	87 ± 29	flexion	52 ± 8
Combing hair	54 ± 27	abduction	112 ± 10
	Horizontal Abduction ROM (degrees)[†]		
Reaching maximally up back	69 ± 11	extension	56 ± 13
Reaching perineum	86 ± 13	extension	38 ± 10

*Values are mean ± SD for eight normal subjects.

[†]The 0° start position for establishing the degrees of horizontal adduction and horizontal abduction is 90° shoulder abduction (see Fig. 3-51).

and 3-5, as compiled from the works of Namdari,[24] Khadilkar,[25] Matsen,[26] and their colleagues. The shoulder ROM required to perform these ADL was less than the full available ROM at the shoulder complex with the exception of horizontal abduction and internal rotation ROM that required full ROM to reach the perineum, or maximally up the back.[24–26] The ROM values in Tables 3-4 and 3-5 can be used as a guide for ADL requirements keeping in mind many variables contribute to the manner in which ADL are performed. Khadilkar and coworkers[25] reported high interindividual variability in performing the specified ADL when subjects were instructed to perform these tasks in their usual manner.

The functional movements of the shoulder complex are described to emphasize the interdependence of the components of the shoulder complex and trunk throughout movement.

Elevation of the Arm Over the Head

This functional motion of elevation to 170° to 180° may be achieved through forward flexion in the sagittal plane or abduction in the frontal plane. Owing to the position of the scapula, which lies 30° to 45° anterior to the frontal plane,[3] many daily functional activities are performed in the plane of the scapula. The plane of the scapula is the plane of reference for diagonal movements of shoulder elevation (Fig. 3-5). Scaption[4] is the term given to this midplane elevation. The plane used by an individual depends on the motion requirements of the activity and the position of the hand required for the task (Table 3-5).

To attain the full 180° of elevation through flexion or abduction, movement of the glenohumeral joint is accompanied by movement at the sternoclavicular, acromioclavicular, and scapulothoracic joints. The final degrees of motion can be achieved only through contribution of the spinal movement of trunk extension and/or contralateral lateral flexion.[3,5,19] The total shoulder complex functions in a coordinated way to provide smooth movement and to gain a large excursion of movement for the upper extremity. The coordinated movement pattern achieved through scapulothoracic and glenohumeral movement is described as a "scapulohumeral rhythm".[3,8,19,21]

There are individual variations as to the contribution of all joints to the movement of elevating the arm overhead. Variation depends on the plane of elevation, the arc of elevation, the amount of load on the arm, and individual anatomical differences.[23] Recognizing these variations, it is generally noted that the range of glenohumeral to scapular motion throughout elevation is in the ratio of 2:1; that is, 2° of glenohumeral motion to every 1° of scapular motion.[8,21,22,27] The scapulohumeral rhythm is described for elevation through flexion and for elevation through abduction. An understanding of the scapulohumeral rhythm is essential in understanding the significance of limitations in joint ROM at the shoulder complex.

Scapulohumeral Rhythm

During the initial 60° of shoulder flexion in the sagittal plane or the initial 30° of abduction in the frontal plane, there is an inconsistent scapulohumeral rhythm. It is during this phase that the scapula is seeking stability in relationship to the humerus.[27–29] The scapula is in a setting phase where it may remain stationary, or it may rotate slightly medially (downward) or laterally (upward)[27]

(Fig. 3-77). The glenohumeral joint is the main contributor to movement in this phase. Feeding activities that are performed within this phase of shoulder elevation include using a spoon or a fork and drinking from a cup. These activities are carried out within the ranges of 5° to 45° shoulder flexion and 5° to 30° shoulder abduction.[30]

Following the setting phase, there is a predictable scapulohumeral rhythm throughout the remaining arc of movement to 170° (Fig. 3-78). For every 15° of movement between 30° abduction or 60° flexion and 170° of abduction/flexion, 10° occurs at the glenohumeral joint and 5° occurs at the scapulothoracic joint. Movement of the scapula following the setting phase consists of the primary scapular movement of lateral (upward) rotation, accompanied by secondary rotations of posterior tilting (sagittal plane) and posterior rotation (transverse plane) as the humeral angle is increased with elevation of the arm in the scapular plane.[31]

Range to 170° through abduction depends on a normal scapulohumeral rhythm and the ability to externally rotate the humerus fully through elevation. When the abducted arm reaches a position of 90°, movement through full range of elevation cannot continue because the greater tuberosity of the humerus contacts the superior margin of the glenoid fossa and the coracoacromial arch.[5,29,32] External rotation of the humerus (in the range of approximately 25° to 50°[2]) places the greater tuberosity posteriorly, allowing the humerus to move freely under the coracoacromial arch. Full shoulder elevation through flexion depends on scapulohumeral rhythm and the ability to rotate the humerus internally through range.[33]

The final degrees of elevation are achieved through contralateral trunk lateral flexion (Fig. 3-79) and/or trunk extension. From the discussion of scapulohumeral rhythm, it becomes apparent that restriction in movement at any of the joints of the shoulder complex will limit the ability to position the hand for function.

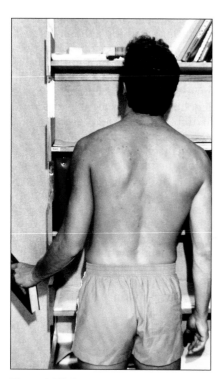

Figure 3-77 Setting phase of the scapula during elevation of the arm through abduction. The scapula remains stationary.

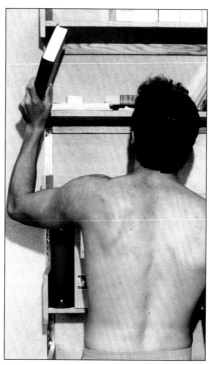

Figure 3-78 Scapulohumeral rhythm: during elevation beyond 60° of flexion or 30° of abduction, the scapula abducts and laterally (upward) rotates.

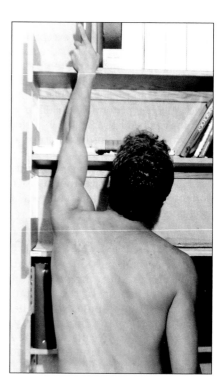

Figure 3-79 Full elevation through abduction: full range is achieved through contralateral trunk lateral flexion.

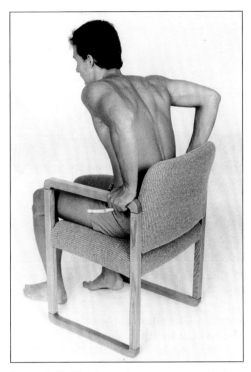

Figure 3-80 Shoulder extension accompanied by scapular adduction and medial (downward) rotation.

Shoulder Extension

The range of 60° of shoulder extension is primarily obtained through the glenohumeral joint.[32] In the performance of functional activities, extension is often accompanied by adduction and medial (downward) rotation of the scapula (Fig. 3-80). A consistent scapulohumeral rhythm is not present in this movement.

Forty-three to 69° of shoulder extension are required to reach maximally up the back[26] (e.g., when hooking a bra; see Fig. 3-81), and 28° to 48° shoulder extension is

necessary to reach the perineum[26] when performing toilet hygiene.

Horizontal Adduction and Abduction

The movements of horizontal adduction and abduction allow the arm to be moved around the body at shoulder level for such activities as washing the axilla or the back (Fig. 3-82), writing on a blackboard (Fig. 3-83), and sliding a window horizontally open or closed. Although by definition horizontal adduction and abduction movements take place in the transverse plane, many ADL require similar motions in planes located above or below shoulder level. These movements may also be referred to as horizontal adduction and abduction until the frontal plane is approached; the movements are then referred to as either adduction or abduction. Table 3-5 provides examples of the ROM required for selected ADL, to bring the arm in front of the body (horizontal adduction) or behind the body (horizontal abduction) and position the arm for other shoulder movements needed to perform these activities.

Internal and External Rotation

Internal and external rotation range of movement varies with the position of the arm. Both internal and external rotation ranges average 68° when the arm is at the side, whereas when the arm is abducted to 90°, 70° of internal rotation and 90° of external rotation can be achieved.[11] Full external rotation is required to place the hand behind the neck when performing self-care activities such as

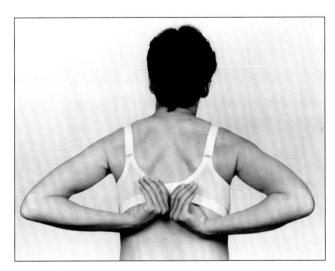

Figure 3-81 Functional extension and internal rotation of the shoulders.

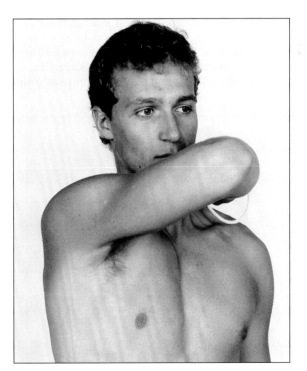

Figure 3-82 Horizontal adduction.

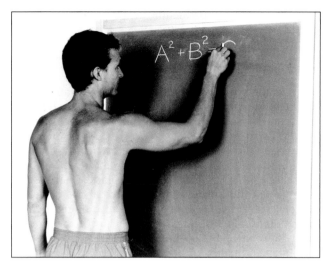

Figure 3-83 Horizontal abduction.

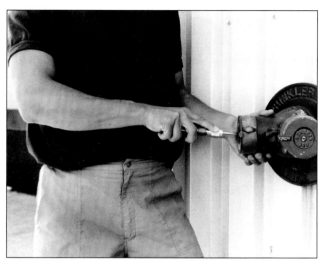

Figure 3-85 Functional association: shoulder internal rotation and forearm pronation.

combing the hair (Fig. 3-84) and manipulating the clasp of a necklace.

Shoulder internal rotation is needed to do up the buttons on a shirt. Five degrees to 25° of shoulder internal rotation are required to use a spoon or fork and to drink from a cup.[30] Full glenohumeral joint internal rotation, augmented by scapulothoracic and elbow joint motion, positions the hand behind the back to reach into a back pocket, perform toilet hygiene, tuck in a shirt, and hook a bra (see Fig. 3-81). Mallon and colleagues[34] analyzed joint motions that occurred at the shoulder complex and elbow in placing the arm behind the back. The analysis revealed the presence of a coordinated pattern of motion occurring between scapular and glenohumeral joint motion. At the beginning of the ROM, internal rotation occurs almost exclusively at the glenohumeral joint as the hand is brought across in front of the body and to a position alongside the ipsilateral hip. As the movement continues and the hand is brought behind the low back, motion at the scapulothoracic joint augments glenohumeral joint

internal rotation. The elbow is then flexed to reach up the spine to the level of the thorax.

Shoulder rotations have a functional link with forearm rotation.[19] When the arm is away from the side, rotation at both joints is concerned with turning the palm to face either the floor or the ceiling. Shoulder internal rotation is linked with pronation of the forearm, as both actions occur simultaneously with performance of many activities and prona-

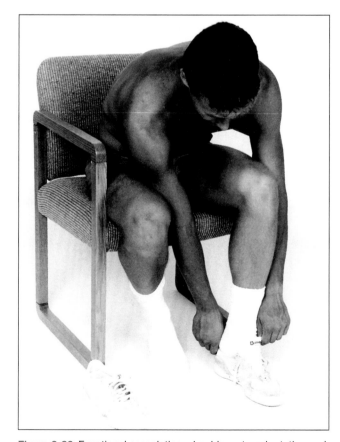

Figure 3-86 Functional association: shoulder external rotation and forearm supination.

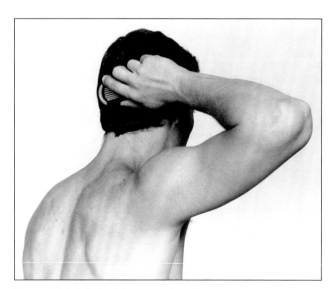

Figure 3-84 Full shoulder external rotation.

tion can be amplified by internal rotation of the shoulder (Fig. 3-85). Shoulder external rotation has a functional link with supination of the forearm when the elbow is extended. Examples of activities that illustrate this combined action are inserting a light bulb into a ceiling socket, releasing a bowling ball from the extended arm, and manipulating the foot into a shoe (Fig. 3-86).

References

1. Standring S, ed. *Gray's Anatomy: The Anatomical Basis of Clinical Practice.* 39th ed. London, UK: Elsevier Churchill Livingstone; 2005.

2. Neumann DA. *Kinesiology of the Musculoskeletal System: Foundations for Rehabilitation.* 2nd ed. St Louis, MO: Mosby Elsevier; 2010.

3. Soderberg GL. *Kinesiology: Application to Pathological Motion.* 2nd ed. Baltimore, MD: Williams & Wilkins; 1997.

4. Perry J. Shoulder function for the activities of daily living. In: Matsen FA, Fu FH, Hawkins RJ, eds. *The Shoulder: A Balance of Mobility and Stability.* Rosemont, IL: American Academy of Orthopaedic Surgeons; 1993.

5. Kapandji IA. *The Physiology of the Joints.* Vol. 1. *The Upper Limb.* 6th ed. New York, NY: Churchill Livingstone Elsevier; 2007.

6. Norkin CC, White DJ. *Measurement of Joint Motion: A Guide to Goniometry.* 4th ed. Philadelphia, PA: FA Davis; 2009.

7. Daniels L, Worthingham C. *Muscle Testing: Techniques of Manual Examination.* 5th ed. Philadelphia, PA: WB Saunders; 1986.

8. Levangie PK, Norkin CC. *Joint Structure & Function: A Comprehensive Analysis.* 3rd ed. Philadelphia, PA: FA Davis; 2001.

9. Woodburne RT. *Essentials of Human Anatomy.* 5th ed. London, UK: Oxford University Press; 1973.

10. Magee DJ. *Orthopedic Physical Assessment.* 5th ed. St Louis, MO: Saunders Elsevier; 2008.

11. American Academy of Orthopaedic Surgeons. *Joint Motion: Method of Measuring and Recording.* Chicago, IL: AAOS; 1965.

12. Berryman Reese N, Bandy WD. *Joint Range of Motion and Muscle Length Testing.* Philadelphia, PA: WB Saunders; 2002.

13. Cyriax J. *Textbook of Orthopaedic Medicine, Vol. 1. Diagnosis of Soft Tissue Lesions.* 8th ed. London, UK: Bailliere Tindall; 1982.

14. Gajdosik RL, Hallett JP, Slaughter LL. Passive insufficiency of two-joint shoulder muscles. *Clin Biomech.* 1994;9: 377-378.

15. Kebaetse M, McClure P, Pratt NA. Thoracic position effect on shoulder range of motion, strength, and three-dimensional scapular kinematics. *Arch Phys Med Rehabil.* 1999;80:945-950.

16. Boon AJ, Smith J. Manual scapular stabilization: its effect on shoulder rotational range of motion. *Arch Phys Med Rehabil.* 2000;81:978-983.

17. Evjenth O, Hamberg J. *Muscle Stretching in Manual Therapy A Clinical Manual: The Extremities.* Vol. 1. Alfta, Sweden: Alfta Rehab Forlag; 1984.

18. Rosa DP, Brostad JD, Pires ED, Camargo PR. Reliability of measuring pectoralis minor muscle resting length in subjects with and without signs of shoulder impingement. *Braz J Phys Ther.* 2016;20(2):176-183. http://dx.doi.org/10.1590/bjpt-rbf.2014.0146

19. Smith LK, Lawrence Weiss E, Lehmkuhl LD. *Brunnstrom's Clinical Kinesiology.* 5th ed. Philadelphia, PA: FA Davis; 1996.

20. MacConaill MA, Basmajian JV. *Muscles and Movements.* 2nd ed. New York, NY: RE Kreiger; 1977.

21. Cailliet R. *Shoulder Pain.* 3rd ed. Philadelphia, PA: FA Davis; 1991.

22. Rosse C. The shoulder region and the brachial plexus. In: Rosse C, Clawson DK, eds. *The Musculoskeletal System in Health and Disease.* New York, NY: Harper & Row; 1980.

23. Zuckerman JD, Matsen FA. Biomechanics of the shoulder. In: Nordin M, Frankel VM, eds. *Basic Biomechanics of the Musculoskeletal System.* 2nd ed. Philadelphia, PA: Lea & Febiger; 1989.

24. Namdari S, Yagnik G, Ebaugh DD, et al. Defining functional shoulder range of motion for activities of daily living. *J Shoulder Elbow Surg.* 2012;21:1177-1183. doi:10.1016/j.jse.2011.07.032

25. Khadilkar L, MacDermid JC, Sinden KE, et al. An analysis of functional shoulder movements during task performance using Dartfish movement analysis software. *Int J Shoulder Surg.* 2014;8(1):1-9. doi:10.4103/0973-6042.131847

26. Matsen FA, Lippitt SB, Sidles JA, Harryman DT. *Practical Evaluation and Management of the Shoulder.* Philadelphia, PA: WB Saunders; 1994.

27. Inman VT, Saunders M, Abbot LC. Observations on the function of the shoulder joint. *J Bone Joint Surg.* 1944;26:1-30.

28. Dvir Z, Berme N. The shoulder complex in elevation of the arm: a mechanism approach. *J Biomech.* 1978;11:219-225.

29. Kent BE. Functional anatomy of the shoulder complex: a review. *Phys Ther.* 1971;51:867-888.

30. Safaee-Rad R, Shwedyk E, Quanbury AO, Cooper JE. Normal functional range of motion of upper limb joints during performance of three feeding activities. *Arch Phys Med Rehabil.* 1990;71:505-509.

31. Ludewig PM, Cook TM, Nawoczenski DA. Three-dimensional scapular orientation and muscle activity at selected positions of humeral elevation. *J Orthop Sports Phys Ther.* 1996;24: 57-65.

32. Peat M. The shoulder complex: a review of some aspects of functional anatomy. *Physiother Can.* 1977;29:241-246.

33. Blakey RL, Palmer ML. Analysis of rotation accompanying shoulder flexion. *Phys Ther.* 1984;64:1214-1216.

34. Mallon WJ, Herring CL, Sallay PI, et al. Use of vertebral levels to measure presumed internal rotation at the shoulder: a radiologic analysis. *J Shoulder Elbow Surg.* 1996;5:299-306.

EXERCISES AND QUESTIONS

See the Answer Guide in Appendix E for suggested answers to the following exercises and questions.

1. PALPATION

A. For each anatomical structure or reference listed below, identify the shoulder complex ROM that would be measured using the structure or reference to align the universal goniometer. Also identify the part of the goniometer (i.e., axis, stationary arm, or moveable arm) that would be aligned with the anatomical structure or reference for the purpose of the measurement.

    i. Acromion process

    ii. Lateral midline of the trunk

    iii. Olecranon process

    iv. Longitudinal axis of the humerus

B. Palpate the following anatomical structures on a skeleton and on a partner.

Spine of the scapula	Coracoid process
Inferior angle of the scapula	Lateral epicondyle of the humerus
Vertebral border of the scapula	Clavicle
Acromion process	Sternum
Fourth rib	

2. ASSESSMENT OF AROM AT THE SHOULDER COMPLEX

A. List the articulations that make up the:

    i. Shoulder complex

    ii. Shoulder girdle

    iii. Shoulder joint.

B. Mobility at the sternoclavicular joint is essential to enable scapular motion. True or false?

C. With a partner, demonstrate how a therapist would perform a general scan of the AROM of the upper extremity joints.

D. i. List, define, and demonstrate the motions the therapist would observe when assessing scapular AROM.

    ii. What actions would a therapist instruct the patient to perform to observe scapular medial (downward) rotation and scapular lateral (upward) rotation?

- Instruct a partner to assume the anatomical position and use a grease pencil to mark the inferior angle of the scapula on the skin.
- Instruct the partner to perform the actions to observe scapular rotations.
- At the end of the full AROM of scapular medial (downward) rotation and at the end of full lateral (upward) rotation, again mark the position of the inferior angle of the scapula on the skin. It may be necessary to support your partner's arm at the end of each action, and ask your partner to relax. This will enable you to more easily palpate and mark the inferior angle of the scapula.
- Observe the range of scapular motion.

    iii. Instruct a partner to perform the scapular AROM identified in D.i. above, and observe the movements.

E. For each of the shoulder movements listed below,

- Assume the start position for the assessment and measurement of the ROM.
- Move your arm through half of the full AROM and hold the shoulder joint in this position to mimic a decreased AROM.
- Without allowing further movement of the upper extremity at the shoulder joint, try to give the appearance of further movement or a greater than available AROM.

• Identify the substitute movements used to give the appearance of a greater than available AROM for the movement being assessed. These should be the same substitute movement(s) a patient may use to augment a restricted AROM for each shoulder movement.

Shoulder AROM	Substitute Movement(s)
i. Extension	_____
ii. Abduction	_____
iii. External rotation	_____
iv. Horizontal abduction	_____

3. ASSESSMENT AND MEASUREMENT OF PROM AT THE SHOULDER COMPLEX

For each of the movements listed below, demonstrate the assessment and measurement of PROM on a partner and answer the questions that follow. Have a third partner evaluate your performance using the appropriate practical test form at http://thepoint.lww.com/ClarksonJM2e. Record your findings on the PROM recording form on page 92.

Scapular Elevation

i. Assume your partner presented with decreased AROM and PROM for scapular elevation. Identify the articulation(s) where motion could be decreased.

ii. What movement of the clavicle is associated with scapular elevation?

iii. If the movement of the clavicle identified in ii above is decreased, _____ glide of the medial end of the clavicle at the sternoclavicular joint would be restricted. Explain why the glide would be decreased in the direction indicated?

Shoulder Elevation Through Flexion and Through Abduction

i. What articulations of the shoulder complex participate in the movements of shoulder elevation through either flexion or abduction?

ii. Identify and describe the shape of the articular components that make up the glenohumeral joint and the sternoclavicular joint.

Glenohumeral (GH) Joint Abduction

i. When assessing GH joint abduction PROM, identify the stabilization procedure used by the therapist to isolate motion at the GH joint.

ii. Assume your partner has decreased GH joint abduction PROM and this was the result of decreased glide at the joint. What glide of the humeral head would be decreased? Explain the reason for the glide being decreased in the direction indicated.

Shoulder Extension

i. What position should the elbow be in when assessing shoulder extension ROM? Explain.

Shoulder Horizontal Adduction

i. Identify the two different start positions of the shoulder that a therapist may use when assessing horizontal adduction ROM. What other shoulder ROM would be assessed using these same start positions?

ii. Assume a patient presented with equally decreased shoulder horizontal adduction AROM and PROM. What restricted glide of the humeral head would result in decreased shoulder horizontal adduction ROM? Explain the reason for the glide being decreased in the direction(s) indicated.

Shoulder Internal Rotation

i. Assume a patient presented with decreased shoulder internal rotation PROM. Identify the joint(s) where motion would be decreased.

ii. Would the therapist assess AROM or PROM to determine end feel for shoulder internal rotation?

iii. When you assessed your partner's shoulder internal rotation PROM, was the PROM normal? What end feel was present? Would this end feel be considered normal or abnormal? Explain.

iv. List the normal limiting factor(s) that would create a normal firm end feel for shoulder internal rotation.

Other Questions

A. If, when assessing and measuring ROM of the shoulder complex, the therapist stabilizes the scapula, what movements of the shoulder complex is the therapist able to assess?

B. Assume a patient's shoulder elevation through flexion is assessed in sitting position and the therapist finds:

   i.   an AROM of 80° and a PROM of 130°; why might the AROM be less than the PROM?

   ii. an AROM of 30° and the PROM of 30°; why might the patient present with these findings?

ROM RECORDING FORM

Patient's Name _____   Age _____

Diagnosis _____   Date of Onset _____

Therapist Name _____   AROM or PROM _____

Therapist Signature _____   Measurement Instrument _____

Left Side   **Right Side**

	*		*	Date of Measurement	*		*	
				Scapula				
				Elevation				
				Depression				
				Abduction				
				Adduction				
				Shoulder Complex				
				Elevation through Flexion (0–180°)				
				Elevation through Abduction (0–180°)				
				Shoulder (Glenohumeral) Joint				
				Flexion (0–120°)				
				Abduction (0–90° to 120°)				
				Extension (0–60°)				
				Horizontal abduction (0–45°)				
				Horizontal adduction (0–135°)				
				Internal rotation (0–70°)				
				External rotation (0–90°)				
				Hypermobility:				
				Comments:				

4. MUSCLE LENGTH ASSESSMENT AND MEASUREMENT

For the pectoralis major and the pectoralis minor, demonstrate the assessment and measurement of muscle length on a partner and answer the questions below that pertain to the muscle being assessed. Have a third partner evaluate your performance using the appropriate Summary & Evaluation Form at http://thepoint.lww.com/ClarksonJM2e.

Pectoralis Major

    i.   Identify the origin and insertion of the pectoralis major muscle.

    ii. What movements of the upper extremity would position the origin and insertion of the pectoralis major muscle far apart and thus place the muscle on stretch?

    iii. If the pectoralis major is shortened, what end feel would the therapist note at the limit of the PROM when assessing pectoralis major muscle length?

    iv. If the pectoralis major is shortened, what shoulder joint ROM would be restricted proportional to the decrease in muscle length? To assess this restriction using a universal goniometer, the goniometer axis is placed _____, the stationary arm is aligned _____, and the movable arm is aligned parallel to the _____.

Pectoralis Minor

    i.   Identify the origin and insertion of the pectoralis minor muscle.

    ii. What movement(s) of the scapula would move the origin and insertion of the pectoralis minor muscle farther apart and thus place the muscle on stretch?

    iii. If the pectoralis minor is shortened and the patient is lying supine, what observation would indicate to the therapist that the pectoralis minor is shortened?

5. FUNCTIONAL ROM AT THE SHOULDER COMPLEX

A. What is the function of the shoulder complex?

B. i. Hold your dominant arm at your side in anatomical position to simulate an immobile glenohumeral joint. Maintain this position and attempt to carry out or simulate the following activities using your dominant upper extremity, using **no** compensatory movements of other body parts to assist. Identify those activities that are impossible to perform with an immobile glenohumeral joint fixed in anatomical position. (*Note:* You will not be able to perform shoulder internal or external rotation with the glenohumeral joint fixed in the anatomical position; therefore, while trying these activities, pay particular attention to restricting these motions.)

    • Perform toilet hygiene activities.
    • Reach to the midline of your chest to do up buttons on a shirt.
    • Comb your hair.
    • Brush your teeth.
    • Wash your axilla on the contralateral side.
    • Drink a full cup of water.
    • Eat cold soup with a spoon.

  ii. Repeat the above activities and use compensatory movements of other body parts, as required, and shoulder internal and external rotation if necessary. Identify the tasks that can now be completed, and identify the shoulder rotation and compensatory movement(s) used.

C. For each of the following shoulder movements, identify two examples of ADL that require the movement:

    i.   extension
    ii. elevation through flexion
    iii. flexion below shoulder level
    iv. external rotation
    v. horizontal adduction

D. i. Explain the term "scapulohumeral rhythm."

   ii. What is the generally recognized ratio of glenohumeral motion to scapular motion through the complete range of shoulder elevation?

   iii. Identify the factors that affect variations in the contribution of all joints to the scapulohumeral rhythm.

   iv. List the joints at which movement occurs to attain full 180° elevation through either flexion or abduction.

   v. Explain the main movement pattern(s) of the setting phase of shoulder elevation through flexion or abduction.

   vi. Explain the movement pattern through the ROM of shoulder elevation through abduction and through flexion following the setting phase.

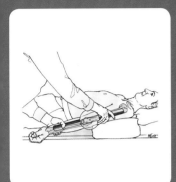

Elbow and Forearm 4

QUICK FIND

ARTICULATIONS AND MOVEMENTS

The elbow, a modified hinge joint (Fig. 4-1), is composed of the humeroulnar and humeroradial joints. The humeroulnar joint is formed proximally by the trochlea of the humerus, which is convex anteroposteriorly,[1] and articulates with the concave surface of the trochlear notch of the ulna. The convex surface of the capitulum of the humerus articulates with the concave proximal aspect of the radial head to form the humeroradial joint.

The elbow may be flexed and extended in the sagittal plane with movement occurring around a frontal axis (Fig. 4-2). The axis for elbow flexion and extension "passes through the center of the arcs formed by the trochlear sulcus and the capitellum"[2 (p. 534)] of the humerus, except at the extremes of motion, when the axis is displaced anteriorly and posteriorly,[2] respectively.

The forearm articulations (Fig. 4-1) consist of the superior and inferior radioulnar joints and the syndesmosis formed by the interosseous membrane between the radius and ulna. The superior radioulnar joint is contained within the capsule of the elbow joint[1] and is a pivot joint formed between the convex surface of the radial head and the concave radial notch on the radial aspect of the proximal ulna. The annular ligament, lined with articular cartilage, encompasses the rim of the radial head.[3] When motion occurs at the superior radioulnar joint, motion also occurs at the humeroradial joint as the head of the radius spins

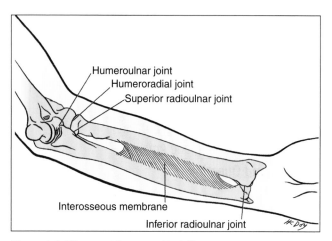

Figure 4-1 Elbow and forearm articulations.

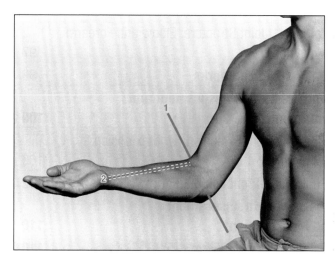

Figure 4-2 Elbow joint and forearm axes: (1) flexion–extension and (2) supination–pronation.

on the capitulum. The inferior radioulnar joint is also a pivot joint, in which the concave ulnar notch on the medial aspect of the distal radius articulates with the convex head of the ulna.

The forearm may be supinated and pronated. These movements occur around an oblique axis that passes through the head of the radius proximally and through the head of the ulna distally[4,5] (Fig. 4-2). With the elbow in anatomical position, the movements of pronation and supination occur in the transverse plane around a longitudinal axis. In supination, the radius lies alongside the ulna (Fig. 4-3A). In pronation, the radius rotates around the relatively stationary ulna (Fig. 4-3B). The movements of the elbow and forearm joints are described in Table 4-1.

TABLE 4-1 Joint Structure: Elbow and Forearm Movements

	Flexion	Extension	Supination	Pronation
Articulation[1,6]	Humeroulnar, Humeroradial	Humeroulnar, Humeroradial	Humeroradial, Superior radioulnar, Inferior radioulnar, Interosseous membrane	Humeroradial, Superior radioulnar, Inferior radioulnar, Interosseous membrane
Plane	Sagittal	Sagittal	Transverse	Transverse
Axis	Frontal	Frontal	Longitudinal	Longitudinal
Normal limiting factors[3,6–8,*] **(see Fig. 4-3A and B)**	Soft tissue apposition of the anterior forearm and upper arm; coronoid process contacting the coronoid fossa and the radial head contacting the radial fossa; tension in the posterior capsule and triceps	Olecranon process contacting the olecranon fossa; tension in the elbow flexors and anterior joint capsule and medial collateral ligament	Tension in the pronator muscles, quadrate ligament, palmar radioulnar ligament of the inferior radioulnar joint, and oblique cord	Contact of the radius on the ulna; tension in the quadrate ligament, the dorsal radioulnar ligament of the inferior radioulnar joint, the distal tract of the interosseous membrane,[9] supinator, and biceps brachii muscles with elbow in extension
Normal end feel[7,10,11,*]	Soft/hard/firm	Hard/firm	Firm	Hard/firm
Normal AROM[12,†] **(AROM**[13]**)**	0°–150° (0°–140°)	0° (0°)	0°–80°–90° (0°–80°)	0°–80°–90° (0°–80°)
Capsular pattern[10,11]	Elbow joint: humeroulnar joint—flexion, extension, and rotation full and painless 　　　　　radiohumeral joint—flexion, extension, supination, pronation Superior radioulnar joint: equal limitation of supination and pronation Inferior radioulnar joint: full rotation with pain at extremes of rotation			

*Note: There is a paucity of definitive research that identifies the normal limiting factors (NLF) of joint motion. The NLF and end feels listed here are based on knowledge of anatomy, clinical experience, and available references.

†AROM, active range of motion.

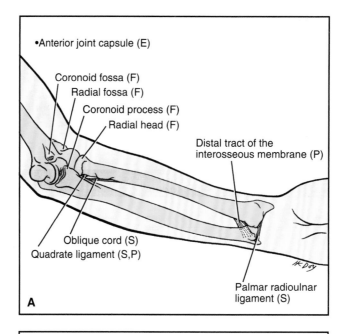

•Anterior joint capsule (E)

Coronoid fossa (F)
Radial fossa (F)
Coronoid process (F)
Radial head (F)

Distal tract of the
interosseous membrane (P)

Oblique cord (S)
Quadrate ligament (S,P)

Palmar radioulnar
ligament (S)

A

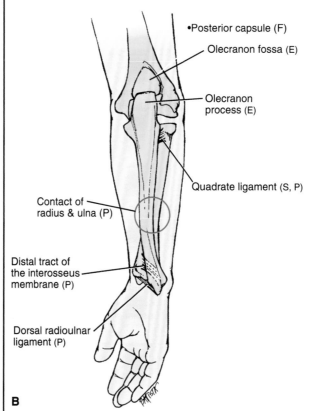

•Posterior capsule (F)

Olecranon fossa (E)

Olecranon
process (E)

Quadrate ligament (S, P)

Contact of
radius & ulna (P)

Distal tract of
the interosseus
membrane (P)

Dorsal radioulnar
ligament (P)

B

Figure 4-3 **Normal Limiting Factors. A.** Anteromedial view of the
elbow and supinated forearm showing noncontractile structures
that normally limit motion. **B.** Posterior view of the elbow with the
forearm pronated showing noncontractile structures that normally
limit motion.

Motion limited by structure is identified in parentheses, using
the following abbreviations: *F*, flexion; *E*, extension; *P*, pronation;
S, supination. Muscles normally limiting motion are not illustrated.

ANATOMICAL LANDMARKS (FIGS. 4-4 TO 4-6)

Anatomical landmarks, numbered 1, 3, 6, 7, and 9 below, are used to align the goniometer axis and arms to measure elbow joint and forearm ROM. Anatomical landmarks, numbered 2, 4, 5, and 8, serve as reference for the location of the landmarks used to evaluate elbow joint and forearm ROM. All anatomical landmarks are described and illustrated below.

Structure	Location
1. Acromion process	Lateral aspect of the spine of the scapula at the tip of the shoulder.
2. Medial epicondyle of the humerus	Medial projection at the distal end of the humerus.
3. Lateral epicondyle of the humerus	Lateral projection at the distal end of the humerus.
4. Olecranon process	Posterior aspect of the elbow; proximal end of the shaft of the ulna.
5. Head of the radius	Distal to the lateral epicondyle of the humerus.
6. Styloid process of the radius	Bony prominence on the lateral aspect of the forearm at the distal end of the radius.
7. Head of the third metacarpal	Bony prominence at the base of the third digit.
8. Head of the ulna	Round bony prominence on the posteromedial aspect of the forearm at the distal end of the ulna.
9. Styloid process of the ulna	Bony projection on the posteromedial aspect of the distal end of the ulna.

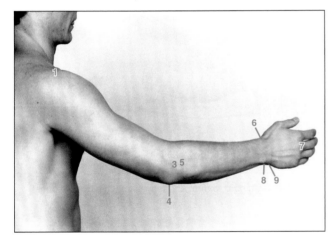

Figure 4-4 Posterolateral aspect of the arm.

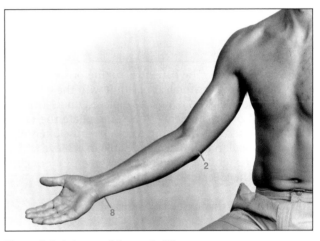

Figure 4-5 Anteromedial aspect of the arm.

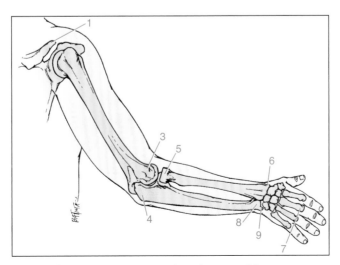

Figure 4-6 Bony anatomy, posterolateral aspect of the arm.

RANGE OF MOTION ASSESSMENT AND MEASUREMENT

 Practice Makes Perfect

To aid you in practicing the skills covered in this section, or for a handy review, use the Summary & Evaluation Forms found at

http://thepoint.lww.com/ClarksonJM2e.

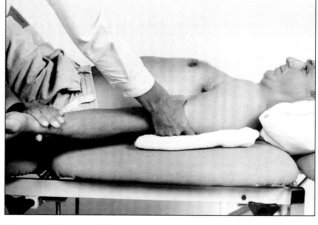

Figure 4-7 Start position for elbow flexion and extension/hyperextension PROM.

Elbow Flexion–Extension/ Hyperextension

AROM Assessment

Substitute Movement. *Flexion*—trunk extension, shoulder flexion, scapular depression, and wrist flexion. *Extension*— trunk flexion, shoulder extension, scapular elevation, and wrist extension.

PROM Assessment

 Start Position. The patient is supine or sitting. The arm is in the anatomical position with the elbow in extension (Fig. 4-7). A towel is placed under the distal end of the humerus to accommodate the range of motion (ROM). Owing to biceps muscle tension, unusually muscular men may not be able to achieve 0°. Up to 15° of hyperextension is common in women[12,14,15] or children because the olecranon is smaller.[15]

Forms 4-1, 4-2

Stabilization. The therapist stabilizes the humerus.

Therapist's Distal Hand Placement. The therapist grasps the distal radius and ulna.

End Positions. The therapist moves the forearm in an anterior direction to the limit of motion of elbow flexion (Fig. 4-8). The therapist moves the forearm in a posterior direction to the limit of elbow extension/hyperextension (Fig. 4-9).

End Feels. *Flexion*—soft/hard/firm; *extension/hyperextension*— hard/firm.

Joint Glides. *Flexion*—concave trochlear notch and concave radial head glide anteriorly on the fixed convexities of the trochlea and capitulum, respectively. *Extension*—concave trochlear notch and concave radial head glide posteriorly on the fixed convexities of the trochlea and capitulum, respectively.

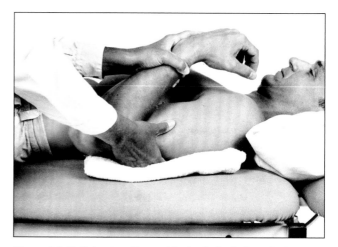

Figure 4-8 Soft, hard, or firm end feel at limit of elbow flexion.

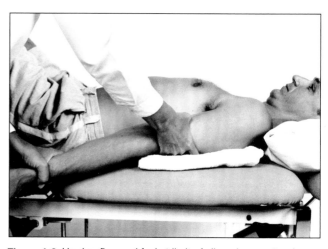

Figure 4-9 Hard or firm end feel at limit of elbow hyperextension.

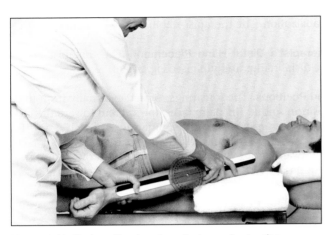

Figure 4-10 Start position for elbow flexion and extension.

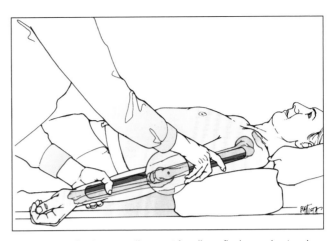

Figure 4-11 Goniometer alignment for elbow flexion and extension.

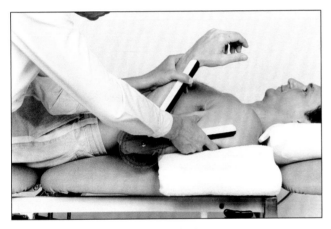

Figure 4-12 End position for elbow flexion.

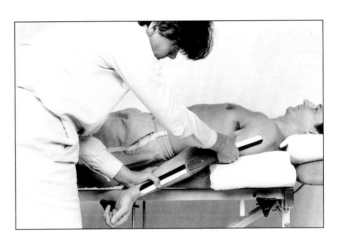

Figure 4-13 End position for elbow hyperextension.

Measurement: Universal Goniometer

Start Position. The patient is supine or sitting. The arm is in the anatomical position with the elbow in extension (0°) (Fig. 4-10). A towel is placed under the distal end of the humerus to accommodate the ROM. Owing to biceps muscle tension, unusually muscular men may not be able to achieve 0°.

Stabilization. The therapist stabilizes the humerus.

Goniometer Axis. The axis is placed over the lateral epicondyle of the humerus (Figs. 4-10 and 4-11).

Stationary Arm. Parallel to the longitudinal axis of the humerus, pointing toward the tip of the acromion process.

Movable Arm. Parallel to the longitudinal axis of the radius, pointing toward the styloid process of the radius.

End Position. From the start position of elbow extension, the forearm is moved in an anterior direction so that the hand approximates the shoulder to the limit of **elbow flexion (150°)** (Fig. 4-12).

Extension/Hyperextension. The forearm is moved in a posterior direction to the limit of **elbow extension (0°)/ hyperextension (up to 15°)** (Fig. 4-13).

Alternate Measurement

The patient is sitting (Figs. 4-14 and 4-15).

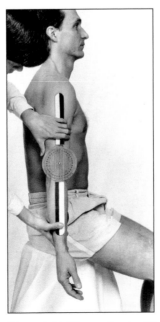

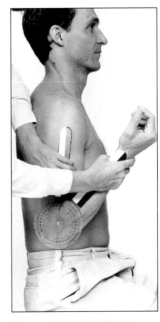

Figure 4-14 Elbow extension 0°.

Figure 4-15 Elbow flexion.

Supination–Pronation

AROM Assessment

Substitute Movement. *Supination*—adduction and external rotation of the shoulder and ipsilateral trunk lateral flexion. *Pronation*—abduction and internal rotation of the shoulder and contralateral trunk lateral flexion.

PROM Assessment

Forms
4-3, 4-4

Start Position. The patient is sitting. The arm is at the side, and the elbow is flexed to 90° with the forearm in midposition (Fig. 4-16A).

Stabilization. The therapist stabilizes the humerus.

Therapist's Distal Hand Placement. The therapist grasps the distal radius and ulna (see Fig. 4-16B).

End Positions. The forearm is rotated externally from midposition so that the palm faces upward and toward the ceiling to the limit of forearm supination (Fig. 4-17A and B). The forearm is rotated internally so that the palm faces downward and toward the floor to the limit of forearm pronation (Fig. 4-18A and B).

End Feels. *Supination*—firm; *pronation*—hard/firm.

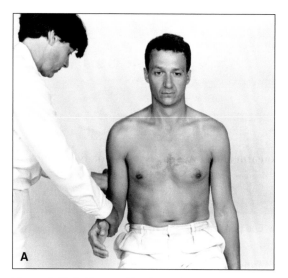
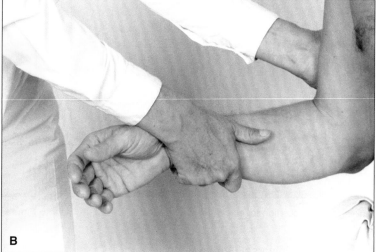

Figure 4-16 A. Start position for supination and pronation. **B.** Therapist's hand position for PROM.

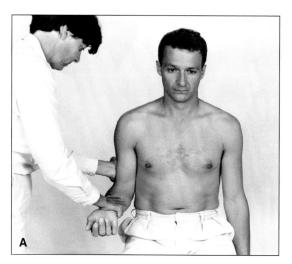
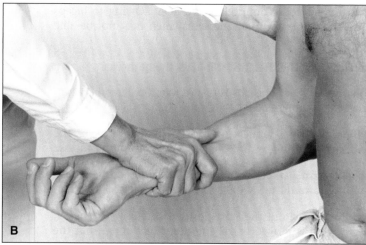

Figure 4-17 A. Firm end feel at limit of supination. **B.** Therapist's hand position.

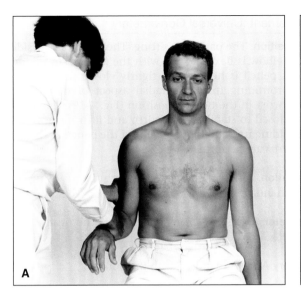
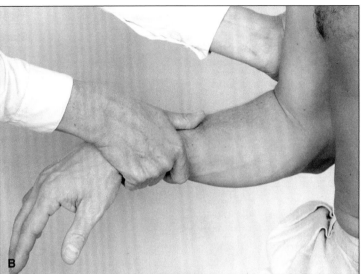

Figure 4-18 **A.** Hard or firm end feel at limit of pronation. **B.** Therapist's hand position.

Joint Glides. *Supination*: (1) The convex radial head rotates within the fibro-osseous ring formed by the annular ligament and the fixed concave radial notch[16] and, according to Baeyens and colleagues,[17] glides anteriorly, contrary to the concave–convex rule. (2) The concave ulnar notch glides posteriorly on the fixed convex ulnar head.[16] *Pronation*: (1) The convex radial head rotates within the fibro-osseous ring formed by the annular ligament and the fixed concave radial notch[16] and, according to Baeyens and colleagues,[17] glides posteriorly, contrary to the concave–convex rule. (2) The concave ulnar notch glides anteriorly on the fixed convex ulnar head.[16] *Humeroradial joint*—the head of the radius spins on the fixed capitulum during supination and pronation.

Five Methods for Measuring Supination and Pronation

Five methods of measuring forearm supination and pronation are presented. Three methods use the universal goniometer and two use the OB "Myrin" goniometer to measure forearm ROM. Most activities of daily living (ADL) combine forearm rotation with hand use (e.g., gripping).[18] Two of the five methods (one using the universal goniometer and one the OB "Myrin" goniometer) measure forearm rotation with the hand in a gripping posture that simulates functional movements (see Figs. 4-19 and 4-29). The measurements performed using the universal goniometer (see Figs. 4-25 to 4-28) and the OB "Myrin" goniometer (see Fig. 4-32) positioned proximal to the wrist measure isolated forearm ROM.

Forearm supination and pronation ROM are affected by change in elbow joint position, that is, as the elbow is flexed, forearm supination ROM increases and forearm pronation ROM decreases, and as the elbow is extended, the converse occurs.[19] The total forearm pronation and supination ROM is greatest between 45° and 90° of elbow flexion.[19] It is therefore important to maintain the elbow in 90° flexion when measuring forearm supination and pronation ROM.

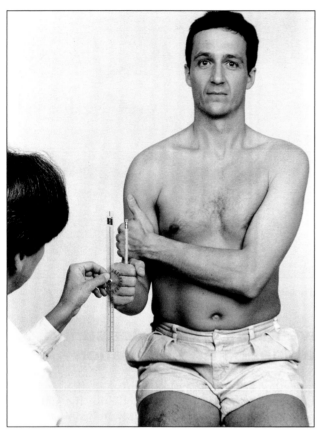

Figure 4-19 Functional measurement method: start position for supination and pronation.

Measurement: Universal Goniometer

Start Position. The patient is sitting. The arm is at the side, and the elbow is flexed to 90° with the forearm in midposition. A pencil is held in the tightly closed fist with the pencil protruding from the radial aspect of the hand,[14] and the wrist in the neutral position (Fig. 4-19). The fist is tightly closed to stabilize the fourth and fifth metacarpals, thus avoiding unwanted movement of the pencil as the test movements are performed.

Stabilization. The patient stabilizes the humerus using the nontest hand.

Goniometer Axis. The axis is placed over the head of the third metacarpal.

Stationary Arm. Perpendicular to the floor.

Movable Arm. Parallel to the pencil.

End Position. The forearm is rotated externally from midposition so that the palm faces upward and toward the ceiling to the limit of **forearm supination (80° to 90° from midposition)** (Fig. 4-20).

Substitute Movement. Altered grasp of the pencil if the fist is not tightly closed during testing, thumb touching and moving the pencil, wrist extension, and/or radial deviation.

End Position. The forearm is rotated internally so that the palm faces downward and toward the floor to the limit of **forearm pronation (80° to 90° from midposition)** (Fig. 4-21).

Substitute Movement. Altered grasp of the pencil, wrist flexion, and/or ulnar deviation.

High intratester[18,20] and intertester[18,21] reliability has been reported for the functional measurement method using the universal goniometer and the pencil held in the hand to measure active supination and pronation ROM.

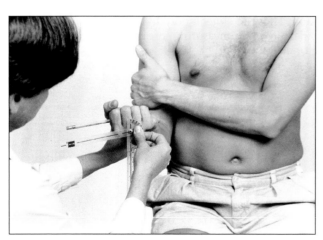

Figure 4-20 Supination.

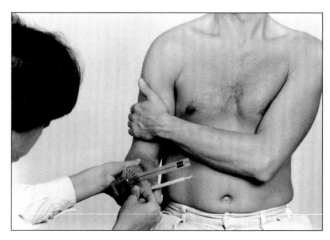

Figure 4-21 Pronation.

Alternate Measurement: Universal Goniometer

This measurement is indicated if the patient cannot grasp a pencil.

Start Position. The arm is at the side, and the elbow is flexed to 90° with the forearm in midposition. The wrist is in neutral, and the fingers are extended (Fig. 4-22).

Stabilization. The patient stabilizes the humerus using the nontest hand.

Goniometer Axis. The axis is placed at the tip of the middle digit.

Stationary Arm. Perpendicular to the floor.

Movable Arm. Parallel to the tips of the four extended fingers.

End Position. The forearm is rotated externally so that the palm faces upward and toward the ceiling to the limit of **forearm supination (80° to 90° from midposition)** (Fig. 4-23).

Substitute Movement. Finger hyperextension, wrist extension, and wrist deviations.

End Position. The forearm is rotated internally so that the palm faces downward and toward the floor to the limit of **forearm pronation (80° to 90° from midposition)** (Fig. 4-24).

Substitute Movement. Finger flexion, wrist flexion, and wrist deviations.

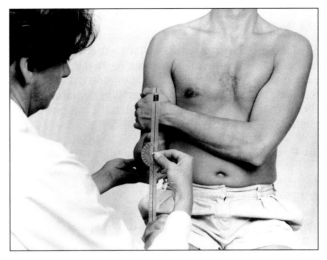

Figure 4-22 Alternate method: start position for supination and pronation.

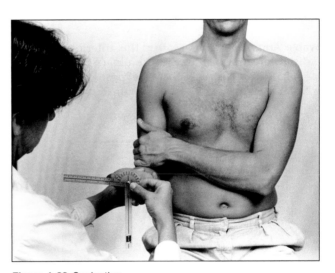

Figure 4-23 Supination.

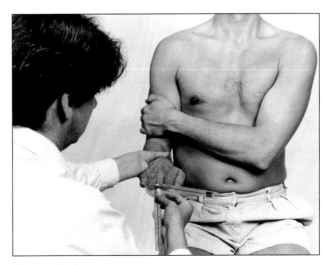

Figure 4-24 Pronation.

Alternate Measurement: Universal Goniometer Proximal to the Wrist

This method eliminates joints distal to the forearm from influencing the measurement and can be used if the patient cannot grasp a pencil. Active range of motion (AROM) measured using this method demonstrated good intratester reliability with the stationary arm parallel to the midline of the humerus.[20]

Start Position. The arm is at the side, and the elbow is flexed to 90° with the forearm in midposition. The wrist is in neutral, and the fingers are relaxed (see Figs. 4-25 and 4-27).

Stabilization. The patient stabilizes the humerus using the nontest hand.

Goniometer Axis. The axis is placed in line with the ulnar styloid process.

Stationary Arm. Perpendicular to the floor.

Movable Arm. *Supination*—against the anterior aspect of the distal forearm in line with the ulnar styloid process (Fig. 4-25). *Pronation*—against the posterior aspect of the distal forearm in line with the ulnar styloid process (Fig. 4-27).

End Position. The forearm is rotated externally so that the palm faces upward and toward the ceiling to the limit of **forearm supination (80° to 90° from midposition)** (Fig. 4-26).

Substitute Movement. Shoulder adduction, shoulder external rotation, and ipsilateral trunk lateral flexion.

End Position. The forearm is rotated internally so that the palm faces downward and toward the floor to the limit of **forearm pronation (80° to 90° from midposition)** (Fig. 4-28).

Substitute Movement. Shoulder abduction, shoulder internal rotation, and contralateral trunk lateral flexion.

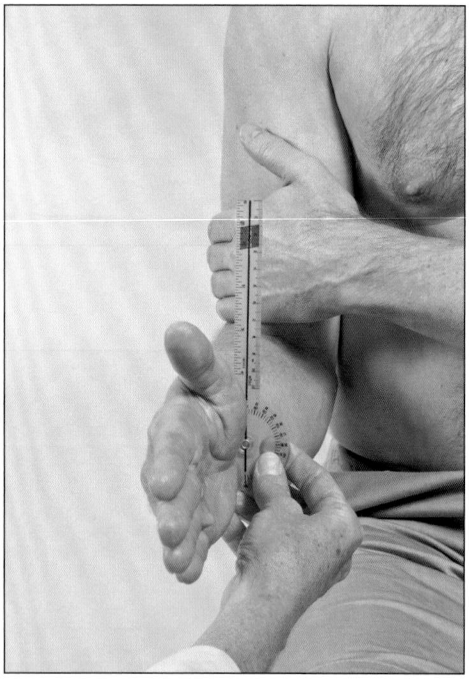

Figure 4-25 Start position for supination.

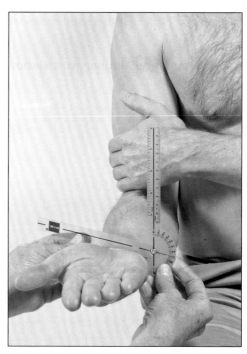

Figure 4-26 End position for supination.

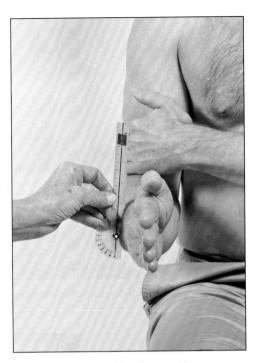

Figure 4-27 Start position for pronation.

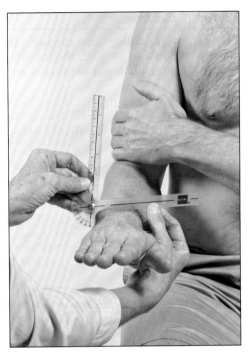

Figure 4-28 End position for pronation.

Measurement: OB "Myrin" Goniometer

Start Position. The patient is sitting. The shoulder is adducted, and the elbow is flexed to 90° with the forearm in midposition. The wrist is in neutral, and the fingers are flexed (Fig. 4-29).

Goniometer Placement. The dial is placed on the right-angled plate. The plate is held between the patient's index and middle fingers.

Stabilization. The therapist stabilizes the humerus.

End Position. The forearm is rotated externally from mid-position to the limit of motion for supination (Fig. 4-30).

Substitute Movement. Wrist extension and deviations, shoulder adduction with external rotation, and ipsilateral trunk lateral flexion.

End Position. The forearm is rotated internally from midposition to the limit of motion for pronation (Fig. 4-31).

Substitute Movement. Wrist flexion and deviations, shoulder abduction with internal rotation, and contralateral trunk lateral flexion.

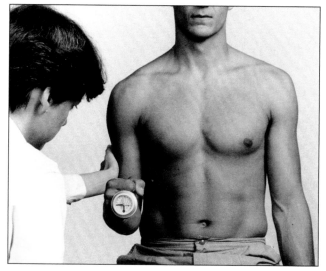

Figure 4-29 Start position for supination and pronation using the OB goniometer.

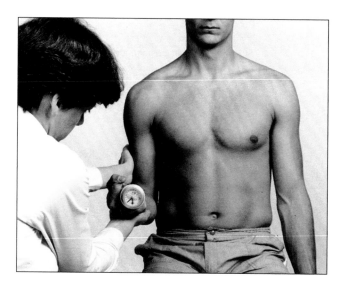

Figure 4-30 End position for supination.

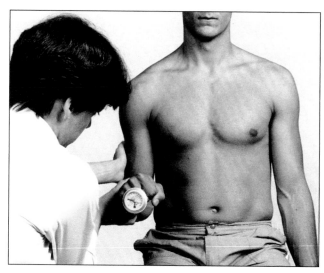

Figure 4-31 End position for pronation.

Alternate Placement: OB "Myrin" Goniometer Proximal to the Wrist

The strap is placed around the distal forearm. The dial is placed on the right-angled plate and attached on the radial side of the forearm (Fig. 4-32). This goniometer placement measures isolated forearm rotation ROM.

Substitute Movement. Using this alternate goniometer placement, substitute movements for supination are limited to shoulder adduction, shoulder external rotation, and ipsilateral trunk lateral flexion. Substitute movements for pronation are limited to shoulder abduction, shoulder internal rotation, and contralateral trunk lateral flexion.

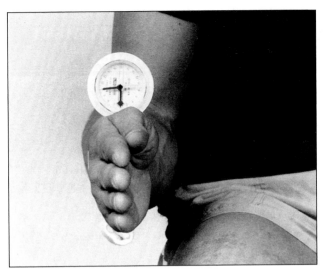

Figure 4-32 Alternate OB goniometer placement for supination and pronation.

MUSCLE LENGTH ASSESSMENT AND MEASUREMENT

 Practice Makes Perfect

To aid you in practicing the skills covered in this section, or for a handy review, use the Summary & Evaluation Forms found at

http://thepoint.lww.com/ClarksonJM2e.

Biceps Brachii

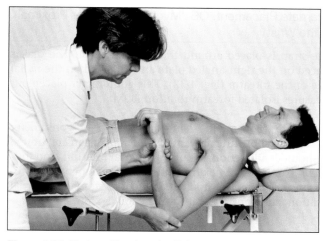

Figure 4-33 Start position: length of biceps brachii.

Origin[1]	Insertion[1]
Biceps Brachii	
a. Short head: apex of the coracoid process of the scapula. b. Long head: supraglenoid tubercle of the scapula.	Posterior aspect of the radial tuberosity and via the bicipital aponeurosis fuses with the deep fascia covering the origins of the flexor muscles of the forearm.

Form 4-5

Start Position. The patient is supine with the shoulder in extension over the edge of the plinth, the elbow is flexed, and the forearm is pronated (Fig. 4-33).

Stabilization. The therapist stabilizes the humerus.

End Position. The elbow is extended to the limit of motion so that the biceps brachii is put on full stretch (Figs. 4-34 and 4-35).

End Feel. Biceps brachii on stretch—firm.

Measurement. The therapist uses a goniometer to measure and record the available elbow extension PROM. If the biceps is shortened, elbow extension PROM will be restricted proportional to the decrease in muscle length.

Universal Goniometer Placement. The goniometer is placed the same as for elbow flexion–extension.

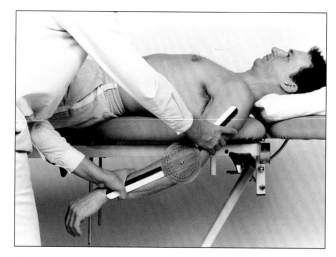

Figure 4-34 Goniometer measurement: length of biceps brachii.

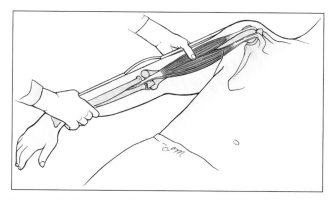

Figure 4-35 Biceps brachii on stretch.

Triceps

Origin[1]	Insertion[1]
Triceps	
a. Long head: infraglenoid tubercle of the scapula.	Posteriorly, on the proximal surface of the olecranon; some fibers continue distally to blend with the antebrachial fascia.
b. Lateral head: posterolateral surface of the humerus between the radial groove and the insertion of teres minor; lateral intermuscular septum.	
c. Medial head: posterior surface of the humerus below the radial groove between the trochlea of the humerus and the insertion of teres major; medial and lateral intermuscular septum.	

Form 4-6

Start Position. The patient is sitting with the shoulder in full elevation through forward flexion and external rotation. The elbow is in extension and the forearm is in supination (Fig. 4-36).

Stabilization. The therapist stabilizes the humerus.

End Position. The elbow is flexed to the limit of motion so that the triceps is put on full stretch (Figs. 4-37 and 4-38).

End Feel. Triceps on stretch—firm.

Measurement. The therapist uses a goniometer to measure and record the available elbow flexion PROM. If the triceps is shortened, elbow flexion PROM will be restricted proportional to the decrease in muscle length.

Goniometer Placement. The goniometer is placed the same as for elbow flexion–extension (Fig. 4-38).

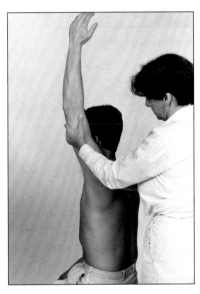

Figure 4-36 Start position: length of triceps.

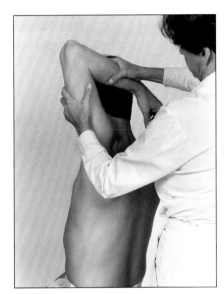

Figure 4-37 End position: triceps on stretch.

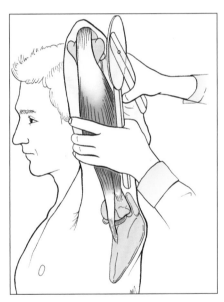

Figure 4-38 Goniometer measurement: length of triceps.

CHAPTER 4

Alternate Measurement: Supine

This position is used if the patient has decreased shoulder flexion ROM.

Start Position. The patient is supine with the shoulder in 90° flexion and the elbow in extension (Fig. 4-39).

Stabilization. The therapist stabilizes the humerus.

End Position. The elbow is flexed to the limit of motion to put the triceps on stretch (Fig. 4-40).

Universal Goniometer Placement. The goniometer is placed the same as for elbow flexion–extension (see Figs. 4-12 and 4-38).

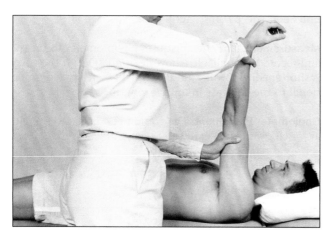

Figure 4-39 Alternate start position: triceps length.

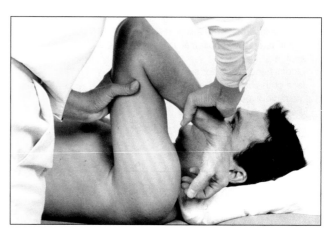

Figure 4-40 End position: triceps on stretch.

FUNCTIONAL APPLICATION

Joint Function

The function of the elbow complex is to serve the hand.[3,6,22] Movement at the elbow joint adjusts the overall functional length of the arm.[16] Elbow extension moves the hand away from the body; elbow flexion moves the hand toward the body. Hand orientation in space and hand mobility are enhanced through supination and pronation of the forearm. The elbow complex, including the forearm, contributes to many skilled and forceful hand movements involved in daily self-care, leisure, and work functions. The elbow complex also provides the power necessary to perform lifting activities[23] and activities involving raising and lowering of the body using the hands.[22]

The elbow and forearm do not function in isolation but link with the shoulder and wrist to enhance hand function.[3] When the elbow is extended, supination and pronation are functionally linked with shoulder external and internal rotation, respectively.[22] These linked movements occur simultaneously during activity. However, when the elbow is flexed, forearm rotation can be isolated from shoulder rotation.[22] This is illustrated in activities such as turning a door handle or using a screwdriver (Fig. 4-41).

Functional Range of Motion

The normal AROM[12] at the elbow is from 0° of extension to 150° of flexion, 80° to 90° of forearm pronation, and 80° to 90° of forearm supination. However, many daily functions are performed with less than these ranges. The ROM required at the elbow and forearm for selected ADL is shown in Table 4-2, as compiled from the works of Morrey,[23] Safaee-Rad,[24] Packer,[25] Magermans,[26] Raiss,[27]

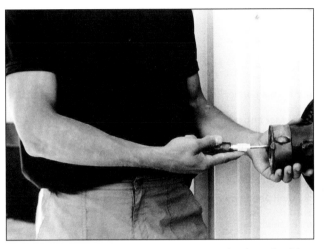

Figure 4-41 Elbow flexion isolates forearm rotation from shoulder rotation.

TABLE 4-2 Elbow and Forearm Range of Motion (ROM) Required for Selected Activities of Daily Living (ADL)[23–28],*

Activity	Flexion ROM (°)		Supination ROM (°)		Pronation ROM (°)	
	Min	Max	Start	End	Start	End
Read a newspaper[23]	78	104	—	—	7	49
Rise from a chair[23]	20	95	—	—	10	34
Sit to stand to sit[25]	15	100	—	—	—	—
Open a door[23]	24	57	—	23	35	—
Open a door[28]	—	—	—	77	—	—
Pour from a pitcher[23]	36	58	22	—	—	43
Pour water into a glass[27]	38	50	20	—	—	55
Drink from a cup[24]	72	129	3	31	—	—
Drink from a glass[27]	42	132	1	23	—	—
Use a telephone[23]	43	136	23	—	—	41
Use a telephone[25]	75	140	—	—	—	—
Use a telephone[27]	69	143	21	—	—	42
Use a telephone[28]	—	146	—	—	—	—
Use a cellular phone[28]	—	147	—	—	—	—
Typing on a computer keyboard[28]	—	—	—	—	—	65
Cut with a knife[23]	89	107	—	—	27	42
Put fork to mouth[23]	85	128	—	52	10	—
Eat with a fork[24]	94	122	—	59	38	—
Eat with a spoon[24]	101	123	—	59	23	—
Eat with a spoon[25]	70	115	—	—	—	—
Eat with a spoon[27]	74	133	—	50	9	—
Comb the hair[26]	112	157	—	—	—	—
Wash axilla[26]	104	132	—	—	—	—
Perineal care[26]	35	100	—	—	—	—

*Mean values from original sources[23,24,27] rounded to the nearest degree. Median values from original source.[25] Minimal and maximal values from the original source[26,28] rounded to the nearest degree.

TABLE 4-3 Elbow and Forearm Positions* of Healthy Subjects Measured During Personal Care and Hygiene Activities[23]

Hand to:	Elbow Flexion (°)	Supination (°)	Pronation (°)
Head–vertex	119	47	—
Head–occiput	144	2	—
Waist	100	12	—
Chest	120	29	—
Neck	135	41	—
Sacrum	70	56	—
Shoe	16	—	19

*Mean values from original source[23] rounded to the nearest degree.

Sardelli,[28] and their colleagues. Positions of the elbow and forearm required to touch different body parts for personal care and hygiene activities are shown in Table 4-3, as based on the work of Morrey and colleagues.[23] The ROM requirements for ADL are influenced by the design of furniture, the placement of utensils, and the patient's posture. In part, these factors could account for the difference in ROM findings between studies for similar ADL shown in Tables 4-2 and 4-3. Thus, the ROM values in Tables 4-2 and 4-3 should be used as a guide for ADL requirements.

Many self-care activities can be accomplished within the arc of movement from 30° to 130° of flexion and from 50° of pronation to 50° of supination.[23] Writing, pouring from a pitcher, reading a newspaper, and performing perineal hygiene are examples of activities performed within these ranges of motion. Feeding activities such as drinking from a cup, using a spoon or fork, and cutting with a knife (Fig. 4-42) may be performed within an arc of movement from about 45° to 136° of flexion and from about 47° pronation to 59° supination.[23,25,29]

Daily functions that may involve extreme ranges of elbow motion include combing or washing the hair (flexion, pronation, and supination) (Fig. 4-43), reaching a back zipper at the neck level (flexion, pronation), using a standard or cellular telephone (approximately 135° to 145° flexion[23,25,27,28] (Fig. 4-44), tying a shoe (16° flexion[23]) (Fig. 4-45), donning a pair of trousers (extension) (Fig. 4-46), throwing a ball (extension), walking with axillary crutches (extension) (Fig. 4-47), using the arms to elevate the body when getting up from a chair (15° flexion[25]), playing tennis (extension), and using a computer mouse or keyboard (65° pronation[28]) (Fig. 4-48).

Less elbow ROM is required to perform most upper extremity activities when elbow flexion and extension ROM is restricted and compensatory motions are allowed at normal adjacent joints. In this case, functional elbow ROM is from 75° to 120° flexion.[30] These compensatory motions occur at the thoracic and lumbar spines, shoulder (primarily scapulothoracic and clavicular joints), and wrist.[31] With the elbow in a fixed position of 90° flexion, although there are limitations in function, in most cases all personal care ADL (i.e., feeding and personal hygiene) can be performed.[30,32] This is supported by the findings of van Andel and colleagues[33] that a minimum of 85° elbow flexion is required to comb hair, reach a back pocket or the contralateral shoulder, or bring the hand to the mouth to drink.

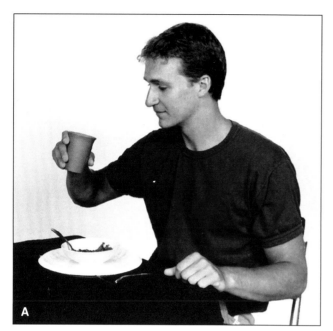

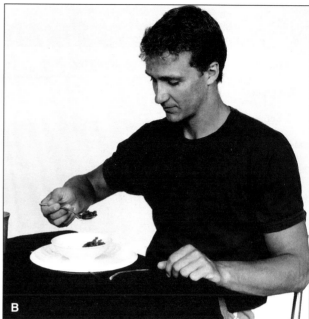

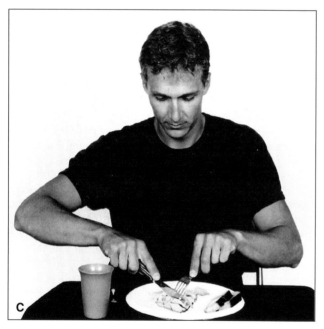

Figure 4-42 Elbow range within the arc of movement from about 45° to 136° of flexion and from about 47° of pronation to 59° of supination. **A.** Drinking from a cup. **B.** Eating using a spoon. **C.** Eating using a knife and fork.

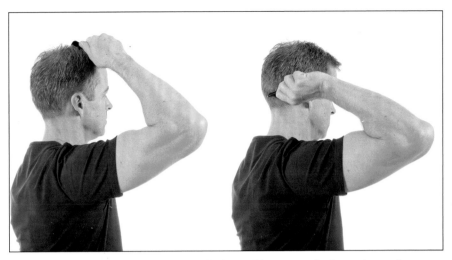

Figure 4-43 Combing hair requires elbow flexion and forearm supination and pronation.

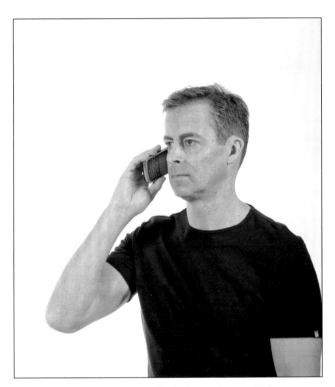

Figure 4-44 Elbow flexion required when using a cell phone.

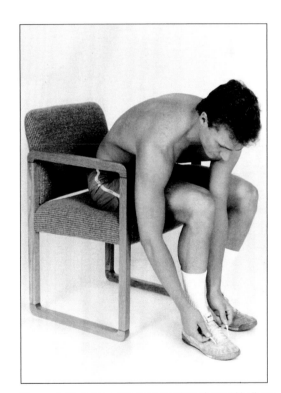

Figure 4-45 Tying a shoelace requires about 16° elbow flexion.

CHAPTER 4

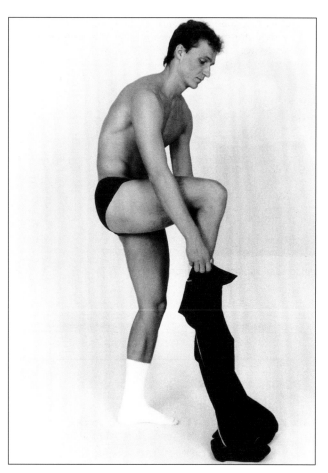

Figure 4-46 Elbow extension when donning a pair of trousers.

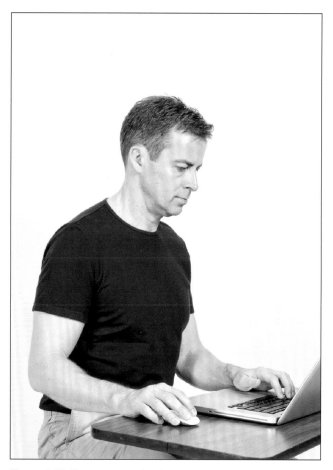

Figure 4-48 Forearm pronation is required when using a computer mouse, trackpad, or keyboard.

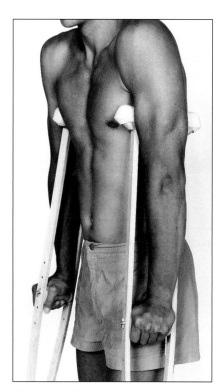

Figure 4-47 Elbow extension required to walk with axillary crutches.

With restriction of elbow ROM, loss of elbow flexion has a greater impact on loss of function than loss of elbow extension in a ratio of about 2:1.[34] Thus, the functional impact of a 5° loss of elbow flexion is approximately equivalent to a 10° loss of elbow extension ROM.

In the presence of restricted forearm ROM, Kasten and associates[35] identified the main compensatory motions at the shoulder and elbow to be shoulder internal/external rotation, followed by shoulder abduction/adduction and elbow flexion/extension, and to a lesser extent shoulder flexion/extension. Compensatory motion also occurs at the wrist joint in the presence of restricted forearm ROM.[36] Kasten and associates[35] concluded that with the forearm fixed in nearly neutral rotation, all of the following ADL tasks, that is, pouring water into a glass, drinking from a glass, eating with a spoon, answering the phone, drawing a large number "8" on a desk, using a keyboard, turning a page, turning a key in a keyhole, combing the hair, and cleaning genitals and buttocks, could be completed with the contribution of shoulder and elbow movements.

References

1. Standring S, ed. *Gray's Anatomy: The Anatomical Basis of Clinical Practice*. 39th ed. London: Elsevier Churchill Livingstone; 2005.
2. London JT. Kinematics of the elbow. *J Bone Joint Surg Am*. 1981;63(4):529-535.
3. Levangie PK, Norkin CC. *Joint Structure and Function: A Comprehensive Analysis*. 4th ed. Philadelphia, PA: FA Davis; 2005.
4. Steindler A. *Kinesiology of the Human Body Under Normal and Pathological Conditions*. Springfield, IL: Charles C Thomas; 1955.
5. Nakamura T, Yabe Y, Horiuchi Y, Yamazaki N. In vivo motion analysis of forearm rotation utilizing magnetic resonance imaging. *Clin Biomech*. 1999;14:315–320.
6. Kapandji IA. *The Physiology of the Joints. Vol. 1. The Upper Limb*. 6th ed. New York, NY: Churchill Livingstone Elsevier; 2007.
7. Norkin CC, White DJ. *Measurement of Joint Motion: A Guide to Goniometry*. 4th ed. Philadelphia, PA: FA Davis; 2009.
8. Nordin M, Frankel VH. *Basic Biomechanics of the Musculoskeletal System*. 3rd ed. Philadelphia, PA: Lippincott Williams & Wilkins; 2001.
9. Gabl M, Zimmermann R, Angermann P, et al. The interosseous membrane and its influence on the distal radioulnar joint. An anatomical investigation of the distal tract. *J Hand Surg Br*. 1998;23(2):179-182.
10. Cyriax J. *Textbook of Orthopaedic Medicine. Vol 1. Diagnosis of Soft Tissue Lesions*. 8th ed. London: Bailliere Tindall; 1982.
11. Magee DJ. *Orthopedic Physical Assessment*. 5th ed. Philadelphia, PA: Saunders Elsevier; 2008.
12. American Academy of Orthopaedic Surgeons. *Joint Motion: Method of Measuring and Recording*. Chicago, IL: AAOS; 1965.
13. Berryman Reese N, Bandy WD. *Joint Range of Motion and Muscle Length Testing*. 2nd ed. Philadelphia, PA: Saunders Elsevier; 2010.
14. Hoppenfeld S. *Physical Examination of the Spine and Extremities*. New York, NY: Appleton-Century-Crofts; 1976.
15. Kaltenborn FM. *Mobilization of the Extremity Joints*. 3rd ed. Oslo, Norway: Olaf Norlis Bokhandel; 1985.
16. Neumann DA. *Kinesiology of the Musculoskeletal System: Foundations for Physical Rehabilitation*. 2nd ed. Philadelphia, PA: Mosby Elsevier; 2010.
17. Baeyens J-P, Van Glabbeek F, Goossens M, Gielen J, Van Roy P, Clarys J-P. In vivo 3D arthrokinematics of the proximal and distal radioulnar joints during active pronation and supination. *Clin Biomech*. 2006;21:S9-S12.
18. Karagiannopoulos C, Sitler M, Michlovitz S. Reliability of 2 functional goniometric methods for measuring forearm pronation and supination active range of motion. *J Orthop Sports Phys Ther*. 2003;33(9):523–531.
19. Shaaban H, Pereira C, Williams R, Lees VC. The effect of elbow position on the range of supination and pronation of the forearm. *J Hand Surg Eur Vol*. 2008;33(1):3-8.
20. Gajdosik RL. Comparison and reliability of three goniometric methods for measuring forearm supination and pronation. *Percept Mot Skills*. 2001;93:353–355.
21. Cimatti B, Marcolino AM, Barbosa RI. A study to compare two goniometric methods for measuring active pronation and supination range of motion. *Hand Ther*. 2013;18(2):57-63.
22. Smith LK, Lawrence Weiss EL, Lehmkuhl LD. *Brunnstrom's Clinical Kinesiology*. 5th ed. Philadelphia, PA: FA Davis; 1996.
23. Morrey BF, Askew LJ, An KN, Chao EY. A biomechanical study of normal functional elbow motion. *J Bone Joint Surg Am*. 1981;63:872-876.
24. Safaee-Rad R, Shwedyk E, Quanbury AO, Cooper JE. Normal functional range of motion of upper limb joints during performance of three feeding activities. *Arch Phys Med Rehabil*. 1990;71:505-509.
25. Packer TL, Peat M, Wyss U, Sorbie C. Examining the elbow during functional activities. *OTJR*. 1990;10:323-333.
26. Magermans DJ, Chadwick EKJ, Veeger HEJ, van der Helm FCT. Requirements for upper extremity motions during activities of daily living. *Clin Biomech*. 2005;20:591-599.
27. Raiss P, Rettig O, Wolf S, Loew M, Kasten P. Range of motion of shoulder and elbow in activities of daily living in 3D motion analysis. *Z Orthop Unfall*. 2007;145:493-498.
28. Sardelli M, Tashjian RZ, MacWilliams BA. Functional elbow range of motion for contemporary tasks. *J Bone Joint Surg Am*. 2011;93:471-477.
29. Cooper JE, Shwedyk E, Quanbury AO, Miller J, Hildebrand D. Elbow joint restriction: effect on functional upper limb motion during performance of three feeding activities. *Arch Phys Med Rehabil*. 1993;74:805-809.
30. Vasen AP, Lacey SH, Keith MW, Shaffer JW. Functional range of motion of the elbow. *J Hand Surg Am*. 1995;20:288-292.
31. O'Neill OR, Morrey BF, Tanaka S, An KN. Compensatory motion in the upper extremity after elbow arthrodesis. *Clin Orthop Relat Res*. 1992;281:89-96.
32. Nagy SM, Szabo RM, Sharkey NA. Unilateral elbow arthrodesis: the preferred position. *J South Orthop Assoc*. 1999;8(2):80-85.
33. van Andel CJ, Wolterbeek N, Doorenbosch CAM, Veeger D, Harlaar J. Complete 3D kinematics of upper extremity functional tasks. *Gait Posture*. 2008;27:120-127.
34. Morrey BF, An KN. Functional evaluation of the elbow. In: Morrey BF, ed. *The Elbow and Its Disorders*. 3rd ed. Philadelphia, PA: WB Saunders; 2000.
35. Kasten P, Rettig O, Loew M, Wolf S, Raiss P. Three dimensional motion analysis of compensatory movements in patients with radioulnar synostosis performing activities of daily living. *J Orthop Sci*. 2009;14:307-312.
36. Ogino T, Hikino K. Congenital radio-ulnar synostosis: compensatory rotation around the wrist and rotation osteotomy. *J Hand Surg Br*. 1987;12(2):173-178.

EXERCISES AND QUESTIONS

See the Answer Guide in Appendix E for suggested answers to the following exercises and questions.

1. PALPATION

A. Identify the anatomical landmarks a therapist would use to align the universal goniometer axis and stationary and moveable arms when measuring the ROM at the elbow and forearm.

   i. Elbow flexion/extension:

     Goniometer axis _____

     Stationary arm _____

     Moveable arm _____

   ii. Forearm supination/pronation measurement with (a) closed fist and pencil, (b) fingers extended, and (c) the goniometer proximal to the wrist:

     Goniometer axis a. _____

                       b. _____

                       c. _____

     Stationary arm   a. _____

                       b. _____

                       c. _____

     Moveable arm   a. _____

                       b. _____

                       c. _____

B. Palpate the anatomical reference points used to align the goniometer when measuring elbow and forearm ROM on a skeleton and on a partner.

2. ASSESSMENT PROCESS

List the 10 main components of the assessment process performed by the therapist to assess pathology located at the elbow and forearm.

3. ASSESSMENT OF AROM AT THE ELBOW AND FOREARM ARTICULATIONS

A. Identify and describe the shape of the articular components that make up the elbow articulation and forearm articulations.

B. Demonstrate, define, and identify the axis and plane of movement, for the following movements:

   i. Elbow joint movements

   ii. Forearm movements with:

     a) Your elbow in 90° flexion

     b) Your elbow in the anatomical position (i.e., 0°), and identify the movements at the shoulder joint that augment each of the forearm movements

C. For each of the movements listed below:
- Assume the start position for the assessment and measurement of the ROM.
- Move the forearm through half of the full AROM, and hold the joint in this position to mimic a decreased AROM.
- Without allowing further movement of the forearm, try to give the appearance of further movement or a greater than available AROM.
- Identify the substitute movements used to give the appearance of a greater than available AROM for the movement being assessed. A patient may use the same substitute movement(s) to augment restricted AROM.

Elbow and Forearm AROM	Substitute Movement(s)
i. Forearm supination	_____
ii. Elbow extension	_____
iii. Elbow flexion	_____
iv. Forearm pronation	_____

D. The therapist assesses a patient's elbow flexion AROM and PROM in sitting and, using a universal goniometer, measures 80° AROM and 130° PROM. Identify possible reasons why the AROM would be less than the PROM for elbow flexion.

4. ASSESSMENT AND MEASUREMENT OF PROM AT THE ELBOW AND FOREARM

For each of the movements listed below, demonstrate the assessment and measurement of PROM on a partner and answer the questions that follow. Record your findings on the PROM Recording Form below. Have a third partner evaluate your performance using the appropriate Summary & Evaluation Form in Appendix B.

ROM RECORDING FORM

Patient's Name _____ Age _____

Diagnosis _____ Date of Onset _____

Therapist Name _____ AROM or PROM _____

Therapist Signature _____ Measurement Instrument _____

			Left Side / **Right Side**				
	*	*	**Date of Measurement**	*		*	
			Elbow and Forearm				
			Flexion (0–150°)				
			Extension (0°)				
			Supination (0–80°–90°)				
			Pronation (0–80°–90°)				
			Hypermobility:				
			Comments:				

Elbow Flexion

    i. What normal end feel(s) is (are) expected when assessing elbow flexion?

    ii. Only one end feel can be identified for each joint motion assessed. True or false?

    iii. What elbow flexion end feel did you identify on your partner?

    iv. Identify the normal limiting factor(s) that could have resulted in the end feel identified on your partner.

Elbow Extension/Hyperextension

    i. Identify the two-joint muscle that crosses the shoulder and elbow joints and if placed on stretch could restrict elbow extension ROM. The muscle is placed on stretch during the assessment of elbow extension ROM if the shoulder is in _____ and the forearm is _____. Therefore, the therapist ensures the forearm is _____ and the shoulder is in the _____ position to avoid passive insufficiency of the two-joint muscle from restricting elbow extension ROM.

    ii. A patient presents with decreased elbow extension PROM caused by decreased movement at the humeroulnar and humeroradial articulations. Identify the direction of the decreased glide of the trochlea of the ulna and the radial head that would cause the decreased elbow extension PROM.

    iii. Explain how a therapist would determine the direction(s) of decreased glide in ii above.

Forearm Supination

    i. Assume a patient presents with decreased forearm supination PROM. Identify the joint(s) where motion could be decreased.

    ii. Identify the motion that occurs between the radial head and the capitulum when the forearm is supinated.

    iii. In the presence of decreased forearm supination ROM, identify the direction of glide of the radial head that could be limited and cause the decreased ROM.

    iv. Explain how a therapist would determine the direction of decreased glide in iii above.

    v. In full supination, the radius lies _____ to the ulna.

Forearm Pronation

    i. What end feel was present when you assessed your partner's forearm pronation PROM?

    ii. What normal end feel(s) can be expected when assessing forearm pronation?

    iii. List the normal limiting factors that would create the normal end feel(s) for forearm pronation.

    iv. Moving from a position of full supination to one of full pronation, the radius _____ around the relatively _____ ulna.

5. MUSCLE LENGTH ASSESSMENT AND MEASUREMENT

Demonstrate the assessment and measurement of muscle length of the biceps brachii and triceps on a partner and answer the questions below that pertain to the triceps muscle. Have a third partner evaluate your performance using the appropriate Summary & Evaluation Form in Appendix B.

Triceps

    i. Identify the origin and insertion of the triceps muscle.

    ii. Identify the movements of the upper extremity that would place the origin and insertion of the triceps muscle farther apart and thus place the triceps on stretch.

    iii. A therapist would identify a _____ end feel at the limit of _____ PROM when assessing triceps muscle length in the presence of an abnormally shortened triceps muscle.

6. FUNCTIONAL ROM AT THE ELBOW AND FOREARM

A. i. With your dominant elbow fixed in 0° extension, identify the regions/parts of your body you would be unable to contact with your dominant hand if you were:

   a) Standing

   b) Sitting

   ii. List personal care ADL that would be impossible to perform using your dominant hand with the elbow fixed in 0° extension.

B. i. With your dominant elbow fixed in 90° flexion, identify the regions/parts of your body you would be unable to contact with your dominant hand if you were:

   a) Standing

   b) Sitting

   ii. List personal care ADL that would be impossible to perform using your dominant hand with the elbow fixed in 90° flexion.

C. Have a partner perform or simulate the following functional activities. Use a universal goniometer and measure the maximum elbow flexion ROM required to successfully complete each of the following activities without using substitute movement(s):

   i. Drinking from a cup

   ii. Holding the telephone to the ear

   iii. Tying a shoe lace

   iv. Combing the hair on the back of the head

   v. Reaching for a wallet in a back pocket

D. Identify the forearm position(s) required to perform the following activities:

   i. Picking up a small object from a tabletop

   ii. Receiving change in the palm of the hand

   iii. Eating with a fork

   iv. Reaching for a wallet in a back pocket

   v. Combing the hair on the vertex of the head

E. According to the findings of Morrey et al.,[1] many self-care activities can be accomplished within the arc of movement from _____° to _____° flexion and from _____° of pronation to _____° of supination.

Reference

1. Morrey BF, Askew LJ, An KN, Chao EY. A biomechanical study of normal functional elbow motion. *J Bone Joint Surg Am.* 1981;63:872-876.

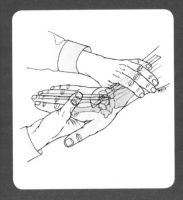

Wrist and Hand 5

QUICK FIND

ARTICULATIONS AND MOVEMENTS

The articulations of the wrist and hand are illustrated in Figures 5-1 and 5-2. The movements of the wrist and hand are summarized in Tables 5-1 to 5-3.

Located between the forearm and hand, the *wrist* is made up of eight small bones (Figs. 5-1 and 5-2A). These bones are arranged in a proximal row (the scaphoid, lunate, triquetrum, and pisiform) and a distal row (the trapezium, trapezoid, capitate, and hamate).

The proximal surface of the proximal row of carpal bones (excluding the pisiform, which articulates solely with the triquetrum) is convex (Fig. 5-2B). This convex surface articulates with the concave surface of the distal aspect of the radius and the articular disc of the inferior radioulnar joint to form the ellipsoidal, *radiocarpal joint.*[2]

The *midcarpal joint* is a compound articulation[2] formed between the proximal and distal rows of carpal bones. The

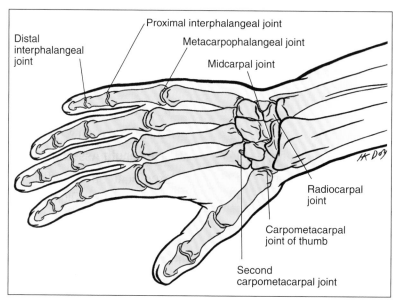

Figure 5-1 Wrist, finger, and thumb articulations.

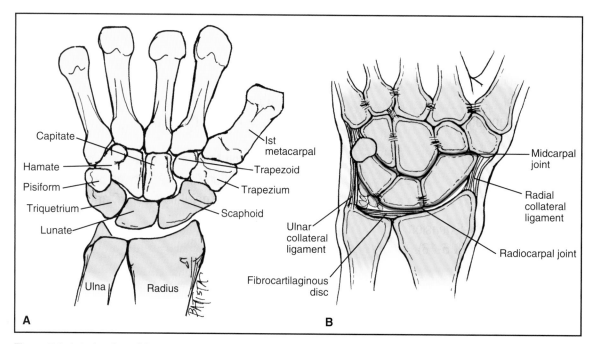

Figure 5-2 Anterior view of the wrist showing **(A)** bony anatomy and **(B)** the concave–convex contours of the midcarpal and radiocarpal joints.

TABLE 5-1 Joint Structure: Wrist Movements

	Flexion	Extension	Radial Deviation	Ulnar Deviation
Articulation[1,2]	Radiocarpal Midcarpal	Midcarpal Radiocarpal	Midcarpal Radiocarpal	Radiocarpal (predominant) Midcarpal
Plane	Sagittal	Sagittal	Frontal	Frontal
Axis	Frontal	Frontal	Sagittal	Sagittal
Normal limiting factors[1,3,4,*] (See Figs. 5-10A and B)	Tension in the posterior radiocarpal ligament and posterior joint capsule	Tension in the anterior radiocarpal ligament and anterior joint capsule; contact between the radius and the carpal bones	Tension in the ulnar collateral ligament, ulnocarpal ligament, and ulnar portion of the joint capsule; contact between the radial styloid process and the scaphoid bone	Tension in the radial collateral ligament and radial portion of joint capsule
Normal end feel[3,5]	Firm	Firm/hard	Firm/hard	Firm
Normal AROM[6] (AROM[7])	0°–80° (0°–80°)	0°–70° (0°–70°)	0°–20° (0°–20°)	0°–30° (0°–30°)
Capsular pattern[5,8]	Flexion and extension are equally restricted			

*There is a paucity of definitive research that identifies the normal limiting factors (NLF) of joint motion. The NLF and end feels listed here are based on knowledge of anatomy, clinical experience, and available references.

TABLE 5-2 Joint Structure: Finger Movements

	Flexion	Extension	Abduction	Adduction
Articulation[1,2]	Metacarpophalangeal (MCP) Proximal interphalangeal (PIP) Distal interphalangeal (DIP)	MCP PIP DIP	MCP	MCP
Plane	Sagittal	Sagittal	Frontal	Frontal
Axis	Frontal	Frontal	Sagittal	Sagittal
Normal limiting factors[1,3,4,*] (See Fig. 5-11)	MCP: tension in the posterior joint capsule, collateral ligaments; contact between the proximal phalanx and the metacarpal; tension in extensor digitorum communis and extensor indicis (when the wrist is flexed)[9] PIP: contact between the middle and proximal phalanx; soft tissue apposition of the middle and proximal phalanges; tension in the posterior joint capsule, and collateral ligaments DIP: tension in the posterior joint capsule, collateral ligaments, and oblique retinacular ligament	MCP: tension in the anterior joint capsule, palmar fibrocartilaginous plate (palmar ligament); tension in flexor digitorum profundus and flexor digitorum superficialis (when the wrist is extended)[9] PIP: tension in the anterior joint capsule, palmar ligament DIP: tension in the anterior joint capsule, palmar ligament	Tension in the collateral ligaments, fascia, and skin of the web spaces	Contact between adjacent fingers
Normal end Feel[3,5]	MCP: firm/hard PIP: hard/soft/firm DIP: firm	MCP: firm PIP: firm DIP: firm	Firm	
Normal AROM[6] (AROM[7])	MCP: 0°–90° (0°–90°) PIP: 0°–100° (0°–100°) DIP: 0°–90° (0°–70°)	MCP: 0°–45° (0°–20°) PIP: 0° (0°) DIP: 0° (0°)		
Capsular pattern[5,8]	Metacarpophalangeal and interphalangeal joints: flexion, extension			

*There is a paucity of definitive research that identifies the normal limiting factors (NLF) of joint motion. The NLF and end feels listed here are based on knowledge of anatomy, clinical experience, and available references.

TABLE 5-3 Joint Structure: Thumb Movements

	Flexion	Extension	Palmar Abduction	Adduction
Articulation[1,2]	Carpometacarpal (CM) Metacarpophalangeal (MCP) Interphalangeal (IP)	CM MCP IP	CM MCP	CM MCP
Plane	CM: oblique frontal MCP: frontal IP: frontal	CM: oblique frontal MCP: frontal IP: frontal	CM: oblique sagittal	CM: oblique sagittal
Axis	CM: oblique sagittal MCP: sagittal IP: sagittal	CM: oblique sagittal MCP: sagittal IP: sagittal	CM: oblique frontal	CM: oblique frontal
Normal limiting factors[1,3,4],* (See Fig. 5-11)	CM: soft tissue apposition between the thenar eminence and the palm; tension in the posterior joint capsule, extensor pollicis brevis, and abductor pollicis brevis MCP: contact between the first metacarpal and the proximal phalanx; tension in the posterior joint capsule, collateral ligaments, and extensor pollicis brevis IP: tension in the collateral ligaments, and posterior joint capsule; contact between the distal phalanx, fibrocartilaginous plate and the proximal phalanx	CM: tension in the anterior joint capsule, flexor pollicis brevis, and first dorsal interosseous MCP: tension in the anterior joint capsule, palmar ligament, and flexor pollicis brevis IP: tension in the anterior joint capsule, palmar ligament	Tension in the fascia and skin of the first web space, first dorsal interosseous, and adductor pollicis	Soft tissue apposition between the thumb and index finger
Normal end feel[3,5,8]	CM: soft/firm MCP: hard/firm IP: hard/firm	CM: firm MCP: firm IP: firm	Firm	Soft
Normal AROM[6] (AROM[7])	CM: 0°–15° (0°–15°) MCP: 0°–50° (0°–50°) IP: 0°–80° (0°–65°)	CM: 0°–20° (0°–20°) MCP: 0° (0°) IP: 0°–20° (0°–10°–20°)	0°–70° (0°–70°)	0° (0°)
Capsular pattern[5,8]	CM joint: abduction and extension MCP and IP joints: flexion, extension			

*There is a paucity of definitive research that identifies the normal limiting factors (NLF) of joint motion. The NLF and end feels listed here are based on knowledge of anatomy, clinical experience, and available references.

proximal aspect of the distal row of carpal bones has a concave surface laterally, formed by the trapezium and trapezoid bones, and a convex surface medially, formed by the capitate and hamate (Fig. 5-2B). These surfaces articulate with the corresponding distal aspect of the proximal row of carpal bones that has a convex surface laterally, formed by the scaphoid bone, and a concave surface medially, formed by the scaphoid, lunate, and triquetrum.

In the clinical setting, it is not possible to independently measure the motion at the radiocarpal and midcarpal joints. Thus, wrist range of motion (ROM) measurements include the combined motion of both joints. Movement at the radiocarpal and midcarpal joints include wrist flexion,

extension, radial deviation, and ulnar deviation. From the anatomical position, wrist flexion and extension occur in the sagittal plane around a frontal axis (Fig. 5-3). Wrist radial deviation and ulnar deviation occur in the frontal plane about a sagittal axis (Fig. 5-4). Maximal wrist flexion and extension active range of motion (AROM) occur with the wrist positioned near 0° radial and ulnar deviation and vice versa.[10]

Movement at the *carpometacarpal (CM) joints* (Fig. 5-1), formed between the distal surfaces of the distal row of carpal bones and the bases of the metacarpal bones, is essential for normal hand function. CM joint movement contributes to the flattening of the palm when the hand is opened fully

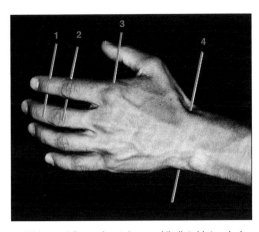

Figure 5-3 Wrist and finger frontal axes: (*1*) distal interphalangeal flexion–extension, (*2*) proximal interphalangeal flexion–extension, (*3*) metacarpophalangeal flexion–extension, and (*4*) wrist flexion–extension.

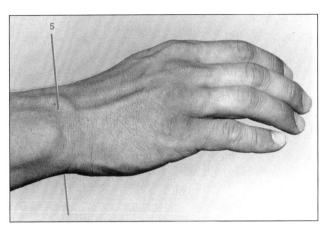

Figure 5-4 Wrist sagittal axis: (*5*) ulnar–radial deviation.

(Fig. 5-5A) and the guttering of the palm when gripping or manipulating objects (Fig. 5-5B). The mobile peripheral metacarpals of the ring and little fingers and the thumb move around the fixed metacarpals of the index and middle fingers. The mobility of the thumb, fourth, and fifth metacarpals around the fixed metacarpals of the index and middle fingers is observed as the open hand is made into a relaxed fist and then into a clenched fist (Fig. 5-6). In the clinical setting, it is not possible to directly measure movements at the CM joints of the second through fifth metacarpals, but it is possible to measure movement at the CM joint of the thumb.

The *CM joint of the thumb* (Fig. 5-7) is a saddle joint formed between the distal surface of the trapezium, which is concave anteroposteriorly and convex mediolaterally, and the corresponding reciprocal surface of the base of the first metacarpal. The movements at the first CM joint include flexion, extension, abduction, adduction, rotation, and opposition. Flexion and extension occur in an oblique

frontal plane about an oblique sagittal axis (Fig. 5-8). During flexion, the thumb is moved from anatomical position (Fig. 5-9A) across the palmar surface of the hand (Fig. 5-9B). Thumb extension (Fig. 5-9C) at the CM joint involves movement of the thumb laterally away from the anatomical position in the opposite direction to flexion. The thumb is abducted when moved from the anatomical position (Fig. 5-9D) in a direction perpendicular to the palm of the hand (Fig. 5-9E). Adduction of the thumb returns the thumb to the anatomical position from the abducted position. Abduction and adduction of the thumb occur in an oblique sagittal plane around an oblique frontal axis. Opposition (Fig. 5-9F) is a sequential movement incorporating abduction, flexion, and adduction of the first metacarpal, with simultaneous rotation.[11]

The *metacarpophalangeal (MCP) joints* of the hand are classified as ellipsoid joints,[2] each formed proximally by the convex head of the metatarsal articulating with the concave base of the adjacent proximal phalanx (Fig. 5-1). The move-

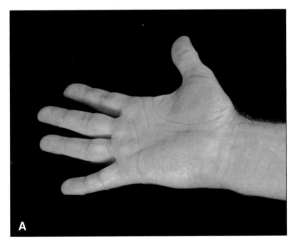

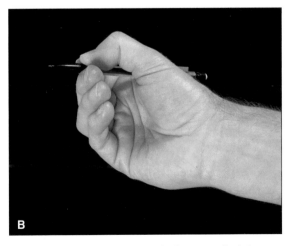

Figure 5-5 A. Flattening of the palm when the hand is opened. **B.** Guttering of the palm when gripping or manipulating an object.

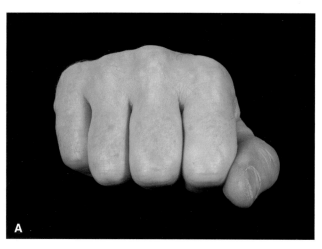 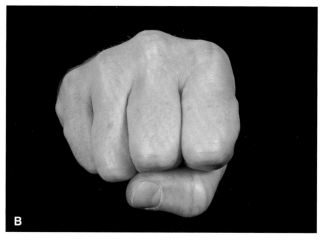

Figure 5-6 Mobility at the fourth and fifth carpometacarpal joints is observed when **(A)** the relaxed fist is compared to **(B)** the clenched fist.

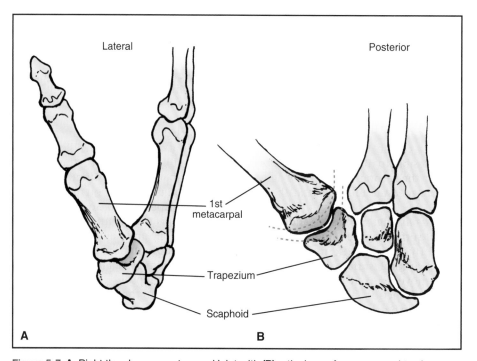

Figure 5-7 A: Right thumb carpometacarpal joint with **(B)** articular surfaces exposed to show concave-convex contours.

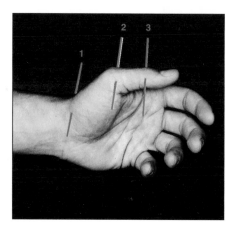

Figure 5-8 Thumb oblique sagittal axes: (*1*) carpometacarpal flexion–extension, (*2*) metacarpophalangeal flexion–extension, and (*3*) interphalangeal flexion–extension.

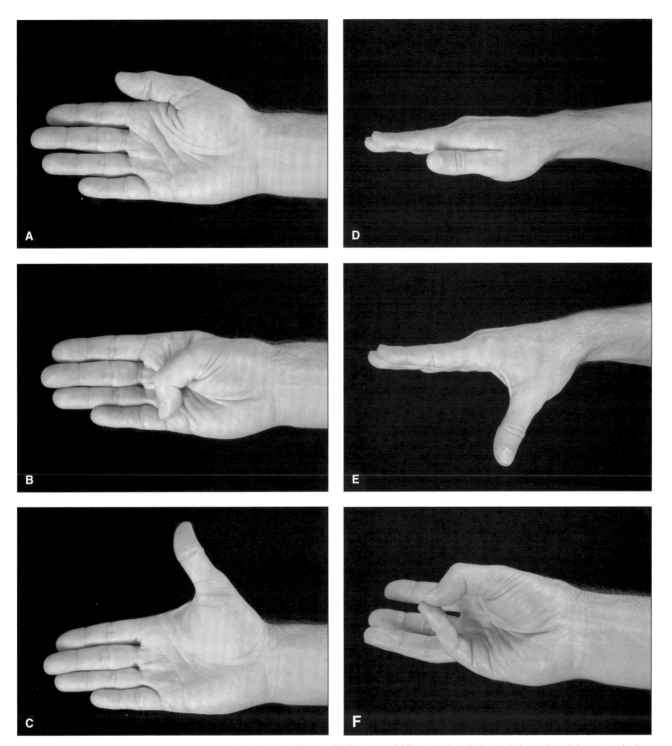

Figure 5-9 A: Anterior view—thumb in anatomical position. Thumb **(B)** flexion and **(C)** extension. **D:** Lateral view—thumb in anatomical position. Thumb **(E)** abduction and **(F)** opposition.

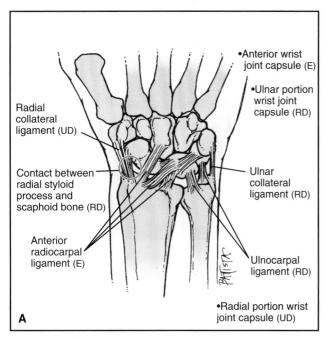

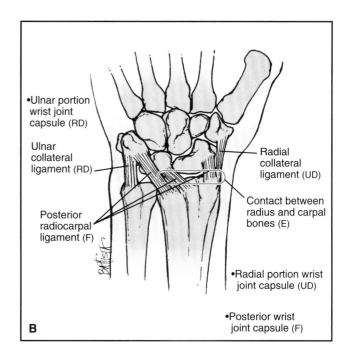

Figure 5-10 Normal limiting factors. A. Anterior view of the wrist showing noncontractile structures that normally limit motion at the wrist. **B.** Posterior view of the wrist showing noncontractile structures that normally limit motion at the wrist. Motion limited by structures is identified in brackets, using the following abbreviations: *F*, flexion; *E*, extension; *UD*, ulnar deviation; *RD*, radial deviation. Muscles normally limiting motion are not illustrated.

ments at the MCP articulations include flexion, extension, abduction, adduction, and rotation. The movements that are measured in the clinical setting are flexion and extension, which occur in the sagittal plane around a frontal axis (see Fig. 5-3), and abduction and adduction, which occur in the frontal plane around a sagittal axis. It is not possible to measure rotation at the MCP joints in the clinical setting.

The *interphalangeal (IP) joints* of the thumb and fingers (see Fig. 5-1) are classified as hinge joints, formed by the convex head of the proximal phalanx articulating with the concave base of the adjacent distal phalanx. The IP joints allow flexion and extension movements of the fingers that occur in the sagittal plane around a frontal axis (Fig. 5-3) and the thumb that occur in the oblique frontal plane about an oblique sagittal axis (Fig. 5-8).

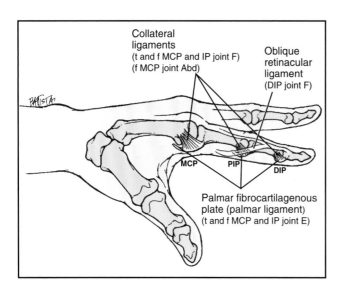

Figure 5-11 Normal limiting factors. Lateral view of the wrist and hand showing noncontractile structures that normally limit motion at the MCP and IP joints of the fingers **(f)** and thumb **(t)**. Other noncontractile structures that normally limit motion at the MCP and IP joints and first CM joint are listed in Table 5-2. Motion limited by structures is identified in brackets, using the following abbreviations: *F*, flexion; *E*, extension; *Abd*, abduction. Muscles normally limiting motion are not illustrated.

ANATOMICAL LANDMARKS (FIGS. 5-12 TO 5-14)

Anatomical landmarks are described and illustrated below. Anatomical landmarks, numbered 1, 3, 4, 6, 7, 8, and 11, are used to assess wrist and hand ROM and/or to align the goniometer axis and arms to measure ROM at the wrist and hand.

Structure	Location
1. Styloid process of the ulna	Bony prominence on the posteromedial aspect of the forearm at the distal end of the ulna.
2. Styloid process of the radius.	Bony prominence on the lateral aspect of the forearm at the distal end of the radius.
3. Metacarpal bones	The bases and shafts are felt through the extensor tendons on the posterior surface of the wrist and hand. The heads are the bony prominences at the bases of the digits.
4. Capitate bone	In the small depression proximal to the base of the third metacarpal bone.
5. Pisiform bone	Medial bone of the proximal row of carpal bones; proximal to the base of the hypothenar eminence.
6. Thumb web space	The web of the skin connecting the thumb to the hand.
7. Distal palmar crease	Transverse crease commencing on the medial side of the palm and extending laterally to the web between the index and middle fingers.
8. Proximal palmar crease	Transverse crease commencing on the lateral side of the palm, extending medially and fading out on the hypothenar eminence.
9. Thenar eminence	The pad on the palm of the hand at the base of the thumb; bound medially and distally by the longitudinal palmar crease.
10. Hypothenar eminence	The pad on the medial side of the base of the palm.
11. First CM joint	At the distal aspect of the anatomical snuffbox, the articulation between the base of the first metacarpal and the trapezium. (*Anatomical snuffbox*: with the thumb held in extension, the triangular area on the postero-lateral aspect of the wrist and hand outlined by the tendons of the extensor pollicis longus laterally and the extensor pollicis brevis medially.)

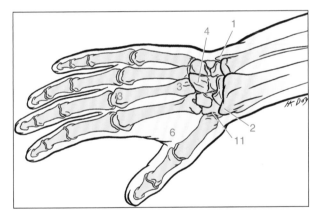

Figure 5-12 Bony anatomy, posterior aspect of the wrist and hand.

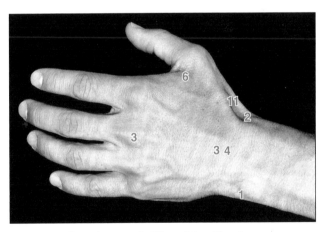

Figure 5-13 Posterior aspect of the wrist and hand.

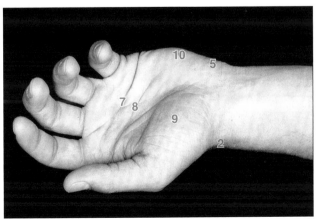

Figure 5-14 Anterior aspect of the wrist and hand.

RANGE OF MOTION ASSESSMENT AND MEASUREMENT

 Practice Makes Perfect

To aid you in practicing the skills covered in this section, or for a handy review, use the Summary & Evaluation Forms found at

http://thepoint.lww.com/ClarksonJM2e.

General Scan: Wrist and Hand Active Range of Motion

The AROM of the wrist and hand is scanned to provide a general indication of the available ROM and/or muscle strength at the wrist and hand. With the patient sitting, the elbow flexed 90°, and the forearm pronated, instruct the patient to:

- Make a fist (Fig. 5-15A). Observe the AROM of finger flexion, thumb flexion and abduction, and wrist extension.
- Open the hand, and maximally spread the fingers (Fig. 5-15B). Observe the AROM for finger extension and abduction, thumb extension, and wrist flexion.
- Supinate the forearm and touch the pad of the thumb to the pad of the fifth finger (Fig. 5-15C). Observe the AROM for opposition of the thumb and fifth finger.

The findings of the scan serve as a guide for detailed assessment of the region.

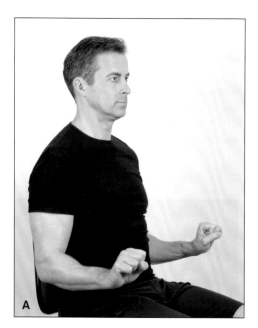

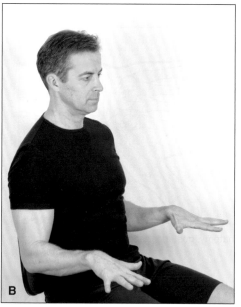

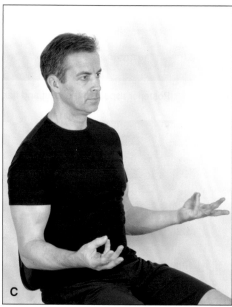

Figure 5-15 General scan of the wrist and hand AROM—the patient **(A)** makes a fist, **(B)** opens the hand, and **(C)** supinates the forearm and touches the pad of the thumb to the pad of the little finger.

Wrist Flexion–Extension

AROM Assessment

Substitute Movement. Wrist ulnar or radial deviation.

PROM Assessment

Start Position. The patient is sitting. The elbow is flexed, the forearm is resting on a table in pronation, the wrist is in neutral position, the hand is over the end of the table, and the fingers are relaxed (Fig. 5-16). Finger position influences wrist ROM; therefore, wrist ROM should be assessed using consistently standardized finger position.[12]

Forms
5-1, 5-2

Stabilization. The therapist stabilizes the forearm.

Therapist's Distal Hand Placement. The therapist grasps the metacarpals.

End Position. The therapist moves the hand anteriorly to the limit of motion to assess wrist flexion (Fig. 5-17). The therapist moves the hand posteriorly to the limit of motion for wrist extension (Fig. 5-18). The fingers should be relaxed when assessing the end feels to avoid restriction of wrist flexion or extension due to stretch of the long finger extensors or flexors, respectively.

End Feels. *Wrist flexion*—firm; *wrist extension*—firm/hard.

Joint Glides. *Flexion. Radiocarpal joint*—the convex surface of the proximal row of carpal bones glides posteriorly on the fixed concave surface of the distal radius and articular disc of the inferior radioulnar joint. *Midcarpal joint*—the concave surface formed by the trapezium and trapezoid glides in an anterior direction on the fixed convex surface of the scaphoid; the convex surface formed by the capitate and hamate glides in a posterior direction on the fixed concave surface formed by the scaphoid, lunate, and triquetrum bones.

Extension. Radiocarpal joint—the convex surface of the proximal row of carpal bones glides anteriorly on the fixed concave surface of the distal radius and articular disc of the inferior radioulnar joint. *Midcarpal joint*—the concave surface formed by the trapezium and trapezoid glides in

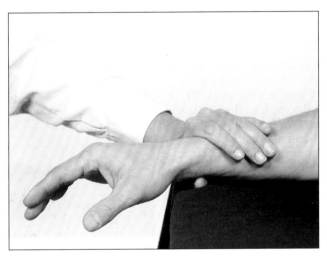

Figure 5-16 Start position for wrist flexion and extension.

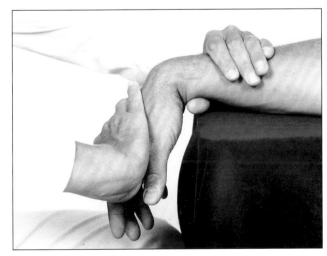

Figure 5-17 Firm end feel at limit of wrist flexion.

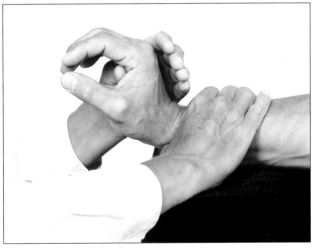

Figure 5-18 Firm or hard end feel at limit of wrist extension.

a posterior direction on the fixed convex surface of the scaphoid; the convex surface formed by the capitate and hamate glides in an anterior direction on the fixed concave surface formed by the scaphoid, lunate, and triquetrum bones.

The above represents a simplified explanation of wrist arthrokinematics with application of the concave–convex rule during wrist movement.

Measurement: Universal Goniometer

Start Position. The patient is sitting. The elbow is flexed, the forearm is resting on a table in pronation, the wrist is in a neutral position, and the hand is over the end of the table (Fig. 5-19). The fingers are relaxed to avoid restriction of wrist flexion or extension due to stretch of the long finger extensors or flexors, respectively.

Stabilization. The therapist stabilizes the forearm.

Goniometer Axis. The axis is placed at the level of the ulnar styloid process (Fig. 5-20).

Stationary Arm. Parallel to the longitudinal axis of the ulna.

Movable Arm. Parallel to the longitudinal axis of the fifth metacarpal.

End Positions. The wrist is moved in an anterior direction to the limit of **wrist flexion (80°)** (Figs. 5-20 and 5-21). The wrist is moved in a posterior direction to the limit of **wrist extension (70°)** (Fig. 5-22). For both movements, ensure that the mobile fourth and fifth metacarpals are not moved away from the start position throughout the assessment procedure, and ensure that no wrist deviation occurs if full range cannot be obtained.

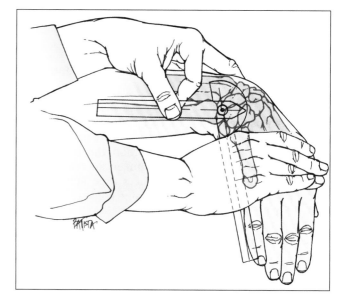

Figure 5-20 Goniometer alignment for wrist flexion and extension, illustrated at limit of wrist flexion.

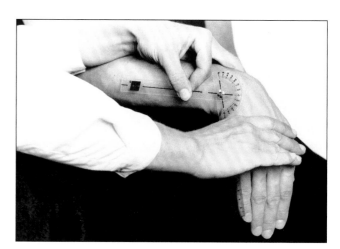

Figure 5-21 End position for wrist flexion.

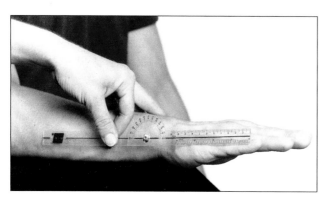

Figure 5-19 Start position for wrist flexion and extension.

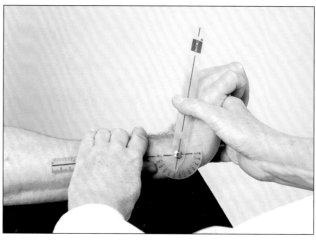

Figure 5-22 End position for wrist extension.

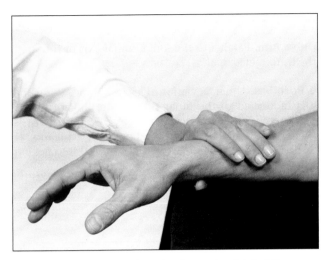

Figure 5-23 Start position for wrist ulnar and radial deviation.

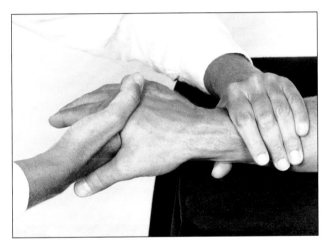

Figure 5-24 Firm end feel at limit of wrist ulnar deviation.

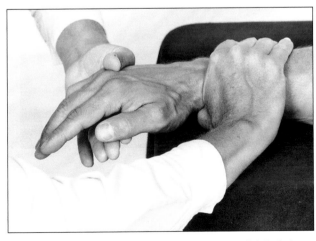

Figure 5-25 Firm or hard end feel at limit of wrist radial deviation.

Wrist Ulnar and Radial Deviation

AROM Assessment

Substitute Movement. Ulnar or radial deviation of the fingers, wrist flexion, and wrist extension.

PROM Assessment

Forms 5-3, 5-4

Start Position. The patient is sitting. The forearm is resting on a table in pronation, the wrist is in neutral position, the hand is over the end of the table, and the fingers are relaxed (see Fig. 5-23). Finger position influences wrist ROM; therefore, wrist ROM should be assessed using consistently standardized finger position.[12]

Stabilization. The therapist stabilizes the forearm.

Therapist's Distal Hand Placement. The therapist grasps the metacarpals from the radial aspect of the hand to assess wrist ulnar deviation (Fig. 5-24). The therapist grasps the metacarpals from the ulnar aspect of the hand to assess wrist radial deviation (Fig. 5-25).

End Positions. The therapist moves the hand in an ulnar direction to the limit of motion to assess wrist ulnar deviation (Fig. 5-24). The therapist moves the hand in a radial direction to the limit of motion for wrist radial deviation (Fig. 5-25).

End Feels. *Ulnar deviation*—firm; *radial deviation*—firm/hard.

Joint Glides.[13] *Ulnar deviation. Radiocarpal joint*—the convex surface of the proximal row of carpal bones glides laterally on the fixed concave surface of the distal radius and articular disc of the inferior radioulnar joint. *Midcarpal joint*—the convex surface formed by the capitate and hamate glides in a lateral direction on the fixed concave surface formed by the scaphoid, lunate, and triquetrum bones.

Radial deviation. Radiocarpal joint—the convex surface of the proximal row of carpal bones glides medially on the fixed concave surface of the distal radius and articular disc of the inferior radioulnar joint. *Midcarpal joint*—the convex surface formed by the capitate and hamate glides in a medial direction on the fixed concave surface formed by the scaphoid, lunate, and triquetrum bones.

The above represents a simplified explanation of wrist arthrokinematics with application of the concave–convex rule during wrist movement.

CHAPTER 5

Measurement: Universal Goniometer

Start Position. The patient is sitting. The elbow is flexed, the forearm is pronated, and the palmar surface of the hand is resting lightly on a table. The wrist remains in a neutral position and the fingers are relaxed (Fig. 5-26) to avoid restriction of wrist ulnar deviation due to finger constraints.[12]

Stabilization. The therapist stabilizes the forearm.

Goniometer Axis. The axis is placed on the posterior aspect of the wrist joint over the capitate bone (Fig. 5-27).

Stationary Arm. Along the midline of the forearm.

Movable Arm. Parallel to the longitudinal axis of the shaft of the third metacarpal.

End Positions. Ulnar deviation (Figs. 5-27 and 5-28): the wrist is adducted to the ulnar side to the limit of **ulnar deviation (30°)**. Radial deviation (Fig. 5-29): the wrist is abducted to the radial side to the limit of **radial deviation (20°)**. Ensure that the wrist is not moved into flexion or extension.

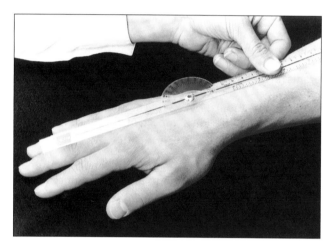

Figure 5-26 Start position for ulnar and radial deviation of the wrist.

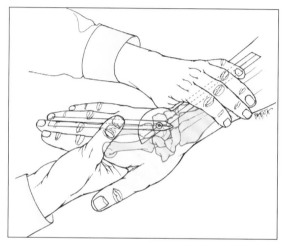

Figure 5-27 Goniometer alignment for wrist ulnar deviation and radial deviation, illustrated at limit of ulnar deviation.

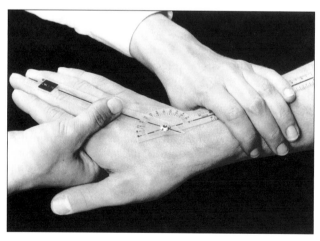

Figure 5-28 End position: ulnar deviation.

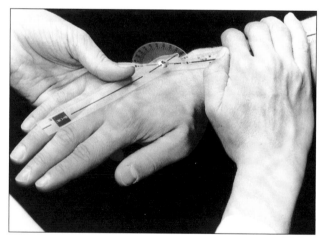

Figure 5-29 End position: radial deviation.

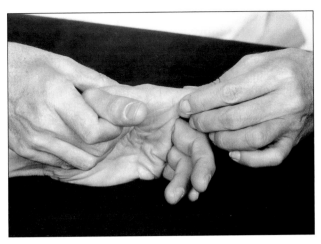

Figure 5-30 Start position: MCP joint flexion and extension.

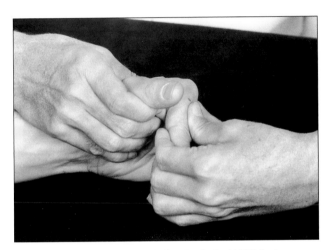

Figure 5-31 Firm or hard end feel at the limit of MCP flexion.

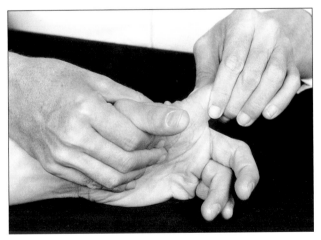

Figure 5-32 Firm end feel at the limit of MCP extension.

Finger MCP Flexion–Extension

PROM Assessment

Forms
5-5, 5-6

Start Position. The patient is sitting. The forearm is resting on a table in midposition, the wrist is in neutral position, and the fingers are relaxed (Fig. 5-30).

Stabilization. The therapist stabilizes the metacarpal.

Therapist's Distal Hand Placement. The therapist grasps the proximal phalanx.

End Positions. The therapist moves the proximal phalanx in an anterior direction to the limit of motion to assess MCP joint flexion (Fig. 5-31). The therapist moves the proximal phalanx in a posterior direction to the limit of motion for MCP joint extension (Fig. 5-32).

End Feels. *MCP joint flexion*—firm/hard; *MCP joint extension*—firm.

Joint Glides. *MCP joint flexion*—the concave base of the proximal phalanx glides in an anterior direction on the fixed convex head of the adjacent metacarpal. *MCP joint extension*—the concave base of the proximal phalanx glides in a posterior direction on the fixed convex head of the adjacent metacarpal.

Measurement: Universal Goniometer

Finger MCP Flexion

Start Position. The patient is sitting. The forearm is resting on a table, the elbow is flexed, the wrist is slightly extended, and the MCP joint of the finger being measured is in 0° of extension (Fig. 5-33).

Stabilization. The therapist stabilizes the metacarpal.

Goniometer Axis. The axis is placed on the posterior aspect of the MCP joint being measured.

Stationary Arm. Parallel to the longitudinal axis of the shaft of the metacarpal.

Movable Arm. Parallel to the longitudinal axis of the proximal phalanx.

End Position. All fingers are moved toward the palm to the limit of **MCP joint flexion (90°)** (Fig. 5-34). Range increases progressively from the index to the fifth finger.[1] The IP joints are allowed to extend so that flexion at the MCP joint is not restricted due to tension of the long finger extensor tendons.

Alternate Goniometer Placement. The index and fifth MCP joints may be measured on the lateral aspect of the joint (Figs. 5-35 and 5-36). Should joint enlargement prevent measurement on the posterior aspect, the index and fifth fingers may be measured and the range estimated for the middle and fourth fingers.[14]

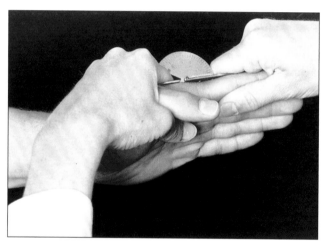

Figure 5-33 Start position for MCP flexion.

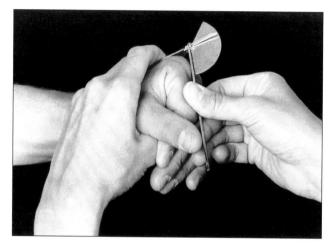

Figure 5-34 End position: MCP flexion.

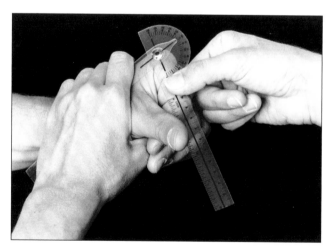

Figure 5-35 Alternate goniometer placement for MCP flexion.

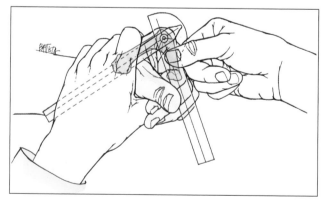

Figure 5-36 Goniometer alignment on the lateral aspect of the joint for MCP joint flexion and extension, illustrated with the MCP joint in flexion.

Measurement: Universal Goniometer

Finger MCP Extension

Start Position. The patient is sitting. The forearm is resting on a table, the elbow is flexed, the wrist is slightly flexed, and the MCP joint of the finger being measured is in 0° of extension (Fig. 5-37).

Stabilization. The therapist stabilizes the metacarpal.

Goniometer Axis. The axis is placed on the anterior surface of the MCP joint being measured.

Stationary Arm. Parallel to the longitudinal axis of the shaft of the metacarpal.

Movable Arm. Parallel to the longitudinal axis of the proximal phalanx.

End Position. The finger is moved in a posterior direction to the limit of **MCP joint extension (45°)** (Fig. 5-38). The IP joints are allowed to flex so that extension at the MCP joint is not restricted due to tension of the long finger flexor tendons.

Alternate Goniometer Placement. The index and fifth MCP joints may be measured on the lateral aspect of the MCP joint (Fig. 5-39).

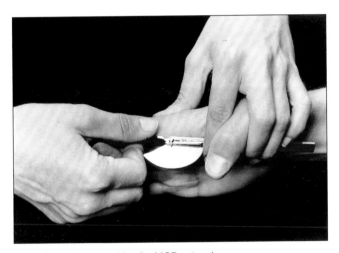

Figure 5-37 Start position for MCP extension.

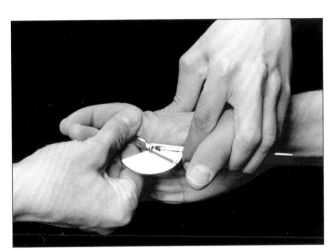

Figure 5-38 End position: MCP extension.

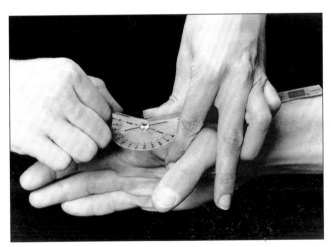

Figure 5-39 Alternate goniometer placement for MCP extension.

Finger MCP Abduction–Adduction

AROM Assessment

MCP Abduction

To gain a composite measure of finger spread and thumb web stretch, finger abduction and thumb extension can be measured in centimeters. A sheet of paper is placed under the patient's hand. The therapist stabilizes the wrist and metacarpals. The patient spreads all fingers and thumb and the therapist traces the contour of the hand (Fig. 5-40). The patient's hand is removed, and a linear measure of the distances between the midpoint of the tip of each finger and the index finger and thumb is recorded in centimeters (Fig. 5-41). *Note* that the ROM at the IP, MCP, and CM joints of the thumb influences the measurement of thumb extension ROM using this method.

PROM Assessment

MCP Abduction

Start Position. The patient is sitting. The forearm is resting on a table, the wrist is in neutral position, and the fingers are in the anatomical position (Fig. 5-42).

Forms 5-7, 5-8

Stabilization. The therapist stabilizes the metacarpal.

Therapist's Distal Hand Placement. The therapist grasps the sides of the proximal phalanx.

End Position. The therapist moves the proximal phalanx to the limit of motion to assess MCP joint abduction (Fig. 5-43).

End Feel. MCP joint abduction—firm.

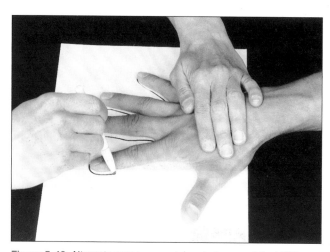

Figure 5-40 Alternate measurement: hand placement for MCP abduction and thumb extension.

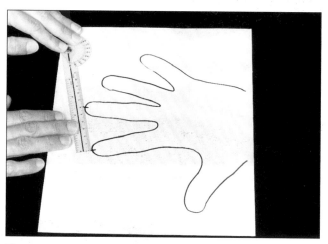

Figure 5-41 Ruler measurement: finger MCP abduction and thumb extension.

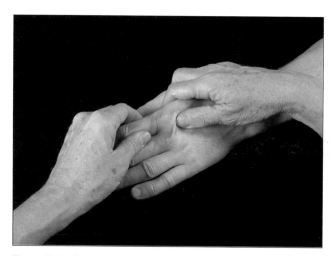

Figure 5-42 Start position: MCP joint abduction (index finger).

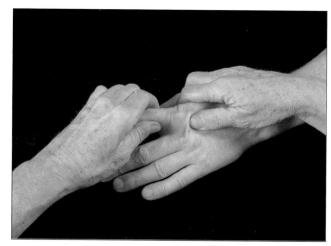

Figure 5-43 Firm end feel at the limit of MCP abduction (index finger).

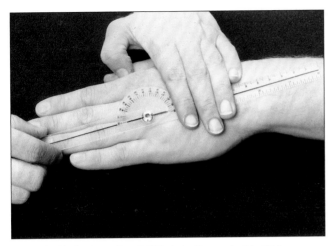

Figure 5-44 Start position: MCP abduction and adduction.

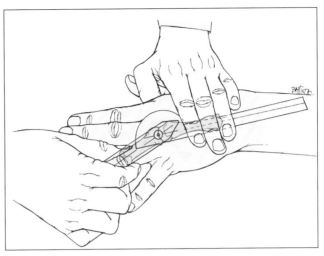

Figure 5-45 Goniometer alignment for MCP joint abduction/adduction, shown with the ring finger in abduction.

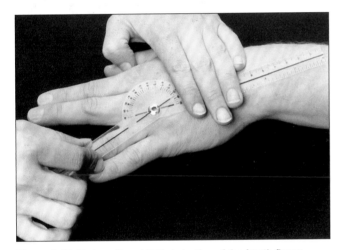

Figure 5-46 End position: MCP abduction of the fourth finger.

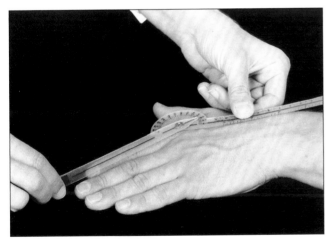

Figure 5-47 End position: MCP adduction of the index finger.

Joint Glides. *MCP joint abduction*—the concave base of the proximal phalanx moves on the fixed convex head of the corresponding metacarpal in the same direction of movement as the shaft of the proximal phalanx. *MCP joint adduction*—the concave base of the proximal phalanx moves on the fixed convex head of the corresponding metacarpal in the same direction of movement as the shaft of the proximal phalanx.

Measurement: Universal Goniometer

MCP Abduction/Adduction

Start Position. The patient is sitting. The elbow is flexed to 90°, the forearm is pronated and resting on a table, the wrist is in neutral position, and the fingers are in the anatomical position (Fig. 5-44).

Stabilization. The therapist stabilizes the metacarpal bones.

Goniometer Axis. The axis is placed on the posterior surface of the MCP joint being measured (Fig. 5-45).

Stationary Arm. Parallel to the longitudinal axis of the shaft of the metacarpal.

Movable Arm. Parallel to the longitudinal axis of the proximal phalanx.

End Position. The finger is moved away from the midline of the hand to the limit of motion in abduction (Figs. 5-45 and 5-46). The finger is moved toward the midline of the hand to the limit of motion in adduction (Fig. 5-47). The remaining fingers are moved to allow full adduction.

Finger IP Flexion–Extension

PROM Assessment

Forms
5-9, 5-10

Start Position. The patient is sitting. The forearm is resting on a table, the wrist is in neutral position, and the fingers are relaxed.

Stabilization. The therapist stabilizes the proximal phalanx for assessment of the proximal interphalangeal (PIP) joint and the middle phalanx for the distal interphalangeal (DIP) joint.

Therapist's Distal Hand Placement. The therapist grasps the middle phalanx to assess the PIP joint and the distal phalanx to assess the DIP joint.

End Positions. The therapist moves the middle or distal phalanx in an anterior direction to the limit of motion to assess PIP (not shown) or DIP joint flexion (Fig. 5-48), respectively. The therapist moves the middle or distal phalanx in a posterior direction to the limit of motion for PIP joint (not shown) or DIP joint extension (Fig. 5-49), respectively.

End Feels. *PIP joint flexion*—hard/soft/firm; *DIP joint flexion*—firm; *PIP joint extension*—firm; *DIP joint extension*—firm.

Joint Glides. *IP joint flexion*—the concave base of the distal phalanx glides in an anterior direction on the fixed convex head of the adjacent proximal phalanx. *IP joint extension*—the concave base of the distal phalanx glides in a posterior direction on the fixed convex head of the adjacent proximal phalanx.

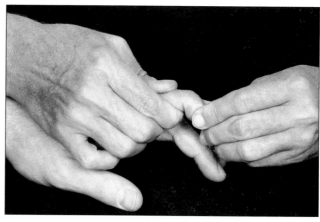

Figure 5-48 Firm end feel at limit of DIP joint flexion.

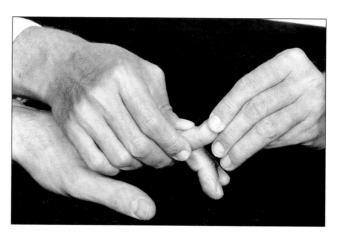

Figure 5-49 Firm end feel at limit of DIP joint extension.

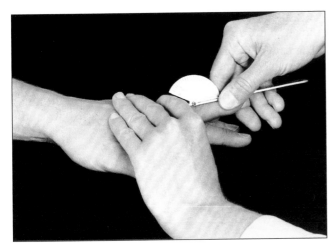

Figure 5-50 Start position: PIP joint flexion.

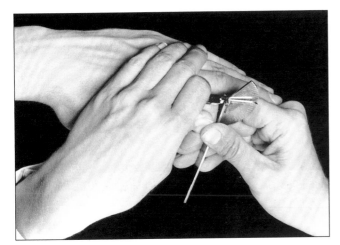

Figure 5-51 End position: PIP joint flexion.

Measurement: Universal Goniometer

Start Position. The patient is sitting. The forearm is resting on a table in either midposition or pronation. The wrist and fingers are in the anatomical position (0° extension at the MCP and IP joints) (Fig. 5-50).

Stabilization. The therapist stabilizes the proximal phalanx for measurement of the PIP joint and the middle phalanx for the DIP joint.

Goniometer Axis. To measure IP joint flexion, use a goniometer with at least one short arm and place the axis over the posterior surface of the PIP (Figs. 5-50 and 5-51) or DIP joint being measured. To measure IP joint extension, the axis is placed over the anterior surface of the PIP or DIP joint being measured.

Kato and colleagues[15] studied the accuracy of goniometric measurements for PIP joint flexion ROM in cadaver hands using three types of goniometer. The researchers recommend the use of goniometers with short arms when measuring the ROM with the goniometer placed over the dorsal aspect of the PIP joint.

Stationary Arm. PIP joint: parallel to the longitudinal axis of the proximal phalanx. DIP joint: parallel to the longitudinal axis of the middle phalanx.

Movable Arm. PIP joint: parallel to the longitudinal axis of the middle phalanx. DIP joint: parallel to the longitudinal axis of the distal phalanx.

End Positions. The PIP joint (Figs. 5-51 and 5-52) or DIP joint (not shown) is flexed to the limit of **PIP or DIP joint flexion (100° or 90°, respectively).** The PIP joint (Fig. 5-53) or DIP joint (not shown) is extended to the limit of **PIP or DIP joint extension (0°).**

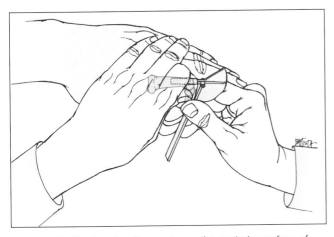

Figure 5-52 Goniometer alignment over the posterior surface of PIP joint to assess flexion.

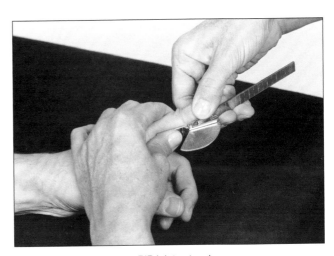

Figure 5-53 End position: PIP joint extension.

Finger MCP and IP Flexion

When evaluating impairment of hand function, a linear measurement of finger flexion should be used in conjunction with goniometry. This measure is particularly relevant in evaluating the extent of impairment[16] associated with grasp. The patient is sitting. The elbow is flexed and the forearm is resting on a table in supination. Two measurements are taken.

1. The patient flexes the IP joints while maintaining 0° of extension at the MCP joints (Fig. 5-54). A ruler measurement is taken from the pulp or tip of the middle finger to the distal palmar crease.

2. The patient flexes the MCP and IP joints (Fig. 5-55), and a ruler measurement is taken from the pulp of the finger to the proximal palmar crease.

Note: Long fingernails limit the flexion ROM at the finger joints (MCP joint flexion being the most affected) when the fingernails contact the palm.[17]

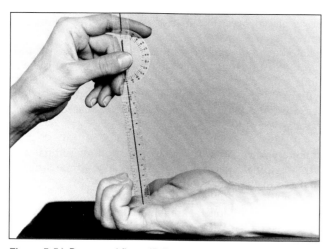

Figure 5-54 Decreased finger IP flexion.

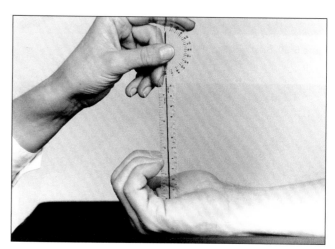

Figure 5-55 Decreased finger MCP and IP flexion.

Thumb CM Flexion–Extension

PROM Assessment

Forms
5-11, 5-12

Start Position. The patient is sitting. The elbow is flexed with the forearm in midposition and resting on a table. The wrist is in neutral position, the fingers are relaxed, and the thumb is in the anatomical position.

Stabilization. The therapist stabilizes the trapezium, wrist, and forearm (see Fig. 5-56).

Therapist's Distal Hand Placement. The therapist grasps the first metacarpal (Fig. 5-57).

End Positions. The therapist moves the first metacarpal in an ulnar direction to the limit of motion to assess thumb CM joint flexion (Fig. 5-58). The therapist moves the first metacarpal in a radial direction to the limit of motion for thumb CM joint extension (Fig. 5-59).

End Feels. *Thumb CM joint flexion*—soft/firm; *thumb CM joint extension*—firm.

Joint Glides.[13] *Thumb CM joint flexion*—the concave surface of the base of the first metacarpal glides in a medial direction (i.e., in the same direction to the movement of the shaft of the first metacarpal) on the convex surface of the trapezium. *Thumb CM joint extension*—the concave surface of the base of the first metacarpal glides in a lateral direction (i.e., in the same direction to the movement of the shaft of the first metacarpal) on the convex surface of the trapezium.

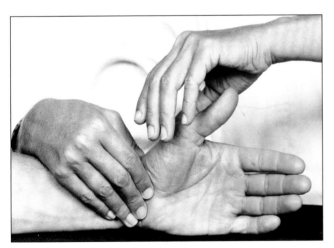

Figure 5-56 Start position: thumb CM flexion and extension. The therapist stabilizes the trapezium between the left thumb and index finger.

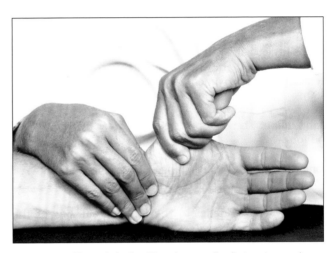

Figure 5-57 Therapist's distal hand grasps the first metacarpal.

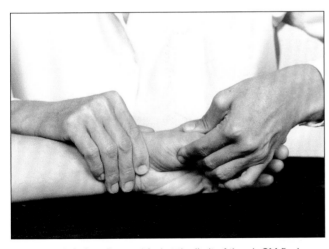

Figure 5-58 Soft or firm end feel at the limit of thumb CM flexion.

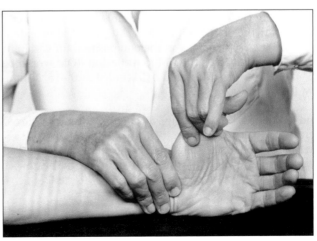

Figure 5-59 Firm end feel at the limit of thumb CM extension.

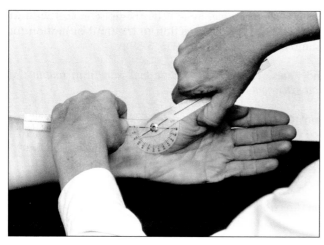

Figure 5-60 Start position: thumb CM flexion and extension.

Measurement: Universal Goniometer

Start Position. The patient is sitting. The elbow is flexed with the forearm in midposition and resting on a table. The wrist is in neutral position, the fingers assume the anatomical position, and the thumb maintains contact with the metacarpal and proximal phalanx of the index finger (Fig. 5-60).

Stabilization. The therapist stabilizes the trapezium, wrist, and forearm.

Goniometer Axis. The axis is placed over the CM joint (Fig. 5-61).

Stationary Arm. Parallel to the longitudinal axis of the radius.

Movable Arm. Parallel to the longitudinal axis of the thumb metacarpal. *Note* that although the goniometer arms are not aligned at 0° in this start position, this position is recorded as the 0° start position. The number of degrees the metacarpal is moved away from this 0° start position is recorded as the ROM for the movement. For example, if the goniometer read 30° at the start position for CM joint flexion–extension (see Fig. 5-60) and 15° at the end position for CM joint flexion (see Fig. 5-62), the CM joint flexion ROM would be 15° (i.e., 30° − 15° = 15°) and be recorded as 0°–15° thumb CM flexion.

End Positions. Flexion (Fig. 5-62): the thumb is flexed across the palm to the limit of **thumb CM joint flexion (15°)**. Extension (Fig. 5-63): the thumb is extended away from the palm to the limit of **thumb CM joint extension (20°)**.

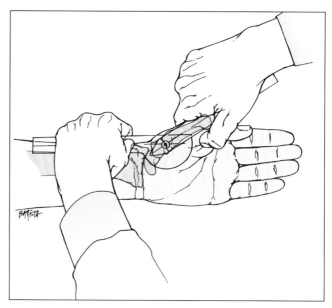

Figure 5-61 Goniometer alignment thumb CM joint flexion and extension.

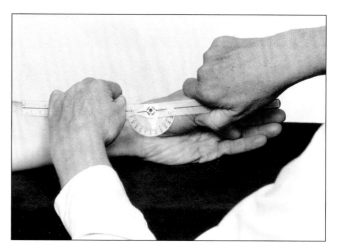

Figure 5-62 End position: thumb CM flexion.

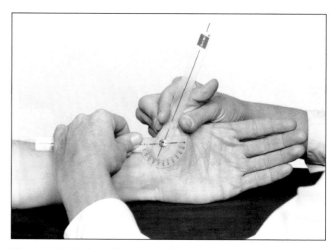

Figure 5-63 End position: thumb CM extension.

Thumb MCP and IP Flexion–Extension

PROM Assessment

Start Position. The patient is sitting. The elbow is flexed and the forearm is resting on a table in mid-position. The wrist is in the neutral position and the fingers are relaxed. The MCP and IP joints of the thumb are in extension (0°).

Forms 5-13 to 5-16

Stabilization. First MCP joint: the therapist stabilizes the first metacarpal. IP joint: the therapist stabilizes the proximal phalanx.

Therapist's Distal Hand Placement. First MCP joint: the therapist grasps the proximal phalanx. IP joint: the therapist grasps the distal phalanx.

End Positions. First MCP joint: the therapist moves the proximal phalanx across the palm to the limit of motion to assess thumb MCP flexion (Fig. 5-64) and to the limit of motion in a radial direction for thumb MCP extension (Fig. 5-65). IP joint: the therapist moves the distal phalanx in an anterior (Fig. 5-66) or a posterior (Fig. 5-67) direction to the limit of motion for thumb IP flexion or extension, respectively.

End Feels. *Thumb MCP flexion—hard/firm; thumb IP flexion—hard/firm; thumb MCP and IP extension—firm.*

Joint Glides. *Thumb MCP flexion*—the concave base of the proximal phalanx moves in an anterior direction on the fixed convex head of the first metacarpal. *Thumb IP joint flexion*—the concave base of the distal phalanx glides in an anterior direction on the fixed convex head of the proximal phalanx. *Thumb MCP extension*—the concave base of the proximal phalanx moves in a posterior direction on the fixed convex head of the first metacarpal. *Thumb IP joint extension*—the concave base of the distal phalanx glides in a posterior direction on the fixed convex head of the proximal phalanx.

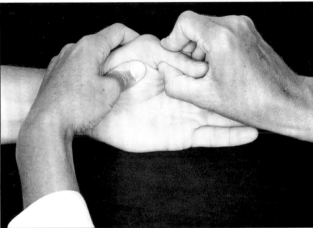

Figure 5-64 Hard or firm end feel at the limit of thumb MCP flexion.

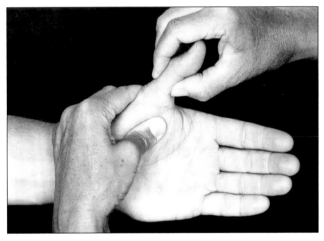

Figure 5-65 Firm end feel at the limit of thumb MCP extension.

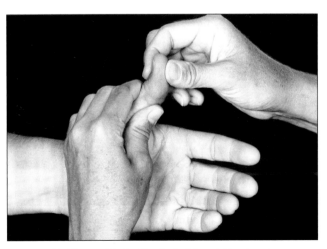

Figure 5-66 Hard or firm end feel at the limit of thumb IP flexion.

Figure 5-67 Firm end feel at the limit of thumb IP extension.

CHAPTER 5

Measurement: Universal Goniometer

Start Position. The patient is sitting. The elbow is flexed and the forearm is resting on a table in midposition. The wrist and fingers are in the anatomical position. The MCP and IP joints are in extension (0°).

Stabilization. MCP joint: the therapist stabilizes the first metacarpal. IP joint: the therapist stabilizes the proximal phalanx.

Goniometer Axis. The axis is placed over the posterior or lateral aspect of the MCP joint (Fig. 5-68) or IP joint (Fig. 5-69) of the thumb.

Stationary Arm. MCP joint: parallel to the longitudinal axis of the shaft of the thumb metacarpal. IP joint: parallel to the longitudinal axis of the proximal phalanx.

Movable Arm. MCP joint: parallel to the longitudinal axis of the proximal phalanx. IP joint: parallel to the longitudinal axis of the distal phalanx.

End Positions. The MCP joint is flexed so that the thumb moves across the palm to the limit of **thumb MCP joint flexion (50°)** (Fig. 5-70). The IP joint is flexed to the limit of **thumb IP joint flexion (80°)** (Fig. 5-71). The goniometer is positioned on the lateral or anterior surface of the thumb to assess MCP and IP joint extension. The MCP joint is extended to the limit of **thumb MCP joint extension (0°)**.

Hyperextension. Hyperextension of the IP joint of the thumb occurs beyond 0° of extension. The **thumb IP joint can actively be hyperextended to 10° and passively to 30°[1]** (Fig. 5-67).

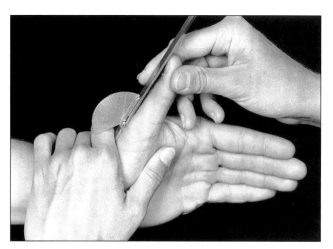

Figure 5-68 Start position: thumb MCP flexion.

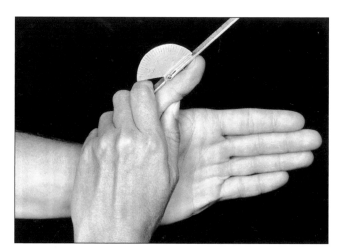

Figure 5-69 Start position: thumb IP flexion.

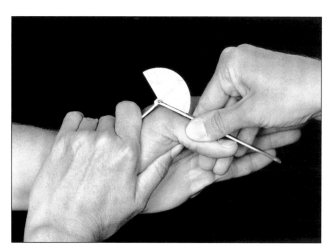

Figure 5-70 End position: thumb MCP flexion.

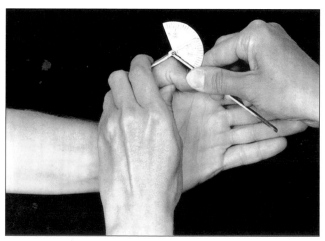

Figure 5-71 End position: thumb IP flexion.

Thumb CM Abduction

PROM Assessment

Form 5-17

Start Position. The patient is sitting. The forearm is in midposition resting on a table, the wrist is in neutral position, and the fingers and thumb are relaxed (Fig. 5-72).

Stabilization. The therapist stabilizes the second metacarpal.

Therapist's Distal Hand Placement. The therapist grasps the first metacarpal.

End Position. The therapist moves the first metacarpal away from the second metacarpal in an anterior direction perpendicular to the plane of the palm to the limit of motion to assess CM joint abduction (Fig. 5-73).

End Feel. CM joint abduction—firm.

Joint Glide.[13] *CM joint abduction*—the convex surface of the base of the first metacarpal glides in a posterior direction (i.e., in the opposite direction as the shaft of the first metacarpal) on the fixed concave surface of the trapezium.

Measurement: Universal Goniometer

Start Position. The patient is sitting. The elbow is flexed and the forearm is resting on a table in midposition. The wrist and fingers are in the anatomical position. The thumb maintains contact with the metacarpal and proximal phalanx of the index finger (Fig. 5-74).

Stabilization. The therapist stabilizes the second metacarpal.

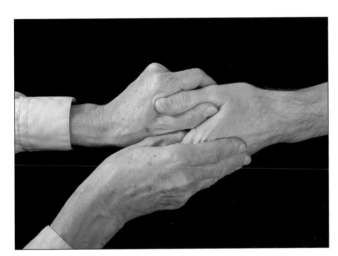

Figure 5-72 Start position: thumb abduction.

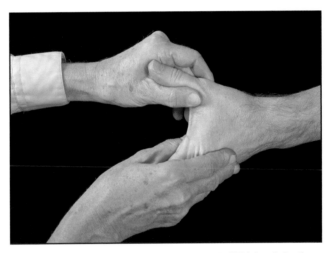

Figure 5-73 Firm end feel at the limit of thumb CM joint abduction.

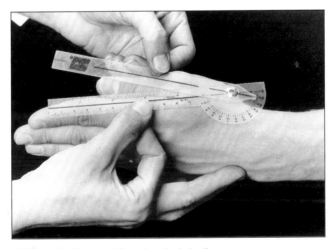

Figure 5-74 Start position: thumb abduction.

Goniometer Axis. The axis is placed at the junction of the bases of the first and second metacarpals (Fig. 5-75).

Stationary Arm. Parallel to the longitudinal axis of the second metacarpal.

Movable Arm. Parallel to the longitudinal axis of the first metacarpal. In the start position described, the goniometer will indicate 15° to 20°. This is recorded as 0°.[14] For example, if the goniometer read 15° at the start position for CM joint abduction (see Fig. 5-74) and 60° at the end position for CM joint abduction (Fig. 5-76), the first CM joint abduction ROM would be 45° (i.e., 60° − 15° = 45°) and be recorded as 0°–45° thumb CM abduction.

End Position. The thumb is abducted to the limit of **thumb CM joint abduction (70°)** so that the thumb column moves in the plane perpendicular to the palm (see Fig. 5-76).

Measurement: Ruler

As an alternate measurement to goniometry, thumb abduction may be measured by using a ruler or tape measure. With the thumb in the abducted position, a ruler measurement is taken from the lateral aspect of the midpoint of the MCP joint of the index finger to the posterior aspect of the midpoint of the MCP joint of the thumb (Fig. 5-77).

Measurement: Caliper

As an alternate, more reliable measurement method to conventional goniometry, thumb abduction is assessed using calipers to measure the intermetacarpal distance (IMD) method.[18] With the thumb in the abducted position, a caliper measurement (Fig. 5-78) is taken with the caliper points positioned on the middorsal points marked on the heads of the first and second metacarpals and is recorded in millimeters. However, unlike angular measurements, the IMD method is affected by changes in hand size that may not permit results to be comparable either between patients or in children when hand size changes.[18]

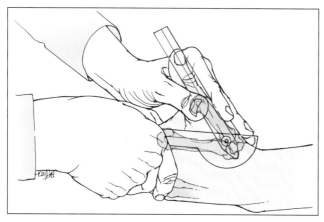

Figure 5-75 Goniometer alignment for end position thumb CM joint abduction.

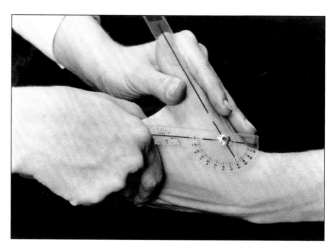

Figure 5-76 End position: thumb abduction.

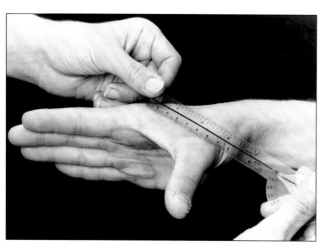

Figure 5-77 Ruler measurement: thumb abduction.

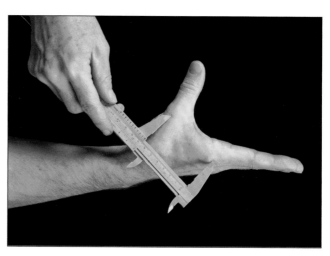

Figure 5-78 Caliper measurement: thumb abduction.

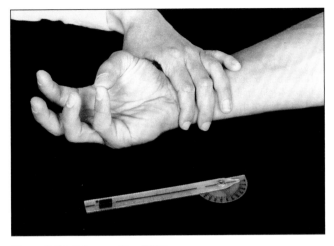

Figure 5-79 Full opposition ROM.

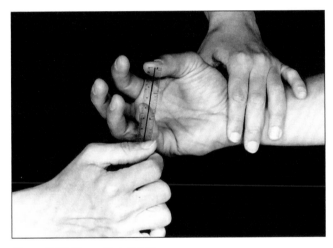

Figure 5-80 Opposition deficit.

Thumb Opposition

Measurement: Ruler

Form 5-18

On completion of full range of opposition between the thumb and fifth finger (Fig. 5-79), it is normally possible to place the pads of the thumb and fifth finger in the same plane.[19] An evaluation of a deficit in opposition (Fig. 5-80) can be obtained by taking a linear measurement between the center of the tip of the thumb pad and the center of the tip of the fifth finger pad.

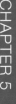

MUSCLE LENGTH ASSESSMENT AND MEASUREMENT

 Practice Makes Perfect

To aid you in practicing the skills covered in this section, or for a handy review, use the Summary & Evaluation Forms found at

http://thepoint.lww.com/ClarksonJM2e.

Flexor Digitorum Superficialis, Flexor Digitorum Profundus, Flexor Digiti Minimi, and Palmaris Longus

Form 5-19

Start Position. The patient is in supine or sitting with the elbow in extension, the forearm supinated, wrist in neutral position, and the fingers extended (Fig. 5-81).

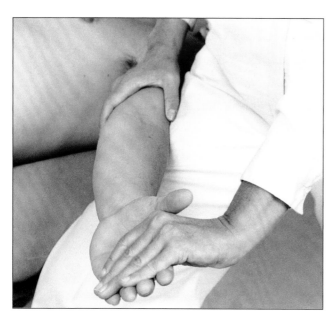

Figure 5-81 Start position: length of flexor digitorum superficialis, flexor digitorum profundus, and flexor digiti minimi.

Origin[2]	Insertion[2]
Flexor Digitorum Superficialis	
a. Humeroulnar head: common flexor origin on the medial epicondyle of the humerus, the anterior band of the ulnar collateral ligament, and the medial aspect of the coronoid process.	Anterior surface of the middle phalanges of the index, middle, ring, and little fingers.
b. Radial head: anterior border of the radius from the radial tuberosity to the insertion of pronator teres.	
Flexor Digitorum Profundus	
Upper three-fourths of the anterior and medial aspects of the ulna; medial aspect of the coronoid process; by an aponeurosis on the upper three-fourths of the posterior border of the ulna; anterior surface of the medial half of the interosseous membrane.	Palmar aspect of the bases of the distal phalanges of the index, middle, ring, and little fingers.
Flexor Digiti Minimi	
Hook of hamate; flexor retinaculum.	Ulnar aspect of the base of the proximal phalanx of the little finger.
Palmaris Longus (Vestigial)	
Common flexor origin on the medial epicondyle of the humerus.	Palmar aspect of the flexor retinaculum; the palmar aponeurosis.

Stabilization. The therapist manually stabilizes the humerus. The radius and ulna are stabilized against the therapist's thigh.

End Position. The therapist maintains the fingers in extension and extends the wrist to the limit of motion so that the long finger flexors are put on full stretch (Figs. 5-82 and 5-83).

Assessment and Measurement. If the finger flexors are shortened, wrist extension ROM will be restricted proportional to the decrease in muscle length. The therapist either observes the available PROM or uses a goniometer (Fig. 5-84) to measure and record the available wrist extension PROM. A second therapist may be required to measure the ROM using a goniometer.

End Feel. Finger flexors on stretch—firm.

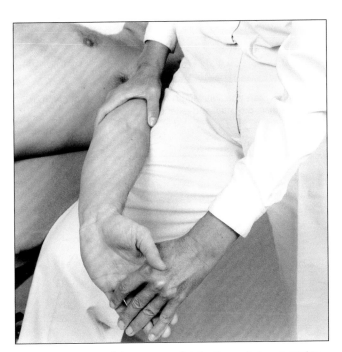

Figure 5-82 Flexor digitorum superficialis, flexor digitorum profundus, and flexor digiti minimi on stretch.

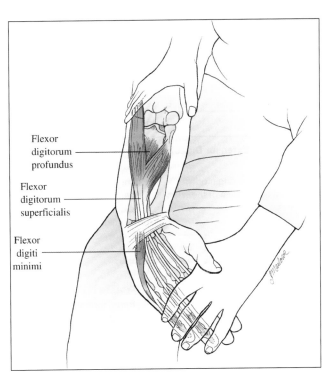

Flexor digitorum profundus

Flexor digitorum superficialis

Flexor digiti minimi

Figure 5-83 Flexor digitorum superficialis, flexor digitorum profundus, and flexor digiti minimi on stretch.

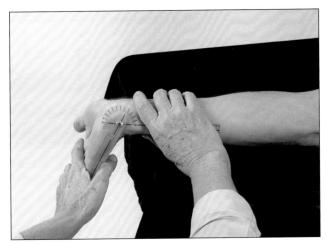

Figure 5-84 Goniometer measurement: length of long finger flexors.

Extensor Digitorum Communis, Extensor Indicis Proprius, and Extensor Digiti Minimi

Form 5-20

Start Position. The patient is in supine or sitting. The elbow is extended, the forearm is pronated, the wrist is in the neutral position, and the fingers are flexed (Fig. 5-85).

Stabilization. The therapist stabilizes the radius and ulna.

End Position. The therapist flexes the wrist to the limit of motion so that the long finger extensors are fully stretched (Figs. 5-86 and 5-87).

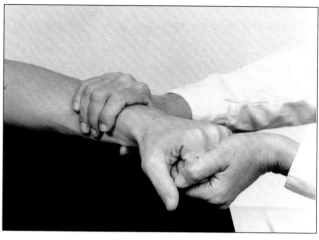

Figure 5-85 Start position: length of extensor digitorum communis, extensor indicis proprius, and extensor digiti minimi.

Origin[2]	Insertion[2]
Extensor Digitorum Communis	
Common extensor origin on the lateral epicondyle of the humerus.	Posterior surfaces of the bases of the distal and middle phalanges of the index, middle, ring, and little fingers.
Extensor Indicis Proprius	
Posterior surface of the ulna distal to the origin of extensor pollicis longus; posterior aspect of the interosseous membrane.	Ulnar side of the extensor digitorum tendon to the index finger at the level of the second metacarpal head.
Extensor Digiti Minimi	
Common extensor origin on the lateral epicondyle of the humerus.	Dorsal digital expansion of the fifth digit.

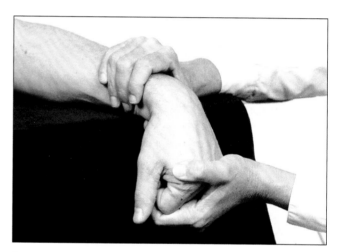

Figure 5-86 Extensor digitorum communis, extensor indicis proprius, and extensor digiti minimi on stretch.

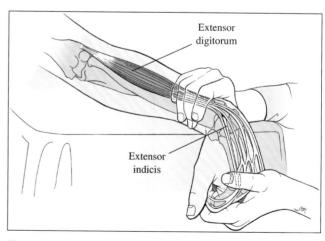

Extensor digitorum

Extensor indicis

Figure 5-87 Long finger extensors on stretch.

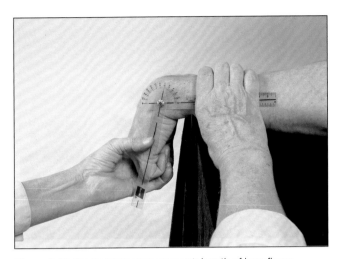

Figure 5-88 Goniometer measurement: length of long finger extensors.

Assessment and Measurement. If the finger extensors are shortened, wrist flexion PROM will be restricted proportional to the degree of muscle shortening. The therapist either observes the available PROM or uses a goniometer (Fig. 5-88) to measure and record the available wrist flexion PROM.

End Feel. Long finger extensors on stretch—firm.

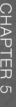

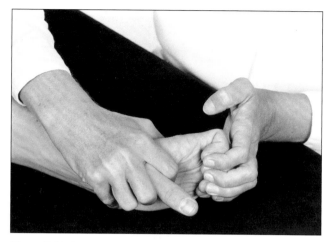

Figure 5-89 Start position: length of lumbricals.

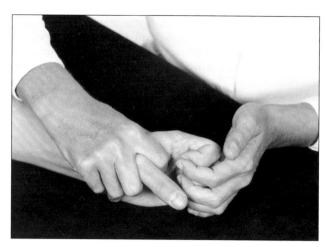

Figure 5-90 Lumbricals on stretch.

Lumbricals

Form 5-21

Start Position. The patient is in sitting or supine with the elbow flexed, forearm in midposition or supination, and the wrist in extension. The IP joints of the fingers are flexed (Fig. 5-89).

Stabilization. The therapist stabilizes the metacarpals.

End Position. The therapist simultaneously applies overpressure to flex the IP joints and extends the MCP joints of the fingers to the limit of motion so that lumbricals are put on full stretch (Figs. 5-90 and 5-91). The lumbricals may be stretched as a group or individually.

Assessment and Measurement. If the lumbricals are shortened, MCP joint extension ROM will be restricted proportional to the degree of muscle shortness. The therapist either observes the available PROM or uses a goniometer (Fig. 5-92) to measure and record the available MCP joint extension PROM.

End Feel. Lumbricals on stretch—firm.

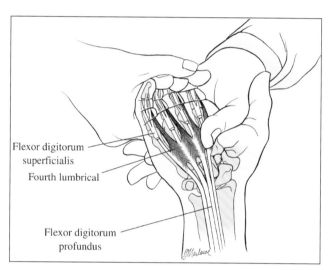

Flexor digitorum superficialis

Fourth lumbrical

Flexor digitorum profundus

Figure 5-91 Wrist extension, MCP joint extension, and IP joint flexion to place lumbricals on stretch.

Origin[2]	Insertion[2]
Lumbricals	
Tendons of flexor digitorum profundus:	Radial aspect of the dorsal digital expansion of the corresponding index, middle, ring, and little fingers.
a. First and second lumbricals: radial sides and palmar surfaces of the tendons of the index and middle fingers.	
b. Third: adjacent sides of the tendons of the middle and ring fingers.	
c. Fourth: adjacent sides of the tendons of the ring and little fingers.	

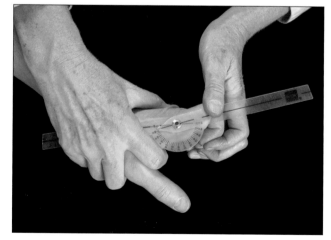

Figure 5-92 Goniometer measurement: length of lumbricals.

FUNCTIONAL APPLICATION

Joint Function: Wrist

The wrist optimizes the function of the hand to touch, grasp, or manipulate objects. Wrist motion positions the hand in space relative to the forearm and serves to transmit load between the hand and forearm.[20] Because of wrist motion and static positioning, the wrist serves to control the length–tension relations of the extrinsic muscles of the hand.

Wrist position affects finger ROM. Moving the wrist from a flexed position into extension causes synergistic finger flexion at the MCP, PIP, and DIP joints of the fingers due to passive tension in the long finger flexors.[21] As the wrist moves from an extended position into flexion, the fingers extend due to passive tension in the long finger extensors and the hand opens.

Functional Range of Motion: Wrist

Wrist extension and ulnar deviation are the most important positions or movements[22] for activities of daily living (ADL). In most daily activities, the wrist assumes a position of extension for the purpose of stabilization of the hand and flexion of the distal joints (Fig. 5-93). However, in the performance of perineal hygiene activities and dressing activities at the back (Fig. 5-94), the wrist assumes a flexed posture.

Two approaches have been used to determine the wrist ROM required to successfully perform ADL:

In *one approach*, the wrist ROM was assessed as normal subjects performed ADL. Brumfield and Champoux[23] evaluated 15 ADL and found the normal functional range of wrist motion for most activities was between 10° flexion and 35° extension. Palmer and coworkers,[24] evaluating 52

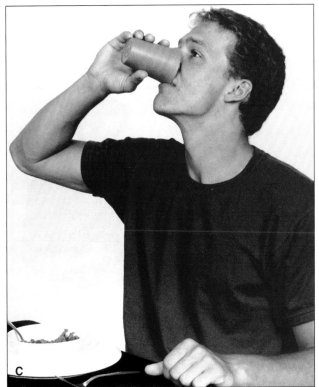

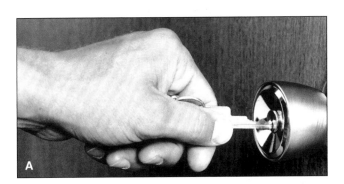

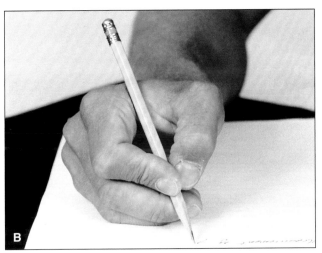

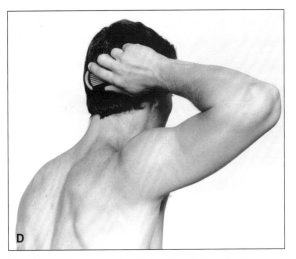

Figure 5-93 In most ADL, the wrist assumes a position of extension. **A.** Unlocking a door with a key. **B.** Writing. **C.** Drinking from a cup. **D.** Brushing one's hair.

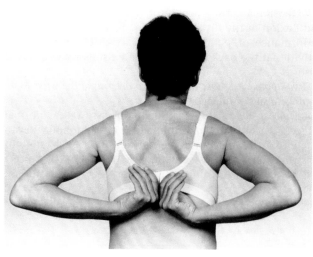

Figure 5-94 The wrist is flexed in performing dressing activities at the back.

standardized tasks, found comparable required ranges of 5° flexion and 30° extension. Normal functional range for ulnar deviation was 15° and radial deviation 10°.[24]

Higher values (54° flexion, 60° extension, 40° ulnar deviation, and 17° radial deviation) for the maximum wrist motion required for ADL were reported by Ryu and colleagues[22] in evaluating 31 activities. The authors suggested differing methods of data analysis and the design and application of the goniometer as possible reasons for these values being higher compared to other studies.

More specific ROM requirements for feeding activities (Fig. 5-95) (i.e., drinking from a cup or glass, eating using a fork or spoon, and cutting using a knife) are from approximately 3° wrist flexion to 35° wrist extension[23,25] and from 20° ulnar deviation to 5° radial deviation.[25]

Using *another approach*, wrist ROM was artificially restricted and the ability to complete ADL was assessed. Nelson[26] evaluated the ability to perform 125 ADL (activities of work or recreation were not included) with the wrist

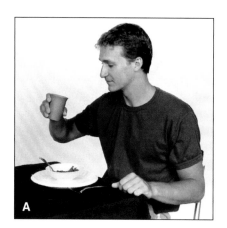

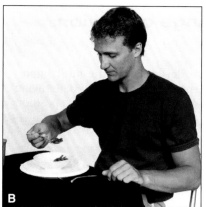

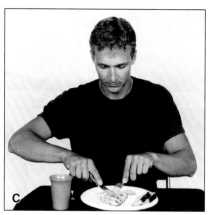

Figure 5-95 Wrist ROM from approximately 3° flexion to 35° extension[23,25] and from 20° ulnar deviation and 5° radial deviation[25] is required for feeding activities. **A.** Drinking from a cup. **B.** Eating using a spoon. **C.** Eating using a knife and fork.

splinted to allow for only 5° flexion, 6° extension, 7° radial deviation, and 6° ulnar deviation. With the wrist splinted in this manner, 123 ADL could be completed. Therefore, marked loss of wrist ROM may not significantly hinder a patient's ability to carry out ADL.

Franko and colleagues[27] used objective ROM parameters, an objective timed test, and subjective surveys to evaluate functional differences between unrestricted (100%), partially (42%), and highly (15%) restricted normal wrist ROM conditions. The objective timed test included contemporary ADL not studied previously, such as the use of a computer mouse, cell phone, and typing on a computer keyboard and handheld device. The researchers concluded that as wrist ROM decreased, objective and subjective functional limitation increased; however, "all subjects in both highly and partially restricted motion conditions had a surprisingly high degree of functional motion, suggesting that a direct correlation does not exist between loss of motion and loss of function"[27 (p. 495.e6)].

Coupled Wrist Motion[11,28]

Wrist movements are coupled during dynamic tasks. Wrist radial deviation occurs with maximal wrist extension, and ulnar deviation occurs with maximal wrist flexion.

Finger Position Effects Wrist ROM

Gehrmann and coworkers[12] assessed wrist ROM with the fingers unconstrained and held in three different flexed positions. With increased finger flexion angles, wrist flexion and ulnar deviation ROM significantly decreased. Flexed finger positions occur when gripping a handle or tool and in these situations wrist ROM may be reduced.

Joint Function: Hand

The hand has multiple functions associated with ADL. The primary functions are to grasp, manipulate objects, communicate, and receive sensory information from the environment. The grasping function is isolated for presentation in this section.

Functional Range of Motion: Hand

Full opening of the hand is not required for grasping tasks in daily self-care activities but may be required for grasp in leisure or occupational tasks. When grasping an object, the shape, size, and weight of the object influence the degree of finger flexion, the area of palmar contact, and the thumb position (Fig. 5-96). The thumb may or may not be included in the grip[10] (see Fig. 5-96A). When grasping different-sized cylinders, the DIP joint angle remains constant and the fingers adjust to the new cylinder size through changes in the joint angles at the MCP and PIP joints.[29]

Pieniazek and colleagues[30] evaluated the flexion and extension ROM at the MCP, PIP, and DIP joints of the hand during three ADL, combing the hair, closing a zip fastener,

and answering a telephone call. The ROM values were about midrange and never reach maximal flexion–extension values. The pattern of relative mobility was similar in all fingers, being greatest at the MCP joints and decreasing from the PIP to the DIP joints, except for the index finger where PIP joint motion was greater than that at the MCP joint.

Hume and coworkers[31] reported the MCP and IP joint flexion ROM needed to perform 11 ADL. No significant differences in the functional positions of the individual fingers were found; therefore, the finger positions were reported as one. The mean functional flexion postures at the joints of the fingers were MCP joint 61°, PIP joint 60°, and DIP joint 39°. The mean functional flexion postures of the thumb MCP and IP joints were 21° and 18°, respectively.

Three other research teams, Hayashi and Shimizu,[32] Murai and associates,[33] and Bain and colleagues,[34] investigated functional joint ROM of the hand as study subjects performed various ADL. These research groups recruited healthy young male and female subjects and used electric goniometers to record the subjects' dominant hand joint ROM during performance of activities of daily living. Each research team utilized a different set of ADL for their research.

Hayashi and Shimizu[32] recorded maximum MCP joint extension and flexion angles of the index, middle, ring, and little fingers as subjects performed 19 ADL. The ADL included personal care and hygiene, housework, and recreational activities based on the Disabilities of the Arm, Shoulder, and Hand (DASH) Outcome Measure. The mean ROM values for extension–flexion at the MCP joints of each finger ranged from −10° to 60°, −10° to 75°, −10° to 80°, and −10° to 85° for the index, middle, ring, and little fingers, respectively. *Note* that the negative values signify flexion angles that represent the joint extension ROM. The majority of the ADL were completed using only flexion angles at the MCP joints of the fingers. However, 3 of the 19 ADL required MCP joint extension ROM of all fingers, with extension angles ranging from 1° to 15°. These tasks included putting on a pullover sweater, making a bed, and heavy household chores represented by the washing of walls. Significant differences were found in the maximum MCP joint flexion ROM between the fingers as MCP flexion ROM increased from the index to the little finger.

Murai and associates[33] measured the finger and thumb MCP joint ROM required to complete 16 ADL, which included typing on a keyboard and using a computer mouse. The functional ROM at the MCP joints, rounded to the nearest degree, for the thumb was −8° to 35°, the index finger 11° to 68°, the middle finger 4° to 80°, the ring finger 3° to 84°, and the little finger 3° to 91°. *Note* that in this study, negative ROM values signify extension ROM and positive values signify flexion ROM. The total arc of functional MCP joint ROM for the thumb and for the index finger, was found to be significantly less than that of the ulnar three fingers and the ulnar two fingers, respectively. Both Murai and associates[33] and Hayashi and Shimizu[32] found the majority of the ADL were completed using only flexion ROM at the MCP joints of the fingers. Murai and associates[33] also reported the same to be true for the MCP joint of the thumb.

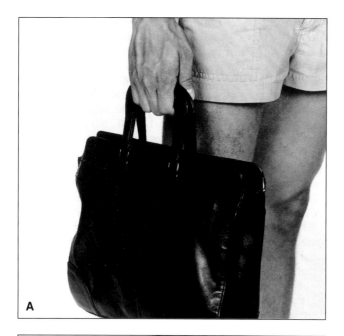

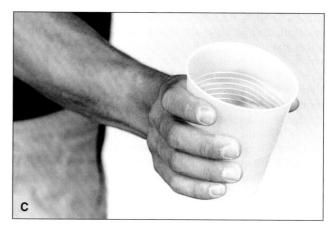

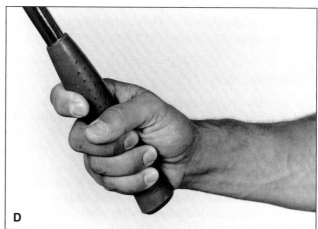

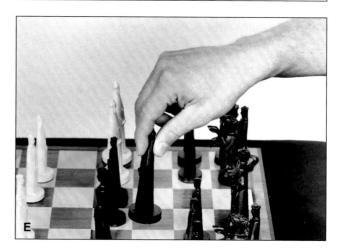

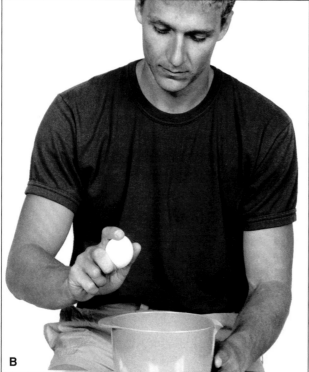

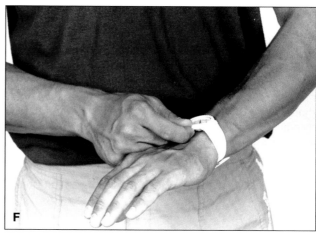

Figure 5-96 When grasping an object, the shape, size, and/or weight of the object influence the degree of finger flexion, the area of palmar contact, and the thumb position, as observed when **(A)** carrying a briefcase, **(B)** cracking an egg, **(C)** holding a large cup, **(D)** gripping the handle of a hammer, **(E)** moving a chess piece, and **(F)** winding a watch.

TABLE 5-4 **Arches of the Hand**[19]

Arch	Location	Keystone	Mobility
Carpal arch	Distal row of carpal bones	Capitate	Fixed
	Proximal row of carpal bones	—	Mobile
Metacarpal arch	Level of metacarpal heads	Third metacarpal head	Mobile
Longitudinal arches	Carpals and each of the five rays*	MCP joints	Mobile; fixed (index and middle metacarpal)

*Ray: the metacarpal and phalanges of one finger or the thumb.

Bain and colleagues[34] measured the functional ROM required at the MCP, PIP, and DIP joints of the fingers to perform 20 ADL as defined by the Sollerman test of hand grip function based on common handgrips used in ADL. For each activity, the MCP, PIP, and DIP joint ROM was assessed at each finger. ROM was measured at the pregrasp position of relative finger extension, as the hand opened and prepared to grasp the object, and also at the grasp position of relative flexion when the fingers were flexed to hold the object. Bain's team[34] recorded functional ranges of motion (i.e., the ROM required to complete 90% of the 20 ADL) at the MCP, PIP, and DIP joints of 19° to 71°, 23° to 87°, and 10° to 64° flexion, respectively. To complete 100% of the 20 ADL studied, much greater MCP joint extension ROM was required to accommodate greater opening of the hand when grasping larger objects, but no significant differences in ROM requirements were identified for the PIP and DIP joints to grasp larger objects. Bain's team[34] reported that functional ROM differed between the fingers. The mean functional ROM of the MCP joints was greatest on the ulnar side of the hand and least on the radial side. The mean functional ROM of the PIP joints was greatest at the little and index fingers, and that of the DIP joint was greatest at the index finger during pinch activities.

Arches of the Hand

The arches of the hand are described in Table 5-4. The arches are observed with the forearm supinated and the hand resting on a table (Fig. 5-97).

The carpal arch, a relatively fixed segment, is covered by the flexor retinaculum. This arrangement functions to maintain the long finger flexors close to the wrist joint, thus reducing the ability of these muscles to produce wrist flexion and enhancing the synergistic action of the wrist flexors and extensors in power grip.[19]

In the relaxed position of the hand, a gently cupped concavity is normally observed. When gripping or manipulating objects, the palmar concavity becomes deeper and more gutter-shaped. When the hand is opened fully, the palm flattens. The guttering and flattening of the palm result from the mobility available at the rays of the ring and little fingers and thumb. Each ray consists of the metacarpal and phalanges of a finger or the thumb. These rays flex, rotate, and move toward the center of the palm, so the pads of the fingers and thumb are positioned to meet. This motion occurs at the CM joints. The mobile peripheral rays move around the fixed metacarpals of the index and middle fingers.

References

1. Kapandji IA. *The Physiology of the Joints. Vol 1. The Upper Limb.* 6th ed. New York, NY: Churchill Livingstone Elsevier; 2007.
2. Standring S, ed. *Gray's Anatomy: The Anatomical Basis of Clinical Practice.* 39th ed. London, UK: Elsevier Churchill Livingstone; 2005.
3. Norkin CC, White DJ. *Measurement of Joint Motion: A Guide to Goniometry.* 4th ed. Philadelphia, PA: FA Davis; 2009.
4. Daniels L, Worthingham C. *Muscle Testing: Techniques of Manual Examination.* 5th ed. Philadelphia, PA: WB Saunders; 1986.
5. Magee DJ. *Orthopedic Physical Assessment.* 5th ed. Philadelphia, PA: Saunders Elsevier; 2008.
6. American Academy of Orthopaedic Surgeons. *Joint Motion: Method of Measuring and Recording.* Chicago, IL: AAOS; 1965.
7. Berryman Reese N, Bandy WD. *Joint Range of Motion and Muscle Length Testing.* 2nd ed. Philadelphia, PA: Saunders Elsevier; 2010.
8. Cyriax J. *Textbook of Orthopaedic Medicine, Vol 1. Diagnosis of Soft Tissue Lesions.* 8th ed. London, UK: Bailliere Tindall; 1982.

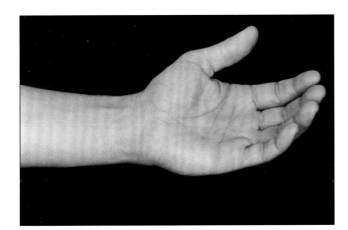

Figure 5-97 Palmar arches. Observe the transverse palmar concavities at the levels of the distal row of carpal bones and the metacarpal bones and the longitudinal concavities along the rays of each finger.

9. Knutson JS, Kilgore KL, Mansour JM, Crago PE. Intrinsic and extrinsic contributions to the passive movement at the metacarpophalangeal joint. *J Biomech*. 2000;33:1675-1681.

10. Li Z-M, Kuxhaus L, Fisk JA, Christophel TH. Coupling between wrist flexion-extension and radial-ulnar deviation. *Clin Biomech (Bristol, Avon)*. 2005;20:177-183.

11. Levangie PK, Norkin CC. *Joint Structure and Function: A Comprehensive Analysis*. 4th ed. Philadelphia, PA: FA Davis; 2005.

12. Gehrmann SV, Kaufmann RA, Li Z-M. Wrist circumduction reduced by finger constraints. *J Hand Surg Am*. 2008;33A:1287-1292.

13. Neumann DA. *Kinesiology of the Musculoskeletal System: Foundations for Physical Rehabilitation*. 2nd ed. St Louis, MO: Mosby Elsevier; 2010.

14. Scott AD, Trombly CA. Evaluation. In: Trombly CA. *Occupational Therapy for Physical Dysfunction*. 2nd ed. Baltimore, MD: Williams & Wilkins; 1983.

15. Kato M, Echigo A, Ohta H, et al. The accuracy of goniometric measurements of proximal interphalangeal joints in fresh cadavers: comparison between methods of measurement, types of goniometers, and fingers. *J Hand Ther*. 2007;20(1):12-18.

16. Swanson AB, Goran-Hagert C, DeGroot Swanson G. Evaluation of impairment of hand function. In: Hunter JM, Schneider LH, Mackin EJ, Bell JA. *Rehabilitation of the Hand*. St Louis, MO: CV Mosby; 1978.

17. Stegink Jansen CW, Patterson R, Viegas SF. Effects of fingernail length on finger and hand performance. *J Hand Ther*. 2000;13:211-217.

18. deKraker M, Selles RW, Schreuders TAR, Stam HJ, Hovius SER. Palmar abduction: reliability of 6 measurement methods in healthy adults. *J Hand Surg Am*. 2009;34A:523-530.

19. Tubiana R, Thomine JM, Macklin E. *Examination of the Hand and Wrist*. 2nd ed. St Louis, MO: Mosby; 1996.

20. Nordin M, Frankel VH. *Basic Biomechanics of the Musculoskeletal System*. 3rd ed. Philadelphia, PA: Lippincott Williams & Wilkins; 2001.

21. Su F-C, Chou YL, Yang CS, Lin GT, An KN. Movement of finger joints induced by synergistic wrist motion. *Clin Biomech (Bristol, Avon)*. 2005;20:491-497.

22. Ryu J, Cooney WP, Askew LJ, et al. Functional ranges of motion of the wrist joint. *J Hand Surg Am*. 1991;16:409-419.

23. Brumfield RH, Champoux JA. A biomechanical study of normal functional wrist motion. *Clin Orthop Relat Res*. 1984;187:23-25.

24. Palmer AK, Werner FW, Murphy DM, Glisson R. Functional wrist motion: a biomechanical study. *J Hand Surg Am*. 1985; 10:39-46.

25. Safaee-Rad R, Shwedyk E, Quanbury AO, Cooper JE. Normal functional range of motion of upper limb joints during performance of three feeding activities. *Arch Phys Med Rehabil*. 1990;71:505-509.

26. Nelson DL. Functional wrist motion. *Hand Clin*. 1997;13:83-92.

27. Franko OI, Zurakowski D, Day CS. Functional disability of the wrist: direct correlation with decreased wrist motion. *J Hand Surg*. 2008;33A:485.e1-485.e9.

28. Wigderowitz CA, Scott I, Jariwala A, Arnold GP, Abboud RJ. Adapting the Fastrak® System for three-dimensional measurement of the motion of the wrist. *J Hand Surg Eur Vol*. 2007;32E(6):700-704.

29. Lee JW, Rim K. Measurement of finger joint angles and maximum finger forces during cylinder grip activity. *J Biomed Eng*. 1991;13:152-162.

30. Pieniazek M, Chwala W, Szczechowicz J, Pelczar-Pieniazek M. Upper limb joint mobility ranges during activities of daily living determined by three-dimensional motion analysis – preliminary report. *Ortop Traumatol Rehabil*. 2007;9(4):413-422.

31. Hume MC, Gellman H, McKellop H, Brumfield RH. Functional range of motion of the joints of the hand. *J Hand Surg Am*. 1990;15:240-243.

32. Hayashi H, Shimizu H. Essential motion of metacarpophalangeal joints during activities of daily living. *J Hand Ther*. 2013;26:69-74.

33. Murai T, Uchiyama S, Nakamura K, Ido Y, Hata Y, Kato H. Functional range of motion in the metacarpophalangeal joints of the hand measured by single axis electric goniometers. *J Orthop Sci*. 2018;23:504-510.

34. Bain GI, Polites N, Higgs BG, Heptinstall RJ, McGrath AM. The functional range of motion of the finger joints. *J Hand Surg Eur Vol*. 2015;40E(4):406-411.

EXERCISES AND QUESTIONS

See the Answer Guide in Appendix E for suggested answers to the following exercises and questions.

1. PALPATION

On a skeleton, and next on a partner, palpate the following anatomical structures. Identify the wrist and hand ROM that can be measured using the anatomical structure to align the universal goniometer.

i.   Styloid process of the ulna   _____

ii. Distal palmar crease   _____

iii. Third metacarpal bone   _____

iv. First carpometacarpal joint   _____

v.   Capitate bone   _____

vi. Lateral aspect of the PIP joint line   _____

2. ASSESSMENT PROCESS

Are the following statements true or false?

i.   AROM is normally assessed prior to assessing PROM at a joint.

ii. End feels are determined when assessing AROM at a joint.

iii. It is important to note the presence or absence of pain when assessing AROM and PROM at a joint.

iv. A goniometer can only be used to measure PROM when assessing a joint.

3. ASSESSMENT OF AROM AT THE WRIST AND HAND ARTICULATIONS

A. Demonstrate the two movement patterns a therapist would have a patient perform when conducting a general scan of the active movements available at the wrist and hand. Identify the ROM the therapist would observe when performing the scan.

B. Identify and describe the shape of the articular components that make up the:

i.   Wrist

ii. CM joint of the thumb

iii. MCP and IP joints of the thumb and fingers

C. Demonstrate, define, and describe* the following movements:

i.   Wrist extension

ii. Thumb abduction

iii. Thumb extension at the CM joint

iv. Finger abduction

v.   Finger flexion at the PIP joint

*Identify the axis/plane of movement.

D. When assessing wrist ulnar deviation, what substitute movements may give the appearance of greater ulnar deviation ROM than is actually present?

CHAPTER 5

4. ASSESSMENT AND MEASUREMENT OF PROM AT THE WRIST AND HAND

For each of the movements listed below, demonstrate the assessment and measurement of PROM on a partner. Use the ROM Recording Form on pages 167 and 168 to record your partner's PROM. Have a third partner, using the appropriate Summary & Evaluation Form at http://thepoint.lww.com/ClarksonJM2e, evaluate your proficiency at assessing and measuring joint ROM, and provide feedback to you. Then, answer the following questions:

Wrist Ulnar Deviation

i.   What normal end feel(s) would be expected when assessing wrist ulnar deviation?

ii. List the normal limiting factor(s) that create the normal end feel(s) for wrist ulnar deviation.

iii. Assess the end feel for wrist ulnar deviation on your partner. Is the end feel normal?

iv. Identify the anatomical structure the axis of the goniometer is aligned with when measuring wrist ulnar deviation ROM.

v.   When measuring wrist ulnar deviation, the movable arm of the goniometer is aligned with the longitudinal axis of the third finger. True or false? Explain.

Wrist Extension

Assume a patient presents with decreased wrist extension PROM.

i.   What glide of the proximal row of carpal bones could be limited at the radiocarpal joint?

ii. Explain the reason for the glide being decreased in the direction indicated in i.

iii. The goniometer alignment for wrist extension is also used to assess wrist _____ ROM and muscle length for the _____ and the _____.

iv. What position should the fingers be in when assessing wrist extension PROM? Why?

MCP Joint Extension of the Fingers and Thumb

i.   A therapist assesses MCP joint extension PROM and notes decreased PROM and a firm end feel. Would the firm end feel be considered a normal end feel? Justify your answer.

ii. A patient has decreased passive thumb MCP joint extension ROM. What glide of the base of the proximal phalanx of the thumb would be decreased in this case? Explain the reason for the glide being decreased in the direction indicated.

iii. Identify the pattern of movement restriction at the MCP joints in the presence of a capsular pattern.

iv. When measuring PROM for finger MCP joint extension, why is the wrist positioned in slight flexion during the procedure?

Finger MCP Joint Abduction

i.   What normal end feel(s) would be expected when assessing MCP joint abduction?

ii. List the normal limiting factor(s) that create the normal end feel(s) for MCP joint abduction.

Thumb CM Joint ROM

i.   Identify the movements that occur at this joint that can be measured using a universal goniometer.

ii. When assessing the PROM at the CM joint of the thumb, identify the segment(s) proximal to the joint that must be stabilized to ensure movement is localized at the CM joint.

Ring Finger PIP Joint Flexion

i.   What normal end feel(s) would be expected when assessing ring finger PIP joint flexion?

ii. List the normal limiting factor(s) that create the normal end feel(s) for ring finger PIP joint flexion.

Thumb Opposition

If your partner has full opposition ROM, have your partner simulate a deficit in opposition so that you can demonstrate the measurement of thumb opposition.

i.   Opposition is a sequential movement that incorporates _____, _____, and _____ of the first metacarpal, with simultaneous _____.

ii. If mobility at the _____ joint is decreased, the motion of the first metacarpal would be restricted and full thumb opposition ROM would not be possible.

ROM RECORDING FORM

Patient's Name _____   Age _____

Diagnosis _____   Date of Onset _____

Therapist Name _____   AROM or PROM _____

Therapist Signature _____   Measurement Instrument _____

Left Side				Right Side			
	*		*	**Date of Measurement**	*		*	
				Wrist				
				Flexion (0–80°)				
				Extension (0–70°)				
				Ulnar deviation (0–30°)				
				Radial deviation (0–20°)				
				Hypermobility: Comments:				
				Thumb				
				CM flexion (0–15°)				
				CM extension (0–20°)				
				abduction (0–70°)				
				MCP flexion (0–50°)				
				IP flexion (0–80°)				
				Opposition				
				Hypermobility: Comments:				
				Fingers				
				MCP digit 2 flexion (0–90°)				
				extension (0–45°)				
				abduction				
				adduction				
				MCP digit 3 flexion (0–90°)				
				extension (0–45°)				
				abduction (radial)				
				adduction (ulnar)				

ROM RECORDING FORM

Patient's Name _____

Therapist _____

Therapist Signature _____

Left Side				Date of Measurement	Right Side			
*			*		*		*	
				Fingers (*continued*)				
				MCP digit 4 flexion (0–90°)				
				extension (0–45°)				
				abduction				
				adduction				
				MCP digit 5 flexion (0–90°)				
				extension (0–45°)				
				abduction				
				adduction				
				PIP digit 2 flexion (0–100°)				
				3 flexion (0–100°)				
				4 flexion (0–100°)				
				5 flexion (0–100°)				
				DIP digit 2 flexion (0–90°)				
				3 flexion (0–90°)				
				4 flexion (0–90°)				
				5 flexion (0–90°)				
				Composite finger abduction/thumb extension—Distance between:				
				Thumb—digit 2				
				Digit 2—digit 3				
				Digit 3—digit 4				
				Digit 4—digit 5				
				Composite flexion—Distance between:				
				Finger pulp—distal palmar crease				
				Finger pulp—proximal palmar crease				
				Hypermobility:				
				Comments:				

5. MUSCLE LENGTH ASSESSMENT AND MEASUREMENT

For the muscles listed below, demonstrate the assessment and measurement of muscle length on a partner and answer the questions. Have a third partner evaluate your performance using the appropriate Summary & Evaluation Form at http://thepoint.lww.com/ClarksonJM2e.

Flexor Digitorum Superficialis, Flexor Digitorum Profundus, Flexor Digiti Minimi, and Palmaris Longus

i.   What position is the elbow in to assess the muscle length of the flexor muscles listed above? Why is the elbow held in this position?

ii. If the length of the finger flexors is decreased, with the elbow extended, the forearm supinated, and the fingers _____, wrist _____ PROM will be restricted proportional to the decrease in muscle length. To assess this PROM restriction using a universal goniometer, the goniometer axis is placed at the _____, the stationary arm is aligned parallel to the _____, and the movable arm is aligned parallel to the _____. The therapist will note a _____ end feel at the end of the restricted wrist PROM.

Lumbricals

i.   Explain why the wrist would be positioned in extension to assess the length of the lumbricals.

ii. If the length of the lumbricals is decreased, with the wrist in extension and the fingers _____, MCP joint _____ PROM will be restricted proportional to the degree of muscle shortness.

Extensor Digitorum Communis, Extensor Indicis Proprius, and Extensor Digiti Minimi

i.   If the length of the long finger extensors is decreased, with the elbow _____, forearm pronated, and fingers _____, wrist _____ PROM will be restricted proportional to the degree of muscle shortness.

6. FUNCTIONAL ROM AT THE WRIST AND HAND

A. What two wrist positions have been identified as the most important positions or movements for ADL?

B. For feeding activities (i.e., drinking from a cup or glass, eating using a fork or spoon, and cutting using a knife), the ROM requirements are approximately _____° wrist flexion to _____° wrist extension and from _____° ulnar deviation to ____° of radial deviation.

C. What are the primary functions of the wrist?

D. What are the primary functions of the hand?

E. Motion at the _____ joints of the ring finger, little finger, and thumb results in the guttering of the palm for gripping and manipulating objects and the flattening of the palm. Explain how the ROM of these joints is measured in the clinic.

F. For each of the following wrist and hand movements, identify two ADL that require the specified movement:

  i.   Wrist flexion

  ii. Wrist extension

  iii. Wrist radial deviation

  iv. Wrist ulnar deviation

  v.   Finger flexion

  vi. Finger extension

  vii. Thumb opposition

G. With the wrist splinted to allow for only 5° flexion, 6° extension, 7° radial deviation, and 6° ulnar deviation, Nelson[1] evaluated the ability to perform 125 ADL and found that 123 ADL could be completed. From these findings, what conclusion was made regarding wrist ROM and the ability to carry out ADL?

H. The majority of ADL require _____ ROM at the MCP joints of the fingers and thumb.

I. The functional ROM of the MCP joints is greatest on the _____ side and least on the _____ side of the hand.

J. Bain and colleagues[2] reported finger PIP and DIP joint _____ ROM was required to perform 20 ADL as defined by the Sollerman test of hand grip function based on common handgrips used in ADL.

References

1. Nelson DL. Functional wrist motion. *Hand Clin.* 1997;13:83-92.

2. Bain GI, Polites N, Higgs BG, Heptinstall RJ, McGrath AM. The functional range of motion of the finger joints. *J Hand Surg Eur Vol.* 2015;40E(4):406-411.

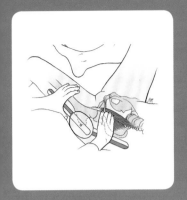

Hip 6

ARTICULATIONS AND MOVEMENTS

The hip joint is a ball-and-socket joint (Fig. 6-1) formed proximally by the cup-shaped, concave surface of the pelvic acetabulum and distally by the ball-shaped, convex head of the femur. Movements at the hip joint include flexion, extension, abduction, adduction, and internal and external rotation.

From the anatomical position, the hip joint may be flexed and extended in the sagittal plane, with movement occurring around a frontal axis, and abducted and adducted in the frontal plane about a sagittal axis (Fig. 6-2). With the hip positioned in 90° of flexion, hip internal and external rotation occurs in the frontal plane about a sagittal axis (Fig. 6-3). Hip rotation can also be performed in the anatomical position, with movement occurring in the transverse plane about a longitudinal (vertical) axis.

Movements at the hip joint can result from movement of the femur on the pelvis, the pelvis on the

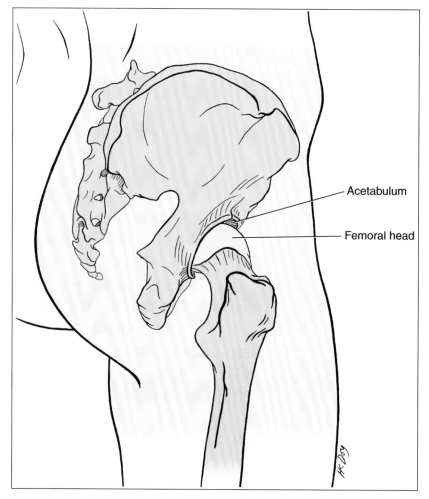

Acetabulum

Femoral head

Figure 6-1 Hip joint: the convex head of the femur articulates with the concave surface of the acetabulum.

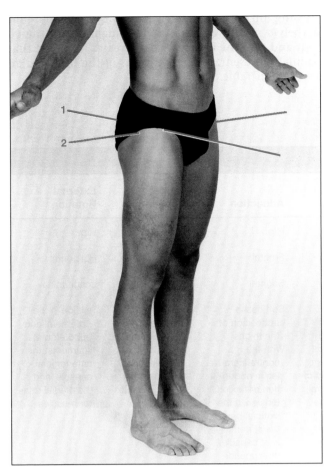

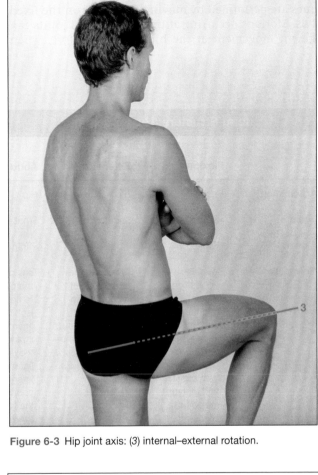

Figure 6-2 Hip joint axes: (*1*) abduction–adduction and (*2*) flexion–extension.

Figure 6-3 Hip joint axis: (*3*) internal–external rotation.

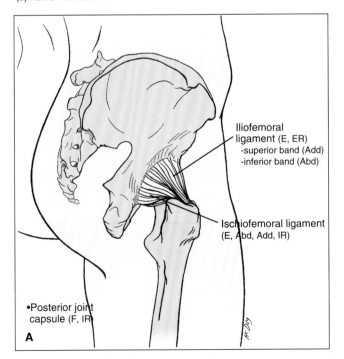

Iliofemoral
ligament (E, ER)
-superior band (Add)
-inferior band (Abd)

Ischiofemoral ligament
(E, Abd, Add, IR)

•Posterior joint
capsule (F, IR)

A

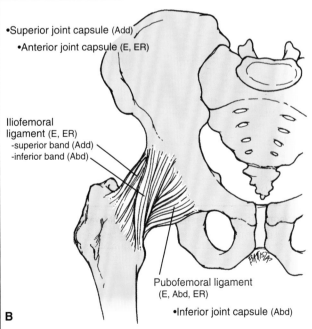

•Superior joint capsule (Add)

•Anterior joint capsule (E, ER)

Iliofemoral
ligament (E, ER)
-superior band (Add)
-inferior band (Abd)

Pubofemoral ligament
(E, Abd, ER)

•Inferior joint capsule (Abd)

B

Figure 6-4 Normal Limiting Factors. A. Posterolateral view of the hip joint showing noncontractile structures that normally limit motion. **B.** Anterolateral view of the hip joint showing noncontractile structures that normally limit motion. *Motion limited by structure is identified in brackets, using the following abbreviations: *F*, flexion; *E*, extension; *Abd*, abduction; *Add*, adduction; *ER*, external rotation; *IR*, internal rotation. Muscles normally limiting motion are not illustrated.

femur, or the femur and pelvis. Hip joint range of motion (ROM) and muscle strength assessment techniques are performed by moving the femur on the fixed pelvis. Motions occurring at the more central joints can augment movement at the hip joint. Therefore, when assessing hip ROM, the pelvis is stabilized to avoid lumbar–pelvic movement that would augment hip movement and give the appearance of greater hip ROM than is actually present. The movements of the hip joint are described in Table 6-1.

TABLE 6-1 Joint Structure: Hip Movements

	Flexion	Extension	Abduction	Adduction	Internal Rotation	External Rotation
Articulation[1,2]	Hip	Hip	Hip	Hip	Hip	Hip
Plane	Sagittal	Sagittal	Frontal	Frontal	Horizontal	Horizontal
Axis	Frontal	Frontal	Sagittal	Sagittal	Longitudinal	Longitudinal
Normal limiting factors[1,3–6,*] (see Fig. 6-4A and B)	Soft tissue apposition of the anterior thigh and the abdomen (the knee is flexed); tension in the posterior hip joint capsule and gluteus maximus	Tension in the anterior joint capsule; the iliofemoral, ischiofemoral, and pubofemoral ligaments; and the iliopsoas	Tension in the pubofemoral and ischiofemoral ligaments, the inferior band of the iliofemoral ligament, the inferior joint capsule, and the hip adductor muscles	Soft tissue apposition of the thighs With the contralateral leg in abduction or flexion; tension in the iliotibial band, the superior joint capsule, the superior band of the iliofemoral ligament, the ischiofemoral ligament, and the hip abductor muscles	Tension in the ischiofemoral ligament, the posterior joint capsule, and the external rotator muscles	Tension in the iliofemoral and pubofemoral ligaments, the anterior joint capsule, and the medial rotator muscles
Normal end feel[3,7]	Soft/firm	Firm	Firm	Soft/firm	Firm	Firm
Normal AROM[8†]	0°–120°	0°–30°	0°–45°	0°–30°	0°–45°	0°–45°
(AROM[9]**)**	(0°–120°)	(0°–20°)	(0°–40°–45°)	(0°–25°–30°)	(0°–35°–40°)	(0°–35°–40°)
Capsular pattern[7,10]	The order of restriction may vary: flexion, abduction, and internal rotation					

Note: Normal hip extension range of motion (ROM) varies between sources, ranging from 10° to 30°.[4,8,9,11–13]

*There is a paucity of definitive research that identifies the normal limiting factors (NLF) of joint range of motion. The NLF and end feels listed here are based on knowledge of anatomy, clinical experience, and available references.

†AROM, active range of motion.

ANATOMICAL LANDMARKS (FIGS. 6-5 THROUGH 6-9)

Anatomical landmarks are described and illustrated below. Anatomical landmarks numbered 2, 6, 8, 9, and 10 are used to assess hip ROM and/or to align the goniometer axis and arms to measure ROM at the hip.

Structure	Location
1. Iliac crest	A convex bony ridge on the upper border of the ilium; the top of the iliac crest is level with the space between the spinous processes of L4 and L5.
2. Anterior superior iliac spine (ASIS)	Round bony prominence at the anterior end of the iliac crest.
3. Tubercle of the ilium	Approximately 5 cm above and lateral to the ASIS along the lateral lip of the iliac crest.
4. Posterior superior iliac spine (PSIS)	Round bony prominence at the posterior end of the iliac crest, felt subcutaneously at the bottom of the dimples on the proximal aspect of the buttocks; the spines are at the level of the spinous process of S2.
5. Ischial tuberosity	With the hip passively flexed, this bony prominence is lateral to the midline of the body and just proximal to the gluteal fold (the deep transverse groove between the buttock and the posterior aspect of the thigh).
6. Greater trochanter	With the tip of the thumb on the lateral aspect of the iliac crest, the tip of the third digit placed distally on the lateral aspect of the thigh locates the upper border of the greater trochanter.
7. Adductor tubercle	Medial projection at the distal end of the femur at the proximal aspect of the medial epicondyle.
8. Lateral epicondyle of the femur	Small bony prominence on the lateral condyle of the femur.
9. Patella	Large triangular sesamoid bone on the anterior aspect of the knee. The base is proximal and the apex distal.
10. Anterior border of the tibia	Subcutaneous bony ridge along the anterior aspect of the leg.

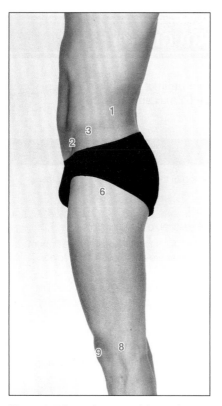

Figure 6-5 Lateral aspect of the trunk and thigh.

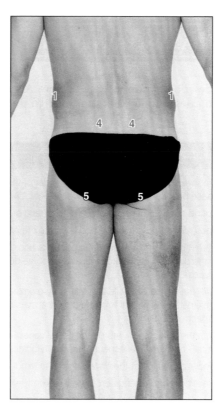

Figure 6-6 Posterior aspect of the trunk and thigh.

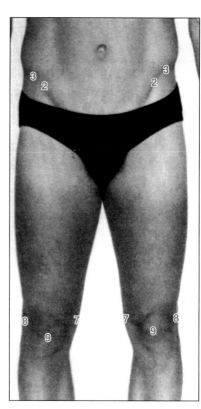

Figure 6-7 Anterior aspect of the trunk and thigh.

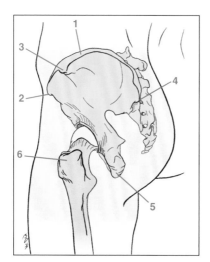

Figure 6-8 Bony anatomy, posterolateral aspect of the pelvis and thigh.

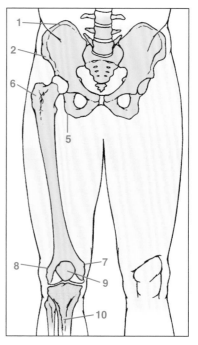

Figure 6-9 Bony anatomy, anterior aspect of the pelvis, thigh, and knee.

RANGE OF MOTION ASSESSMENT AND MEASUREMENT

 Practice Makes Perfect

To aid you in practicing the skills covered in this section, or for a handy review, use the Summary & Evaluation Forms found at

http://thepoint.lww.com/ClarksonJM2e.

General Scan: Lower Extremity Active Range of Motion

Active range of motion (AROM) of the lower extremity joints is scanned with the patient either non–weight-bearing or weight-bearing, as follows:

Non–Weight-Bearing

1. The patient is in the supine position with the legs in the anatomical position. In supine-lying position, the patient extends the toes, dorsiflexes the ankle, and brings the heel toward the contralateral hip (Fig. 6-10A). The therapist observes the AROM of hip flexion, abduction,

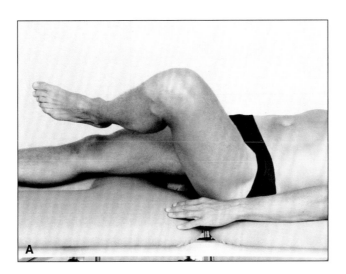

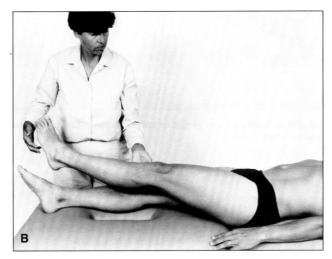

Figure 6-10 **A.** Non–weight-bearing scan: AROM of lower extremity. **B.** Non–weight-bearing scan: AROM of lower extremity.

external rotation, knee flexion, ankle dorsiflexion, and toe extension. As the patient attempts to touch the contralateral hip, the level reached by the heel may be used as a guide of AROM of the hip and knee joints.

2. The patient flexes the toes, plantarflexes the ankle, extends the knee, and adducts, internally rotates, and extends the hip to move the great toe toward the corner on the other side of the plinth (Fig. 6-10B). The therapist observes the AROM of hip adduction, internal rotation, knee extension, ankle plantarflexion, and toe flexion.

Weight-Bearing

1. The patient squats (Fig. 6-11A). The therapist observes bilateral hip flexion, knee flexion, ankle dorsiflexion, and toe extension ROM.

2. Standing, the patient rises onto the toes (Fig. 6-11B). The therapist observes hip extension, knee extension, ankle plantarflexion, and toe extension ROM bilaterally.

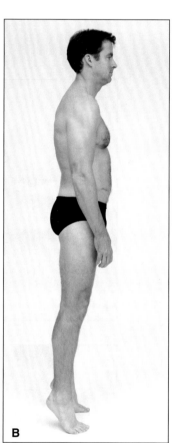

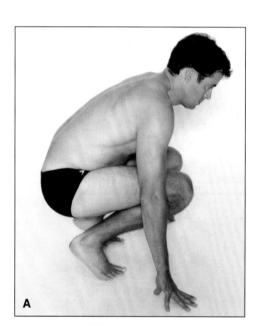

Figure 6-11 A. Weight-bearing scan: AROM of lower extremity. **B.** Weight-bearing scan: AROM of lower extremity.

Hip Flexion

AROM Assessment

Substitute Movement. Posterior pelvic tilt and flexion of the lumbar spine.

PROM Assessment

Start Position. The patient is supine. The hip and knee on the test side are in the anatomical position (Fig. 6-12). The pelvis is in the neutral position; that is, the ASISs and the symphysis pubis are in the same frontal plane, and the right and left ASISs are in the same transverse plane.[11,14]

Stabilization. The therapist stabilizes the ipsilateral pelvis at the ASIS and iliac crest to maintain a neutral position. The trunk is stabilized through body positioning.

Therapist's Distal Hand Placement. The therapist raises the lower extremity off the plinth and grasps the posterior aspect of the distal femur.

End Position. While maintaining pelvic stabilization, the therapist moves the femur anteriorly to the limit of hip flexion (Fig. 6-13). The knee is allowed to flex to prevent the two-joint hamstring muscles from limiting hip flexion ROM.

End Feel. Hip flexion—soft/firm.

Joint Spin.[6] Hip flexion—the convex femoral head spins in the fixed concave acetabulum.

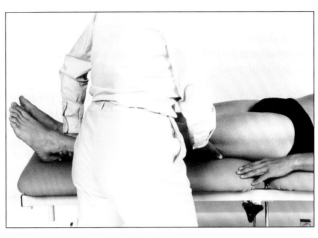

Figure 6-12 Start position: hip flexion.

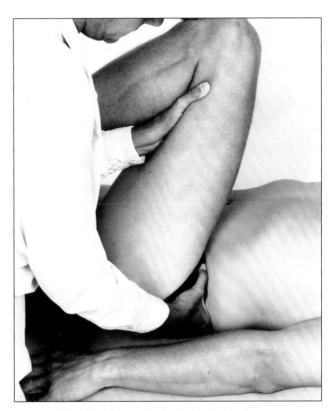

Figure 6-13 Soft or firm end feel at limit of hip flexion.

Measurement: Universal Goniometer

Start Position. The patient is supine. The hip and knee on the test side are in the anatomical position (Fig. 6-14). The pelvis is in the neutral position.

Stabilization. The trunk is stabilized through body positioning and the therapist stabilizes the ipsilateral pelvis.

Goniometer Axis. The axis is placed over the greater trochanter of the femur (Fig. 6-15).

Stationary Arm. Parallel to the midaxillary line of the trunk.

Movable Arm. Parallel to the longitudinal axis of the femur, pointing toward the lateral epicondyle.

End Position. The hip is moved to the limit of **hip flexion (120°)** (Fig. 6-16). The knee is allowed to flex to prevent hamstring muscles from limiting hip flexion ROM.

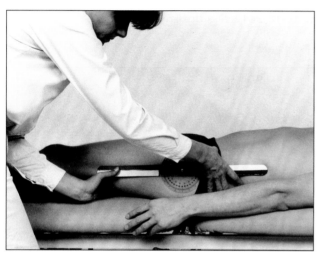

Figure 6-14 Start position: hip flexion.

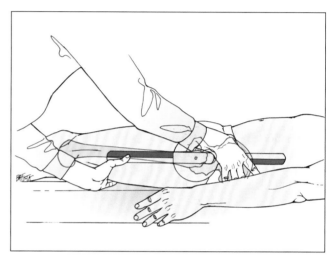

Figure 6-15 Goniometer alignment: hip flexion.

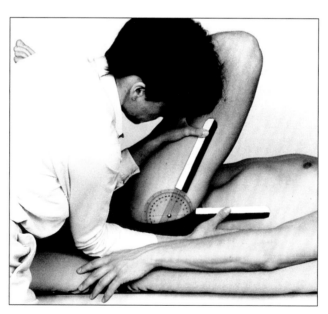

Figure 6-16 End position: hip flexion.

Hip Extension

AROM Assessment

Substitute Movement. Anterior pelvic tilt and extension of the lumbar spine.

PROM Assessment

Form
6-2

Start Position. The patient is prone. Both hips and knees are in the anatomical position. The feet are over the end of the plinth (Fig. 6-17).

Stabilization. The therapist stabilizes the pelvis.

Therapist's Distal Hand Placement. The therapist grasps the anterior aspect of the distal femur.

End Position. The therapist moves the femur posteriorly to the limit of hip extension (Fig. 6-18).

End Feel. Hip extension—firm.

Joint Spin.[6] Hip extension—the convex femoral head spins in the fixed concave acetabulum.

Measurement: Universal Goniometer

Start Position. The patient is prone. The hips and knees are in the anatomical position. The feet are over the end of the plinth (Fig. 6-19).

Stabilization. The pelvis is stabilized through strapping. Alternatively, a second therapist may assist to manually stabilize the pelvis.

Goniometer Axis. The axis is placed over the greater trochanter of the femur.

Stationary Arm. Parallel to the midaxillary line of the trunk.

Movable Arm. Parallel to the longitudinal axis of the femur, pointing toward the lateral epicondyle.

End Position. The patient's knee is maintained in extension to place the rectus femoris on slack. The hip is moved to the limit of **hip extension (30°)** (Fig. 6-20).

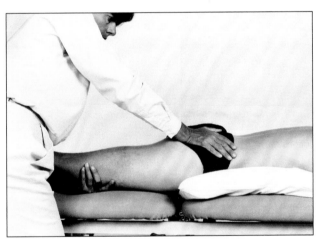

Figure 6-17 Start position: hip extension.

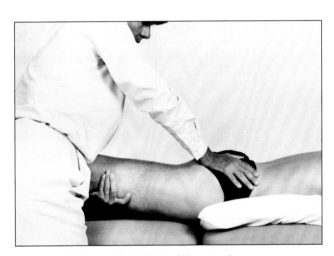

Figure 6-18 Firm end feel at limit of hip extension.

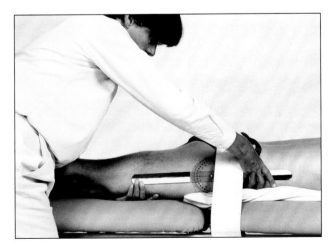

Figure 6-19 Start position: hip extension.

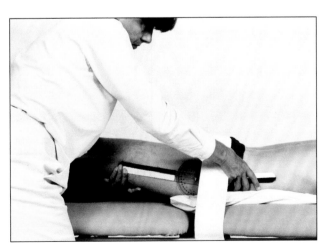

Figure 6-20 End position: hip extension.

Hip Abduction

AROM Assessment

Substitute Movement. External rotation and flexion of the hip, hiking of the ipsilateral pelvis.

PROM Assessment

Start Position. The patient is supine; the pelvis is level and the lower extremities are in the anatomical position (Fig. 6-21).

Form 6-3

Stabilization. The therapist stabilizes the ipsilateral pelvis. If additional stabilization of the trunk and pelvis is required, the contralateral lower extremity may be positioned in hip abduction with the knee flexed over the edge of the plinth and the foot supported on a stool (see Fig. 6-26).

Therapist's Distal Hand Placement. The therapist grasps the medial aspect of the distal femur.

End Position. The therapist moves the femur to the limit of hip abduction motion (Fig. 6-22).

End Feel. Hip abduction—firm.

Joint Glide. Hip abduction—the convex femoral head glides inferiorly on the fixed concave acetabulum.

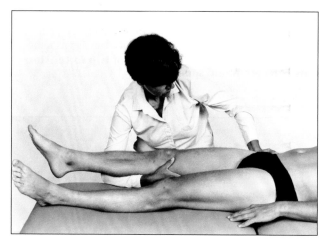

Figure 6-21 Start position for hip abduction.

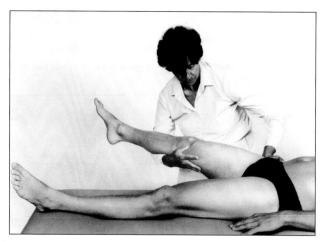

Figure 6-22 Firm end feel at the limit of hip abduction.

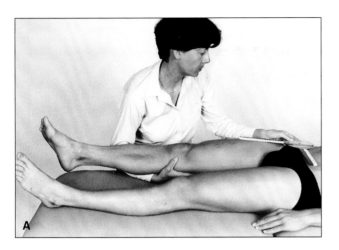

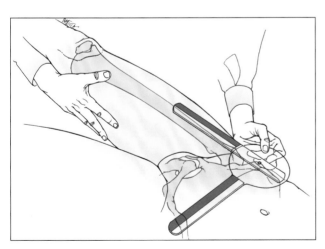

Figure 6-23 A. Start position: hip abduction. **B.** Goniometer alignment.

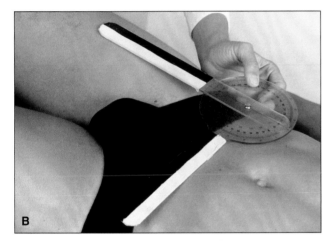

Figure 6-24 Goniometer alignment: hip abduction and adduction.

Measurement: Universal Goniometer

Start Position. The patient is supine with the lower extremities in the anatomical position (Fig. 6-23A). Ensure the pelvis is level.

Stabilization. The therapist stabilizes the ipsilateral pelvis. If additional stabilization of the trunk and pelvis is required, the contralateral lower extremity may be positioned in hip abduction with the knee flexed over the edge of the plinth and the foot supported on a stool (see Fig. 6-26).

Goniometer Axis. The axis is placed over the ASIS on the side being measured (Figs. 6-23B and 6-24).

Stationary Arm. Along a line that joins the two ASISs.

Movable Arm. Parallel to the longitudinal axis of the femur, pointing toward the midline of the patella. In the start position described, the goniometer will indicate 90°. This is recorded as 0°. The number of degrees the femur is moved away from this 0° start position is recorded as the ROM for hip abduction. For example, if the goniometer reads 90° at the start position for hip abduction and 60° at the end position, hip abduction PROM would be 30° (i.e., 90° − 60° = 30°) and be recorded as 0°–30° hip abduction.

End Position. The hip is moved to the limit of **hip abduction (45°)** (Fig. 6-25).

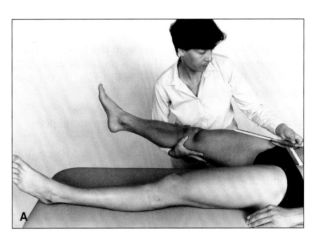

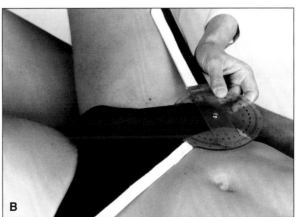

Figure 6-25 A. End position: hip abduction. **B.** Goniometer alignment.

Hip Adduction

AROM Assessment

Substitute Movement. Hip internal rotation, hiking of the contralateral pelvis.

PROM Assessment

Start Position. The patient is supine, the pelvis is level, and the lower extremity is in the anatomical position. The hip on the nontest side is abducted to allow full ROM in adduction on the test side. The abducted nontest limb may remain on the plinth, or the knee may be flexed over the edge of the plinth with the foot supported on a stool (Fig. 6-26).

Stabilization. The therapist stabilizes the ipsilateral pelvis.

Therapist's Distal Hand Placement. The therapist grasps the distal femur.

End Position. The therapist moves the femur to the limit of hip adduction ROM (Fig. 6-27).

End Feel. Hip adduction—soft/firm.

Joint Glide. Hip adduction—the convex femoral head glides superiorly on the fixed concave acetabulum.

Measurement: Universal Goniometer

Start Position. The patient is supine with the lower extremity in the anatomical position. The hip on the nontest side is abducted to allow full range of hip adduction on the test side. The pelvis is level.

Stabilization. The therapist stabilizes the ipsilateral pelvis.

Goniometer Axis. The axis is placed over the ASIS on the side being measured. The goniometer is aligned the same as for hip abduction ROM measurement (see Fig. 6-24).

Stationary Arm. Along a line that joins the two ASISs.

Movable Arm. Parallel to the longitudinal axis of the femur, pointing toward the midline of the patella. In the start position described, the goniometer will indicate 90°. This is recorded as 0°. The number of degrees the femur is moved away from this 0° start position is recorded as the ROM for hip adduction. For example, if the goniometer reads 90° at the start position for hip adduction and 105° at the end position, hip adduction PROM would be 15° (i.e., 105° – 90° = 15°) and be recorded as 0°–15° hip adduction.

End Position. The hip is moved to the limit of **hip adduction (30°)** (Fig. 6-28).

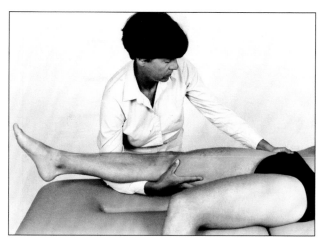

Figure 6-26 Start position: hip adduction.

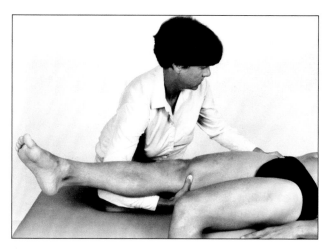

Figure 6-27 Soft or firm end feel at limit of hip adduction.

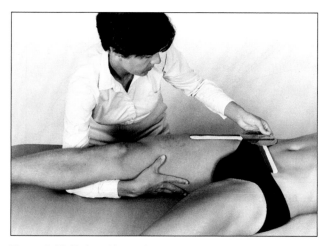

Figure 6-28 End position: universal goniometer measurement for hip adduction.

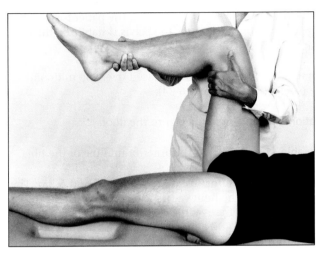

Figure 6-29 Start position: hip internal and external rotation.

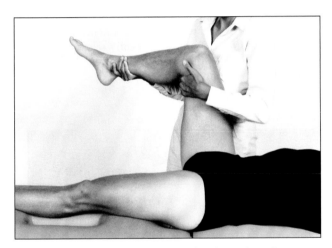

Figure 6-30 Firm end feel at the limit of hip internal rotation.

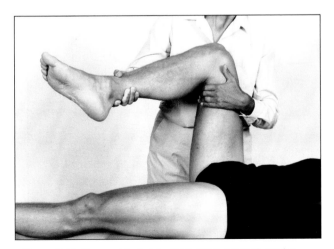

Figure 6-31 Firm end feel at the limit of hip external rotation.

Hip Internal and External Rotation

AROM Assessment

Substitute Movement. Lateral tilting of the pelvis. In sitting, the patient shifts body weight to raise the pelvis and lift the buttocks off the sitting surface.

PROM Assessment

Forms
6-5, 6-6

Start Position. The patient is sitting or supine with the hip and knee flexed to 90° (Fig. 6-29).

Stabilization. The pelvis is stabilized through body positioning. The therapist maintains the position of the femur, without restricting movement.

Therapist's Distal Hand Placement. The therapist grasps the distal tibia and fibula.

End Position. The therapist moves the tibia and fibula in a lateral direction to the limit of hip internal rotation (Fig. 6-30) and in a medial direction to the limit of hip external rotation (Fig. 6-31). The stresses on the knee joint should be considered and caution exercised.

End Feels. *Hip internal rotation*—firm; *hip external rotation*—firm.

Joint Glides. *Hip internal rotation*—the convex femoral head glides on the fixed concave acetabulum in a posterior direction with the hip in anatomical position, and in an inferior direction with the hip in a position of 90° flexion.

Hip external rotation—the convex femoral head glides on the fixed concave acetabulum in an anterior direction with the hip in anatomical position, and in a superior direction with the hip in a position of 90° flexion.

Measurement: Universal Goniometer

Start Position. The patient is sitting. In sitting, the hip being measured is in 90° of flexion and neutral rotation with the knee flexed to 90°. A pad is placed under the distal thigh to keep the thigh in a horizontal position. The contralateral hip is abducted and the foot is supported on a stool (Fig. 6-32).

Alternate Starting Positions.

- Supine with the lower extremities in anatomical position
- Supine with the hip and knee flexed to 90° (see Fig. 6-29)
- Sit-lying (i.e., supine with the knees flexed 90° over the end of the plinth)
- Prone with the knee flexed 90° (see Fig. 6-37)

Hip rotation PROM is greater when measured with the patient prone than sitting.[15] Passive hip rotation measurements also differ when measured in sitting versus supine positions.[16] To accurately evaluate patient progress, the position used to measure hip rotation PROM should be charted,[15] and the same position used on subsequent measurement.

Stabilization. The pelvis is stabilized through body positioning. The therapist maintains the position of the femur without restricting movement. In sitting, the patient grasps the edge of the plinth. In prone, the pelvis is stabilized through strapping (Fig. 6-37).

Goniometer Axis. The axis is placed over the midpoint of the patella (Figs. 6-33 and 6-34).

Stationary Arm. Perpendicular to the floor.

Movable Arm. Parallel to the anterior midline of the tibia.

End Positions. Internal rotation (Figs. 6-34 and 6-35): The hip is moved to the limit of **hip internal rotation (45°)** as the leg and foot move in a lateral direction.

External rotation (Figs. 6-36 and 6-37): The hip is moved to the limit of **hip external rotation (45°)** as the leg and foot move in a medial direction.

Hip rotation PROM measurements may not accurately reflect hip rotation ROM if the measurement technique is influenced by mobility at the knee joint. Harris-Hayes and colleagues[17] measured hip rotation PROM in prone with the knee flexed 90°, with and without the tibiofemoral joint stabilized. The researchers found a clinically relevant increase in hip rotation PROM in women (not men), attributed to motion at the knee joint.

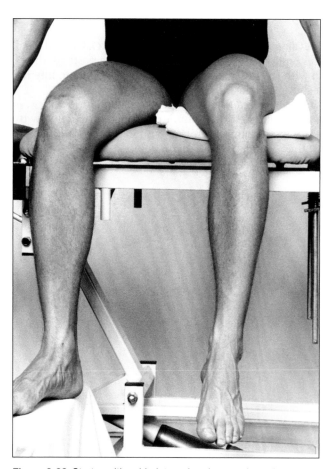

Figure 6-32 Start position: hip internal and external rotation.

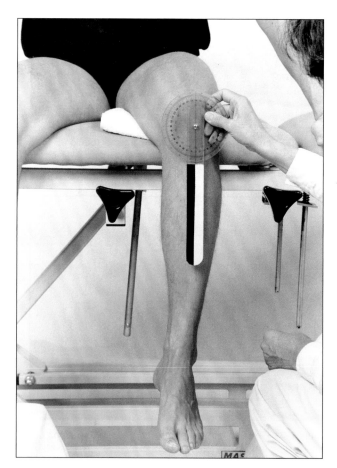

Figure 6-33 Start position: goniometer placement for hip internal and external rotation.

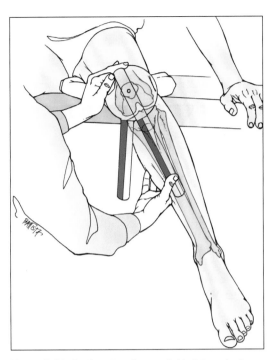

Figure 6-34 Goniometer alignment: hip internal rotation and external rotation. Illustrated with the hip in internal rotation.

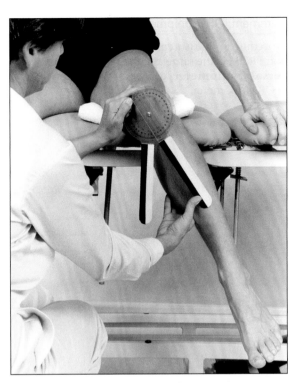

Figure 6-35 End position: internal rotation.

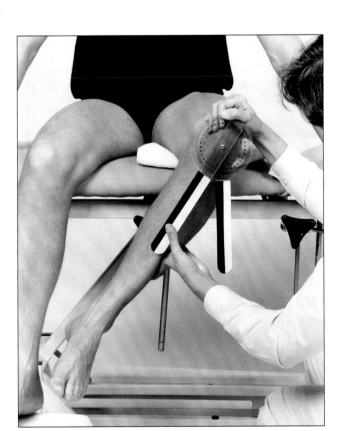

Figure 6-36 End position: external rotation.

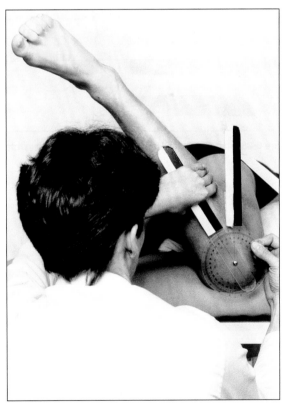

Figure 6-37 Alternate test position: prone with the knee flexed 90° and the hip in external rotation.

Measurement: OB Goniometer

The procedure for measurement of hip internal and external rotation PROM is the same as described for **Measurement: Universal Goniometer**, except for the placement and use of the OB goniometer.

OB Goniometer Placement. The strap is placed around the lower leg proximal to the ankle. The dial is placed on the anterior aspect of the lower leg (Figs. 6-38, 6-39, and 6-40).

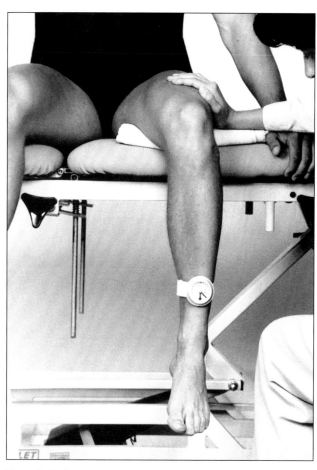

Figure 6-38 Start position: OB goniometer measurement hip rotation.

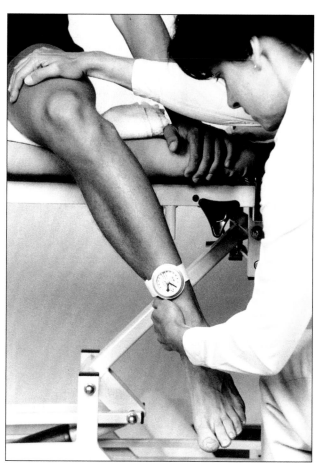

Figure 6-39 Internal rotation.

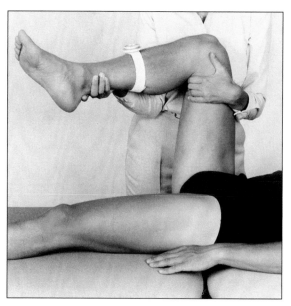

Figure 6-40 External rotation.

MUSCLE LENGTH ASSESSMENT AND MEASUREMENT

 Practice Makes Perfect

To aid you in practicing the skills covered in this section, or for a handy review, use the Summary & Evaluation Forms found at

http://thepoint.lww.com/ClarksonJM2e.

Hamstrings (Semitendinosus, Semimembranosus, Biceps Femoris)

Origins[2]	Insertions[2]
Semitendinosus	
Inferomedial impression on the superior aspect of the ischial tuberosity.	Proximal part of the medial surface of the tibia.
Semimembranosus	
Superolateral aspect of the ischial tuberosity.	Tubercle on the posterior aspect of the medial tibial condyle.
Biceps Femoris	
a. Long head: inferomedial impression of the superior aspect of the ischial tuberosity; lower portion of the sacrotuberous ligament.	Head of the fibula; slip to the lateral condyle of the tibia; slip to the lateral collateral ligament.
b. Short head: lateral lip of the linea aspera and lateral supracondylar line.	

Passive Straight Leg Raise (PSLR)

 Start Position. The patient is supine with the lower extremities in the anatomical position (Fig. 6-41). The low back and sacrum should be flat on the plinth.[11] Ankle dorsiflexion limits the ROM of SLR;[18,19] therefore, the test is performed with the ankle relaxed in plantarflexion.

Form 6-7

Stabilization. It is difficult to stabilize the pelvis when performing PSLR, and pelvic rotation is not eliminated from the movement.[20] However, the therapist must ensure that excessive anterior or posterior pelvic tilt is avoided through the use of a precise start position, adequate stabilization, and observation of pelvic motion. To stabilize the pelvis, the patient's nontest thigh is held on the plinth with the use of a strap (Fig. 6-41), or the therapist's knee is placed over the distal aspect of the anterior surface of the patient's nontest thigh (not shown).

End Position. The hip is flexed to the limit of motion while maintaining knee extension so that the biceps femoris, semitendinosus, and semimembranosus are put on full stretch (Figs. 6-42 and 6-43). The ankle is relaxed in plantarflexion during the test.

End Feel. Hamstrings on stretch—firm.

Measurement. The therapist uses a goniometer to measure and record the available hip flexion PROM (Figs. 6-42, 6-43, and 6-44).

Universal Goniometer Placement. The goniometer is placed the same as for hip flexion. A second therapist may assist to align and read the goniometer. Normal ROM and hamstring length is about 80° hip flexion.[11] Youdas and colleagues[21] assessed the PSLR ROM of 214 men and women, aged 20 to 79 years, and reported mean hip flexion PROM of 76° for women and 69° for men. When interpreting test results, consider that changes in PSLR might also result from changes in the degree of pelvic rotation.[22]

OB Goniometer Placement. This measurement procedure allows the therapist to easily assess PSLR ROM without assistance. The strap is placed around the distal thigh and the dial is placed on the lateral aspect of the thigh (Fig. 6-45).

Alternate Positions—Passive Knee Extension (PKE) Supine and Sitting

These alternate techniques used to evaluate hamstring muscle length are described in Chapter 7, pages 215 and 216.

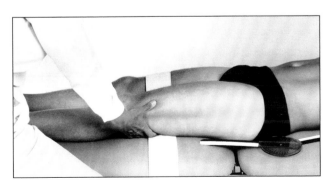

Figure 6-41 Start position: length of hamstrings.

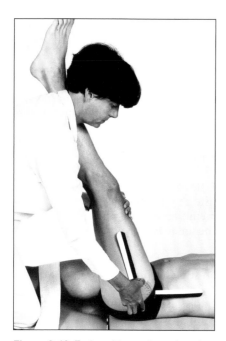

Figure 6-42 End position: universal goniometer measurement of hamstring length.

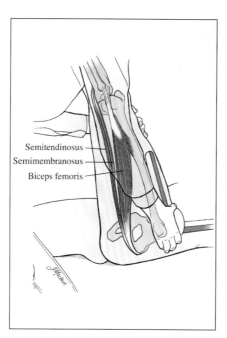

Figure 6-43 Hamstring muscles on stretch.

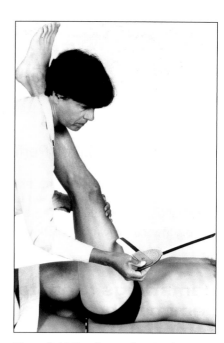

Figure 6-44 Reading goniometer: hamstring length.

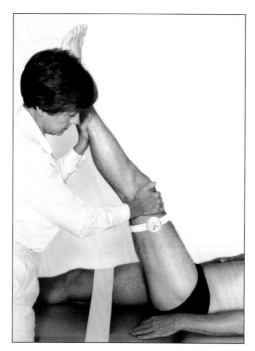

Figure 6-45 End position: OB goniometer measurement of hamstring length.

Hip Flexors[11] (Iliacus, Psoas Major, Tensor Fascia Latae, Sartorius, and Rectus Femoris)

Origins[2]	Insertions[2]
Iliacus	
Superior two-thirds of the iliac fossa, the inner lip of the iliac crest, ventral sacroiliac and iliolumbar ligaments, and the upper surface of the lateral aspect of the sacrum.	Lateral side of the tendon of the psoas major, and into the lesser trochanter.
Psoas Major	
Anterior aspects of the transverse processes of all of the lumbar vertebrae, sides of the bodies and intervertebral discs of T12 and all the lumbar vertebrae.	Lesser trochanter of the femur.
Tensor Fascia Latae	
Anterior aspect of the outer lip of the iliac crest, outer surface and notch below the ASIS, and the deep surface of the fascia latae.	Via the iliotibial tract onto the lateral condyle of the tibia.
Sartorius	
ASIS and the upper half of the notch below it.	Upper part of the medial surface of the tibia (anterior to gracilis and semitendinosus).
Rectus Femoris	
a. Straight head: anterior aspect of the anterior inferior iliac spine. b. Reflected head: groove above the acetabulum and the capsule of the hip joint.	Base of the patella, via the quadriceps tendon into the tibial tuberosity.

Thomas Test

Form 6-8

Start Position. The patient sits at the end of the plinth with the edge of the plinth at midthigh level. From this position, the patient is assisted into supine. Using both hands, the patient holds the hip of the nontest leg in flexion so that the sacrum and lumbar spine are flat on the plinth (Fig. 6-46). Care should be taken to avoid flexion of the lumbar spine due to excessive hip flexion ROM.

(*Note*: In the presence of excessive hip flexor length, the patient's hips are positioned at the edge of the plinth to allow the full available ROM.[11])

Stabilization. The supine position, and the patient holding the nontest hip in flexion, stabilizes the pelvis and lumbar spine. The therapist manually stabilizes and observes the ASIS to ensure there is no pelvic tilting during the test. The therapist's participation to ensure adequate stabilization is especially important when assessing female patients, as Beneck and colleagues[23] observed anterior rotation of the pelvis in female subjects and no movement out of the neutral position in the male subjects as the hip moved into extension using the modified Thomas test.

End Position. The test leg is allowed to fall toward the plinth into hip extension (Fig. 6-47). As the test leg falls toward the plinth, the therapist ensures (1) the knee is free to move into extension to avoid placing the rectus femoris on stretch and (2) the thigh remains in neutral adduction/abduction and rotation.

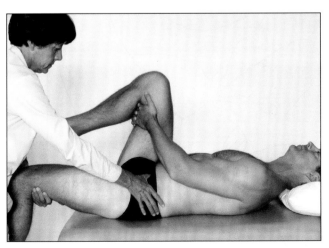

Figure 6-46 Start position: length of hip flexors.

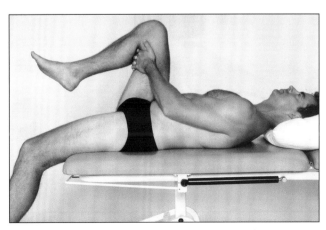

Figure 6-47 End position: thigh touching plinth indicates normal length of hip flexors.

If the thigh touches the plinth (Fig. 6-47), the hip flexors, that is, iliopsoas, is considered to be of normal length.[11]

If the thigh does not touch the plinth (Fig. 6-48), the therapist passively extends the knee and:

1. If the thigh touches the plinth (Fig. 6-49), shortness of rectus femoris restricted the hip extension ROM.

2. If there is no change in the position of the thigh, the therapist applies slight overpressure on the anterior aspect of the thigh to passively move the femur posteriorly to the limit of movement (Figs. 6-50 and 6-51). The end feel is evaluated to determine if iliopsoas shortness is the cause of the hip extension ROM restriction. Note that a flexion deformity at the hip can be obscured by an increased lumbar lordosis.[24]

End Feel. The iliacus and psoas major on stretch—firm.

Measurement. With shortness of the hip flexors, that is, iliopsoas, the angle between the midaxillary line of the trunk and the longitudinal axis of the femur represents the degree of hip flexion contracture (Figs. 6-50 and 6-51).

Universal Goniometer Placement. The same as for hip flexion–extension with the axis over the greater trochanter of the femur (Figs. 6-50 and 6-51).

Additional Considerations. If a restriction of hip joint extension is present (i.e., the thigh does not rest on the plinth) with the knee joint in extension, shortness of the iliopsoas, sartorius, or tensor fascia latae muscles may contribute to the limited ROM. The muscle shortness causing the restriction can be determined using the following criteria:[11]

A. Shortness of the *sartorius* should be suspected if the hip joint assumes a position of external rotation and abduction and/or the knee flexes at the restricted limit of hip extension.

B. Shortness of the *tensor fascia latae* may be suspected if the thigh is observed to abduct as the hip joint extends. If during testing the thigh is abducted as the hip is extended, and this results in increased hip extension, there is shortness of the tensor fascia latae. Specific length testing of tensor fascia latae should be performed to confirm this finding. Van Dillen and colleagues[25] suggest that abducting the hip may place the anterior fibers of the gluteus medius and minimus on slack and thus also contribute to the increase in hip extension. If hip abduction makes no difference to the restricted hip extension ROM, the *iliopsoas* muscle is shortened and preventing the full movement.

If the thigh is prevented from abducting during testing, a shortened tensor fascia latae may also produce hip internal rotation, lateral deviation of the patella, external rotation of the tibia, or knee extension.

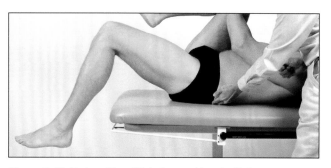

Figure 6-48 End position: thigh does not touch plinth.

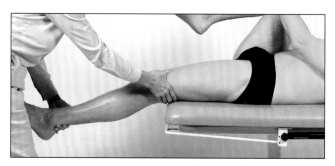

Figure 6-49 Thigh touches plinth with the knee extended.

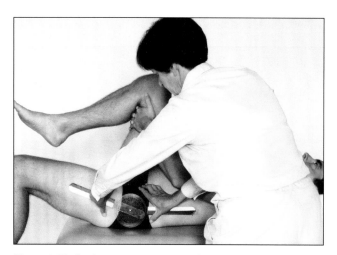

Figure 6-50 Goniometer measurement: length of shortened hip flexors.

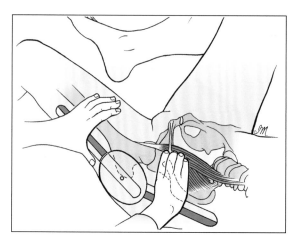

Figure 6-51 Hip flexors on stretch.

Hip Adductors (Adductor Longus, Adductor Brevis, Adductor Magnus, Pectineus, and Gracilis)

Form 6-9

Start Position. The patient is supine with the lower extremity in the anatomical position. On the non-test side, the hip is abducted, the knee is flexed, and the foot rests on a stool beside the plinth (Fig. 6-52).

Stabilization. The therapist stabilizes the ipsilateral pelvis.

End Position. The hip is abducted to the limit of motion so that the hip adductor muscles are put on full stretch (Fig. 6-53).

End Feel. Hip adductors on stretch—firm.

Origins[2]	Insertions[2]
Adductor Longus	
Front of the pubis in the angle between the crest and the symphysis.	Middle third of the linea aspera of the femur.
Adductor Brevis	
External surface of the inferior pubic ramus between the gracilis and obturator externus.	Line between lesser trochanter and linea aspera, upper part of the linea aspera.
Adductor Magnus	
External surface of the inferior ramus of the pubis adjacent to the ischium, the external surface of the inferior ramus of the ischium, and the infero-lateral aspect of the ischial tuberosity.	Medial margin of the gluteal tuberosity of the femur, medial lip of the linea aspera, medial supracondylar line, adductor tubercle.
Pectineus	
The pecten pubis between the iliopectineal eminence and the pubic tubercle.	Line between the lesser trochanter and the linea aspera.
Gracilis	
Lower half of the body of the pubis, the inferior ramus of the pubis and ischium.	Upper part of the medial surface of the tibia (between sartorius and semitendinosus).

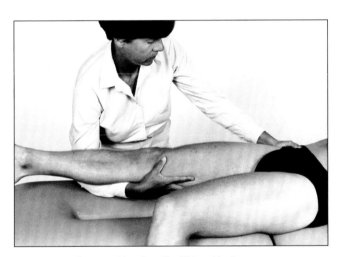

Figure 6-52 Start position: length of hip adductors.

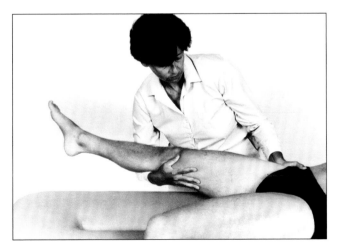

Figure 6-53 Hip adductors on stretch.

Measurement. If the hip adductors are shortened, hip abduction PROM will be restricted proportional to the decrease in muscle length. The therapist uses a goniometer to measure and record the available hip abduction PROM (Figs. 6-54 and 6-55).

Universal Goniometer Placement. The goniometer is placed the same as for hip abduction (Fig. 6-55).

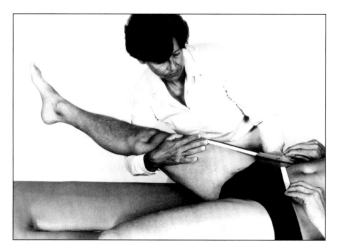

Figure 6-54 Goniometer measurement: length of hip adductors.

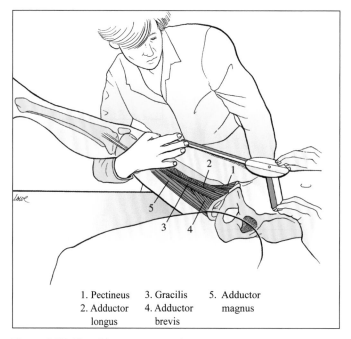

1. Pectineus	3. Gracilis	5. Adductor
2. Adductor longus	4. Adductor brevis	magnus

Figure 6-55 Hip adductors on stretch.

Tensor Fascia Latae (Iliotibial Band)

Origin²	Insertion²
Tensor Fascia Latae	
Anterior aspect of the outer lip of the iliac crest, the outer surface and notch below the ASIS, and the deep surface of the fascia latae.	Via the iliotibial tract onto the anterolateral aspect of the lateral condyle of the tibia.

Ober's Test²⁶

Form 6-10

Start Position. The patient is in the side-lying position on the nontest side and holds the nontest leg in hip and knee flexion to flatten the lumbar spine. The therapist stands behind and against the patient's pelvis to maintain the side-lying position. The hip is positioned in abduction and then extension to stretch the iliotibial band over the greater trochanter. The hip is in neutral rotation and the knee is positioned in 90° flexion (Fig. 6-56).

Stabilization. The position of the nontest leg stabilizes the pelvis and lumbar spine; the therapist stabilizes the lateral pelvis at the superior aspect of the iliac crest.

End Position. The test leg is allowed to fall toward the plinth. The therapist may apply slight overpressure on the lateral aspect of the thigh to passively adduct the hip to the limit of movement (not shown). With shortness of the tensor fascia latae, the hip remains abducted (Figs. 6-57 and 6-58). If the leg cannot be passively adducted to the horizontal, there is maximal tightness; if the horizontal position is reached, there is moderate tightness; and if the leg falls below horizontal but does not completely reach the plinth, there is minimal tightness.²⁷

Note that tightness of the tensor fascia latae at the hip can be obscured by a downward lateral tilt of the pelvis on the test side that may be accompanied by trunk lateral flexion on the opposite side. The position of the test leg must be carefully maintained in hip extension and neutral or slight external rotation to perform an accurate test of tensor fascia latae tightness.

If the rectus femoris muscle is tight or there is a need to decrease stress in the region of the knee, the Ober's test may be modified (Modified Ober's test) and performed with the knee in extension¹¹ (not shown). Note that the degree of hip adduction ROM used to indicate the length of tensor fascia latae will be more restricted with the knee in flexion (Ober's test) than with the knee in extension (Modified Ober's test).²⁸,²⁹ Therefore, these tests should not be used interchangeably²⁹ when assessing tensor fascia latae muscle length.

End Feel. Tensor fascia latae (iliotibial band) on stretch—firm.

Measurement. If the tensor fascia latae is shortened, hip adduction PROM will be restricted proportional to the decrease in muscle length.

Universal Goniometer Placement. The goniometer is placed the same as for hip abduction/adduction. A second therapist is required to assist with the alignment and reading of the goniometer.

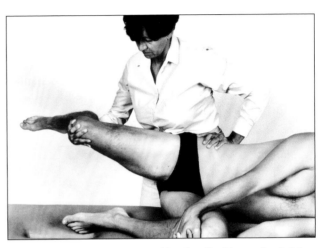

Figure 6-56 Ober's test start position: length of tensor fascia latae.

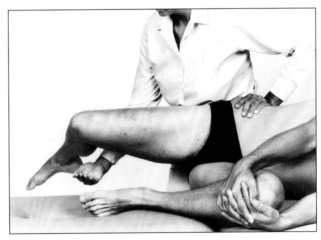

Figure 6-57 Ober's test end position: tensor fascia latae on stretch.

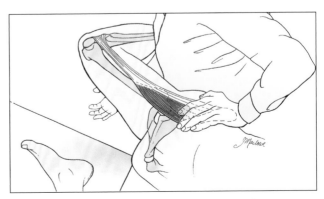

Figure 6-58 Ober's test: tensor fascia latae on stretch.

Alternate Measurement: Ober's Test—Trunk Prone

Form 6-11

Kendall and colleagues[11] describe the "Modified Ober's Test: Trunk Prone" to assess tensor fascia latae muscle length. This test provides better stabilization than the Ober's test.

Start Position. The patient is standing at the end of the plinth and flexes the hips so the trunk is resting on the plinth (Fig. 6-59). The nontest leg is placed under the plinth with the hip and knee flexed. The patient positions the arms overhead and grasps the sides of the plinth. The therapist supports the test leg and, while maintaining the knee in 90° flexion and the hip in neutral rotation, moves the hip into full abduction, followed by full extension to stretch the iliotibial band over the greater trochanter.

Stabilization. The therapist stabilizes the posterior aspect of the ipsilateral pelvis to prevent anterior pelvic tilt. It is also important the therapist stabilize the lateral aspect of the pelvis to prevent elevation of the contralateral pelvis and downward lateral tilt of the ipsilateral pelvis. The patient's arm position aids in preventing lateral pelvic tilt. The weight of the trunk offers stabilization.

End Position. With the hip maintained in full extension and neutral rotation, the hip is adducted to the limit of motion to place the tensor fascia latae on full stretch (Fig. 6-60). If the tensor fascia latae is shortened, hip adduction PROM with the hip in extension will be restricted proportional to the decrease in muscle length.

End Feel. Tensor fascia latae on stretch—firm.

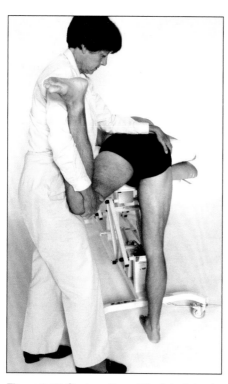

Figure 6-59 Start position—Ober's test: trunk prone.

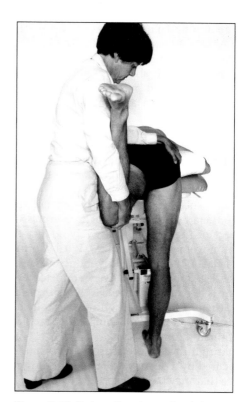

Figure 6-60 End position: tensor fascia latae on stretch.

FUNCTIONAL APPLICATION

Joint Function[30]

The hip joint transmits forces between the ground and the pelvis to support the body weight and acts as a fulcrum during single-leg stance. With the foot fixed on the ground, hip movement enables the body to be moved closer to or farther away from the ground. Hip motion brings the foot closer to the trunk and positions the lower limb in space.

Functional Range of Motion

Common activities of daily living (ADL) can be accomplished in a normal manner with hip ROM of at least 120° flexion, 20° abduction, and 20° external rotation.[31] In performing functional activities, hip movements are accompanied at various points in the ROM by lumbar–pelvic motions.[32] These motions extend the functional range capabilities of the hip joint.

Hip Flexion and Extension

The normal AROM for hip flexion is 0° to 120° and extension is 0° to 30°.[8] Full hip flexion and extension ranges of motion are required for many ADL. Standing requires 0° or slight hip extension.[33] Using electrogoniometric measures, it has been found that without using compensatory movement patterns at other joints, activities such as squatting to pick up an object from the ground, tying a shoe lace with the foot on the ground (Fig. 6-61) or with the foot across the opposite thigh, and rising from a sitting position (Fig. 6-62) require an average of 110° to 120° of hip flexion.[31]

Activities requiring less than 90° of hip flexion include sitting on the floor cross-legged,[34] sitting in a chair of standard height,[31] putting on a pair of trousers (Fig. 6-63), and ascending (Fig. 6-64) and descending stairs.[31,35] Ascending stairs requires an average of 67° hip flexion, and descending stairs requires an average of 36° hip flexion.[31] A maximum of about 1° to 2° hip extension may be required to ascend and descend stairs.[35] Kneeling[34,36] also requires less than 90° of hip flexion; however, this activity may require greater hip flexion of approximately 101° in elderly Chinese people as compared to young Chinese due to kneeling style.

The range required for sitting is determined by the height of the chair. About 84° of hip flexion is required for sitting in a standard chair.[31] To sit from standing requires

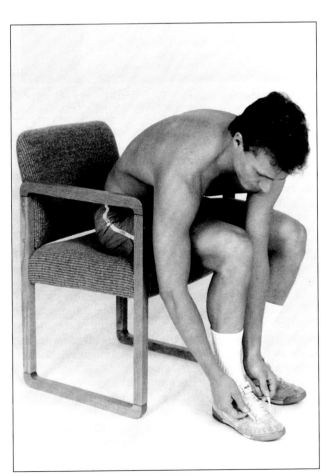

Figure 6-61 Tying a shoelace with the foot flat on the floor requires approximately 120° of hip flexion. (From Johnston RC, Smidt GL. Hip motion measurements for selected activities of daily living. *Clin Orthop Relat Res*. 1970;72:205-15.)

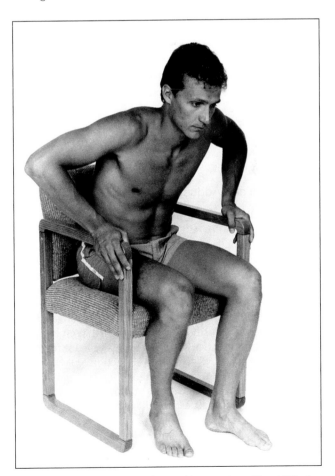

Figure 6-62 Rising from a sitting position requires at least 90° of hip flexion. (From Johnston RC, Smidt GL. Hip motion measurements for selected activities of daily living. *Clin Orthop Relat Res*. 1970;72:205-15.)

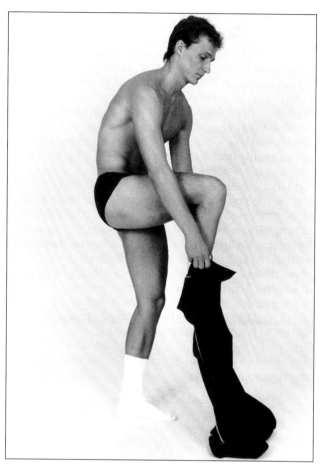

Figure 6-63 Donning a pair of trousers.

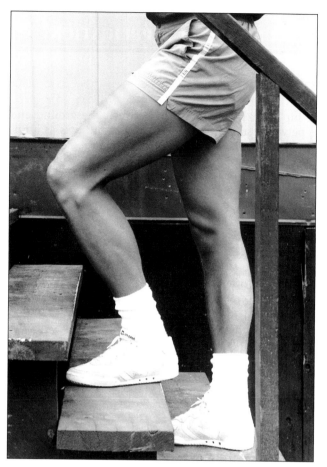

Figure 6-64 Ascending stairs.

an average of 104° hip flexion;[31] to rise from sitting requires an average of 98° to 101° hip flexion ROM.[37] These ranges increase with decreased chair height and decrease with increased chair height.

Hip Abduction and Adduction

The normal AROM at the hip for abduction is 0° to 45°; for adduction, it is 0° to 30°.[8] Most daily functions do not require the full ranges of hip abduction and adduction.

Many ADL can be performed within an arc of 0° to 20° of hip abduction.[31] Squatting to pick up an object and sitting with the foot across the opposite thigh (Fig. 6-65) are examples of activities performed within this ROM. Mounting a men's bicycle (Fig. 6-66) may require the full range of hip abduction bilaterally. Positions essential in ADL used by Asian and Eastern cultures such as squatting, cross-legged sitting, and kneeling require about 30° to 40° abduction ROM.[34,38]

Hip adduction in ADL is illustrated when sitting with the thighs crossed (Fig. 6-67) and when standing on one leg; the leg one stands on adducts as a result of the pelvis dropping on the contralateral side.

Hip Internal and External Rotation

The AROM of hip internal and external rotation is 0° to 45° in both directions.[8] The extremes of these rotational motions are seldom used in ADL. Ranges of 0° to 20° external rotation are required for most ADL.[31] Mounting a bicycle (Fig. 6-66), sitting on a chair with the foot across the opposite thigh (Fig. 6-65), to tie a shoelace, or visually observing the skin on the

sole of the foot when performing foot hygiene activities illustrates the use of hip external rotation. Positions essential in ADL used by Asian and Eastern cultures require full hip external rotation ROM for cross-legged sitting on the floor[34,38] and lesser average hip external rotation ROM for kneeling (25°) and squatting (19°).[34]

Walking and pivoting on one leg to turn are examples of functional activities that utilize hip internal rotation.

Gait

A normal walking pattern requires hip motion in the sagittal, frontal, and horizontal planes. In the sagittal plane, about 10° to 20° of hip extension is required at terminal stance, and 30° of hip flexion is required at the end of swing phase and the beginning of stance phase as the limb is advanced forward to take the next step (from the Rancho Los Amigos gait analysis forms as cited in Levangie and Norkin.)[33]

With the feet fixed on the ground, the femoral heads can act as fulcrums for the pelvis as it tilts anteriorly and posteriorly. The pelvis can also tilt laterally, causing the iliac crests to move either superiorly or inferiorly. Lateral tilting of the pelvis occurs when one leg is off the ground, the hip joint of the supporting leg acts as a fulcrum, and the tilting results in relative abduction and adduction at the hip joints.[33] When walking, there is a lateral tilt of the pelvis inferiorly on the unsupported side during the swing phase of the gait cycle. This dropping of the pelvis on the unsupported side results in ipsilateral hip abduction. As the pelvis drops, the inferior aspect of the pelvis moves toward the

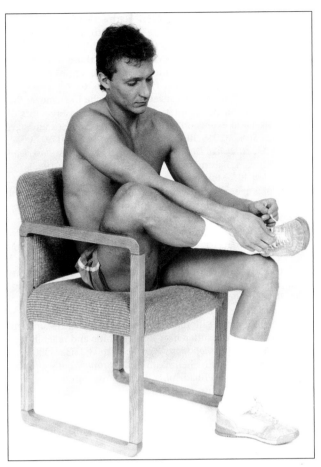

Figure 6-65 Sitting with the foot across the opposite thigh requires hip flexion, abduction, and external rotation.

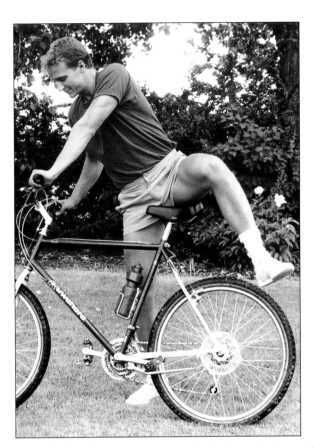

Figure 6-66 Mounting a bicycle requires hip flexion, abduction, and external rotation.

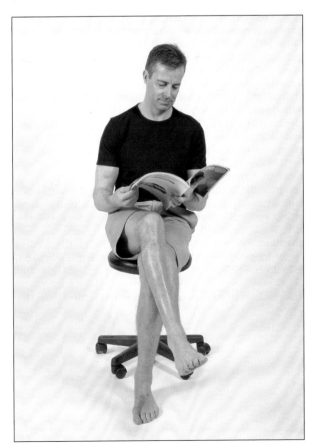

Figure 6-67 Hip adduction.

femur of the stance leg, producing hip adduction on this side. About 7° of hip abduction is required at initial swing, and 5° of hip adduction is required at the end of the stance phase of the gait cycle.[39]

Pelvic rotation occurs in the horizontal plane about a vertical axis. Rotations of the thigh occur relative to the pelvis. As the swinging leg advances during locomotion, the pelvis rotates forward on the same side. The fulcrum for this forward rotation of the pelvis is the head of the femur on the supporting leg. As the supporting or stance leg is fixed on the ground, the pelvis rotates around the femoral head, resulting in internal rotation at the hip joint. As the pelvis moves forward on the swing side, the swinging leg moves forward in the sagittal plane in the line of progression, resulting in external rotation of the hip during the swing phase of the gait cycle. During the normal gait cycle, about 5° of internal rotation and 9° of external rotation are required at the hip joint.[39] External rotation occurs at the end of the stance phase and through most of the swing phase, and internal rotation occurs at terminal swing before initial contact to the end of the stance phase.[39] Refer to Appendix D for further description and illustrations of the positions and motions at the hip joint during gait.

Hip flexion and extension ROM requirements for running are greater than for walking and vary depending on the speed of running. When running, average peak hip flexion ROM is 65° and hip extension ROM is 20°.[33]

References

1. Kapandji IA. *The Physiology of the Joints. Vol 2. The Lower Limb.* 6th ed. New York, NY: Churchill Livingstone Elsevier; 2011.
2. Standring S, ed. *Gray's Anatomy: The Anatomical Basis of Clinical Practice.* 39th ed. London, UK: Elsevier Churchill Livingstone; 2005.
3. Norkin CC, White DJ. *Measurement of Joint Motion: A Guide to Goniometry.* 4th ed. Philadelphia, PA: FA Davis; 2009.
4. Daniels L, Worthingham C. *Muscle Testing: Techniques of Manual Examination.* 5th ed. Philadelphia, PA: WB Saunders; 1986.
5. Norkin CC, Levangie PK. *Joint Structure and Function: A Comprehensive Analysis.* Philadelphia, PA: FA Davis; 1983.
6. Neumann DA. *Kinesiology of the Musculoskeletal System: Foundations for Rehabilitation.* 2nd ed. St. Louis, MO: Mosby Elsevier; 2010.
7. Magee DJ. *Orthopedic Physical Assessment.* 5th ed. St. Louis, MO: Saunders Elsevier; 2008.
8. American Academy of Orthopaedic Surgeons. *Joint Motion: Method of Measuring and Recording.* Chicago, IL: AAOS; 1965.
9. Berryman Reese N, Bandy WD. *Joint Range of Motion and Muscle Length Testing.* 2nd ed. St. Louis, MO: Saunders Elsevier; 2010.
10. Cyriax J. *Textbook of Orthopaedic Medicine. Vol 1. Diagnosis of Soft Tissue Lesions.* 8th ed. London, UK: Bailliere Tindall; 1982.
11. Kendall FP, McCreary EK, Provance PG, Rogers MM, Romani WA. *Muscles Testing and Function with Posture and Pain.* 5th ed. Baltimore, MD: Lippincott Williams & Wilkins; 2005.
12. Cailliet R. *Soft Tissue Pain and Disability.* Philadelphia, PA: FA Davis; 1977.
13. Boone DC, Azen SP. Normal range of motion of joints in male subjects. *J Bone Joint Surg Am.* 1979;61:756-759.
14. Steindler A. *Kinesiology of the Human Body Under Normal and Pathological Conditions.* Springfield, IL: Charles C Thomas; 1955.
15. Hollman JH, Burgess B, Bokermann JC. Passive hip rotation range of motion: effects of testing position and age in runners and non-runners. *Physiother Theor Pract.* 2003;19:77-86.
16. Gradoz MC, Bauer LE, Grindstaff TL, Bagwell JJ. Reliability of hip range of motion in supine and seated positions. *J Sport Rehabil.* 2018;16:1-4. doi:10.1123/jsr.2017-0243.
17. Harris-Hayes M, Wendl PM, Sahrmann SA, Van Dillen LR. Does stabilization of the tibiofemoral joint affect passive prone hip rotation range of motion measures in unimpaired individuals? A preliminary report. *Physiother Theor Pract.* 2007;23:315-323.
18. Gajdosik RL, LeVeau BF, Bohannon RW. Effects of ankle dorsiflexion on active and passive unilateral straight leg raising. *Phys Ther.* 1985;65:1478-1482.
19. Palmer TB, Kazuma Akehi K, Thiele RM, Smith DB, Warren AJ, Thompson BJ. Dorsiflexion, plantar-flexion, and neutral ankle positions during passive resistance assessments of the posterior hip and thigh muscles. *J Athl Train.* 2015;50(5):467-474. doi:10.4085/1062-6050-49.6.04.
20. Bohannon RW. Cinematographic analysis of the passive straight-leg-raising test for hamstring muscle length. *Phys Ther.* 1982;62:1269-1274.
21. Youdas JW, Krause DA, Hollman JH, Harmsen WS, Laskowski E. The influence of gender and age on hamstring muscle length in healthy adults. *J Orthop Sports Phys Ther.* 2005;35:246-252.
22. Bohannon R, Gajdosik R, LeVeau BF. Contribution of pelvic and lower limb motion to increases in the angle of passive straight leg raising. *Phys Ther.* 1985;65:474-476.
23. Beneck GJ, Selkowitz DM, Janzen DS, Malecha E, Tiemeyer BR. The influence of pelvic rotation on clinical measurements of hip flexion and extension range of motion across sex and age. *Phys Ther Sports.* 2018;30:1-7. doi:10.1016/j.ptsp.2017.07.005.
24. Salter RB. *Textbook of Disorders and Injuries of the Musculoskeletal System.* 2nd ed. Baltimore, MD: Williams & Wilkins; 1983.
25. Van Dillen LR, McDonnell MK, Fleming DA, Sahrmann SA. Effect of knee and hip position on hip extension range of motion in individuals with and without low back pain. *J Orthop Sports Phys Ther.* 2000;30:307-316.
26. Ober FR. Back strain and sciatica. *JAMA.* 1935;104:1580-1583.
27. Gose JC, Schweizer P. Iliotibial band tightness. *J Orthop Sports Phys Ther.* 1989;10:399-407.
28. Gajdosik RL, Sandler MM, Marr HL. Influence of knee positions and gender on the Ober test for length of the iliotibial band. *Clin Biomech (Bristol, Avon).* 2003;18:77-79.
29. Berryman Reese N, Bandy WD. Use of an inclinometer to measure flexibility of the iliotibial band using the Ober test and the modified Ober test: differences in magnitude and reliability of measurements. *J Orthop Sports Phys Ther.* 2003;33:326-330.
30. Smith LK, Weiss EL, Lehmkuhl LD. *Brunnstrom's Clinical Kinesiology.* 5th ed. Philadelphia, PA: FA Davis; 1996.
31. Johnston RC, Smidt GL. Hip motion measurements for selected activities of daily living. *Clin Orthop Relat Res.* 1970;72:205-215.
32. Cailliet R. *Low Back Pain Syndrome.* 2nd ed. Philadelphia, PA: FA Davis; 1968.
33. Levangie PK, Norkin CC. *Joint Structure and Function. A Comprehensive Analysis.* 3rd ed. Philadelphia, PA: FA Davis; 2001.
34. Hemmerich A, Brown H, Smith S, Marthandam SSK, Wyss UP. Hip, knee, and ankle kinematics of high range of motion activities of daily living. *J Orthop Res.* 2006;24:770-781.
35. Livingston LA, Stevenson JM, Olney SJ. Stairclimbing kinematics on stairs of differing dimensions. *Arch Phys Med Rehabil.* 1991;72:398-402.
36. Zhou H, Wang DM, Liu TR, Zeng XS, Wang CT. Kinematics of hip, knee, ankle of the young and elderly Chinese people during kneeling activity. *J Zhejiang Univ Sci B.* 2012;13(10):831-838.
37. Ikeda ER, Schenkman ML, Riley PO, Hodge WA. Influence of age on dynamics of rising from a chair. *Phys Ther.* 1991;71:473-481.
38. Kapoor A, Mishra SK, Kewangan SK, Mody BS. Range of movements of lower limb joints in cross-legged sitting posture. *J Arthroplasty.* 2008;23:451-453.
39. Johnston RC, Smidt GL. Measurement of hip-joint motion during walking. Evaluation of an electrogoniometric method. *J Bone Joint Surg Am.* 1969;51:1083-1094.

EXERCISES AND QUESTIONS

See the Answer Guide in Appendix E for suggested answers to the following exercises and questions.

1. PALPATION

A. Palpate the following anatomical structures on a skeleton and on a partner:

Iliac crest	Greater trochanter of the femur
Anterior superior iliac spine (ASIS)	Lateral epicondyle of the femur
Tubercle of the ilium	Adductor tubercle
Posterior superior iliac spine (PSIS)	Patella
Ischial tuberosity	Anterior border of the tibia

B. For each anatomical structure listed below, identify the hip joint ROM that would be measured using the structure to align the universal goniometer. Also, identify the part of the goniometer (i.e., axis, stationary arm, or moveable arm) that would be aligned with the anatomical structure for the purpose of the measurement.

   i. Greater trochanter of the femur

   _____

   ii. Anterior border of the tibia

   _____

   iii. Anterior superior iliac spines (ASISs)

   _____

   iv. Lateral epicondyle of the femur

   _____

   v. Patella

   _____

C. Identify the muscle(s) that attaches to the following structures:

   i. Adductor tubercle

   _____

   ii. Ischial tuberosity

   _____

2. ASSESSMENT OF AROM AT THE HIP JOINT

A. Identify and describe the shape of the articular components that make up the hip articulation.

B. Demonstrate, define, and describe* the following movements of the hip joint and identify the reciprocal movement:

   i. Hip extension
   ii. Hip internal rotation
   iii. Hip abduction
   *Identify the plane and axis of movement.

C. Demonstrate a quick scan of the AROM for the lower extremities on a partner under the following conditions:

   i. Unable to weight-bear
   ii. Able to weight-bear

D. List the active movements a therapist would assess when evaluating the hip joint (i.e., include active movements for the appropriate joints proximal and distal to the hip joint).

E. Identify patient criteria that would have to be met for the therapist to safely assess hip joint AROM in standing.

F. For each of the movements listed below:

- Assume the start position for the assessment and measurement of the ROM.
- Move your hip through half of the full AROM, and hold the joint in this position to mimic a decreased AROM.
- Without allowing further movement of the thigh, try to give the appearance of further hip movement or a greater than available AROM.
- Identify the substitute movements used to give the appearance of a greater than available AROM for the movement being assessed. These should be the same substitute movement(s) a patient may use to augment a restricted AROM for each movement.

Hip AROM	Substitute Movement(s)
i. Hip flexion	_____
ii. Hip abduction	_____
iii. Hip internal rotation	_____

3. ASSESSMENT AND MEASUREMENT OF PROM AT THE HIP JOINT

A. For each of the movements listed below, demonstrate the assessment and measurement of PROM on a partner, record your findings on the ROM Recording Form on page 203, and have a third partner evaluate your performance using the appropriate Practice Makes Perfect—Summary and Evaluation Form in Appendix B.

Answer the following questions:

Hip Flexion

When you correctly assessed and measured the PROM for hip flexion:

i. What position was the knee in on the test side?

ii. Why was the knee maintained in this position during the PROM assessment and measurement of hip flexion?

iii. Identify the normal end feel(s) expected when assessing hip flexion.

iv. What end feel did you identify on your partner for hip flexion?

v. List the normal limiting factors that created the end feel identified on your partner.

Hip Extension

Having correctly assessed and measured the PROM for hip extension:

i. What position was the knee in on the test side?

ii. Why was the knee maintained in this position during the PROM assessment and measurement of hip extension?

iii. If stabilization was inadequate when assessing the PROM for hip extension, the movements of _____ will result in erroneously large PROM values for hip extension.

iv. If a patient presents with decreased hip extension PROM, what arthrokinematic motion (i.e., glide/slide) of the femoral head could be decreased?

Hip Abduction

i. The pelvis should be level when assessing hip abduction PROM. How does the therapist ensure that the pelvis is level?

ii. If a patient presents with decreased hip abduction PROM, what glide of the femoral head could be restricted in this case? Explain the reason for the glide being decreased in the direction indicated.

Hip Internal Rotation

i. What end feel was present when you assessed your partner's hip internal PROM? Would this be considered a normal end feel?

ii. List the normal limiting factors that create a normal end feel for internal rotation.

iii. List the patient start position(s) that could be used to assess and measure the PROM for hip internal rotation. Assess and measure the PROM for hip internal rotation on your partner using each of these positions, and compare the PROM values measured at each position.

iv. If a patient presents with decreased hip internal PROM, what glide of the femoral head could be limited in this case? Explain the reason for the glide being decreased in the direction indicated.

B. A therapist evaluates the hip PROM and finds hip flexion to be the most restricted motion, followed by abduction and then internal rotation. This pattern of restricted motion could be a _____ pattern that would indicate to the therapist the presence of _____.

ROM RECORDING FORM

Patient's Name _____   Age _____

Diagnosis   _____   Date of Onset _____

Therapist Name _____   AROM or PROM _____

Therapist Signature _____   Measurement Instrument _____

Left Side				Right Side			
	*		*	**Date of Measurement**	*		*	
				Hip				
				Flexion (0–120°)				
				Extension (0–30°)				
				Abduction (0–45°)				
				Adduction (0–30°)				
				Internal Rotation (0–45°)				
				External Rotation (0–45°)				
				Hypermobility:				
				Comments:				

4. MUSCLE LENGTH ASSESSMENT AND MEASUREMENT

Demonstrate the assessment and measurement of the length of the following muscles on a partner, have a third partner evaluate your performance using the appropriate Practice Makes Perfect—Summary and Evaluation Form in Appendix E. Answer the following questions:

Hamstrings

   i. When assessing the hamstrings length using the SLR technique, the therapist must ensure the knee is maintained in full extension at the limit of motion and the pelvis is not moving into a _____ tilt position that would decrease the stretch on the hamstrings.

  ii. When using the Passive Knee Extension (PKE) Test, hamstring tightness is indicated if the knee cannot be _____.

 iii. Identify the end feel at the limit of the PROM when the hamstring muscles are put on full stretch.

Hip Flexors

   i. Identify the muscles for which muscle length is being assessed when assessing hip flexor muscle shortness.

  ii. When assessing the hip flexor muscle length, in what position is the nontest hip held, and why?

 iii. An *increased/decreased* (choose one) lumbar lordosis can mask a hip flexion contracture; therefore, this position of the lumbar spine should be avoided when assessing the length of the hip flexors.

  iv. When assessing the hip flexor muscle length, the hip is positioned in abduction to place the _____ on slack.

Tensor Fascia Latae

   i. If a skeleton is available, tape one end of a piece of string to the site of origin of the tensor fascia latae muscle and tape the other end of the string to the site of insertion of the iliotibial tract on the skeleton. If a skeleton is not available, hold the string at the sites of muscle origin and insertion on a partner. With the string in place, position the hip and knee articulations such that the muscle origin and insertion are as far apart as possible so as to maximally stretch the string (i.e., the simulated tensor fascia latae). Identify the positions of the hip and knee that place maximal stretch on the simulated tensor fascia latae.

  ii. Perform both the "Ober's test" and the "Ober's test: trunk prone" on a partner. Identify the test that offers the optimal stability of the pelvis and lumbar spine.

5. FUNCTIONAL ROM AT THE HIP JOINT

A. Have a partner perform the following functional activities. For each activity, use a universal goniometer to measure the position of your partner's hip joint or the maximum hip ROM used for the movement indicated. Record your measurements.

    i. Squatting to pick up an object on the ground—hip flexion

    ii. Sitting in a standard-height chair—hip flexion

    iii. Sitting on a high stool—hip flexion

    iv. Rising from sitting—hip flexion

    v. Ascending a staircase—hip flexion

    vi. Descending a staircase—hip flexion

    vii. Cutting one's toenails—hip flexion and hip abduction

    viii. Walking—hip flexion and hip extension

B. For each hip movement listed below, identify three daily activities that require the specified movement and demonstrate each activity:

    i. Hip abduction ROM

    ii. Hip adduction ROM

    iii. Hip internal rotation ROM

    iv. Hip external rotation ROM

C.   i. Identify the purposes served by the hip joint in performing ADL.

    ii. For each purpose the hip serves in performing ADL, identify an activity that illustrates the purpose.

    iii. According to Johnston and Smidt,[1] common ADL can be accomplished in a normal manner with hip ROM of at least _____° flexion, _____° abduction, and _____° external rotation.

Reference

1. Johnston RC, Smidt GL. Hip motion measurements for selected activities of daily living. *Clin Orthop Relat Res*. 1970;72:205-215.

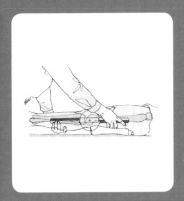

Knee 7

Practice Makes Perfect—Summary & Evaluation Forms ⊜ Forms 7-1 through 7-10 at http://thepoint.lww.com/ClarksonJM2e

ARTICULATIONS AND MOVEMENTS

The knee is made up of the tibiofemoral and patellofemoral articulations (Fig. 7-1). The tibiofemoral articulation is a bicondylar joint formed proximally by the convex condyles of the femur and distally by the concave surfaces of the tibial condyles. The congruency of these surfaces is enhanced by the menisci located between the articulating surfaces.[1] From the anatomical position, the tibiofemoral joint may be flexed and extended in the sagittal plane, with movement occurring around a frontal axis (Fig. 7-2). Rotation also occurs at the tibiofemoral joint and is an essential component of normal range of motion (ROM) at the knee. Rotation occurs in the horizontal plane around a longitudinal axis (Fig. 7-2). At the beginning of knee flexion from full extension, the tibia automatically rotates internally on the femur, and at the end of knee extension, the tibia automatically rotates externally. The external rotation at the end of knee extension locks the knee in full extension and is referred to as the "screw home mechanism." The greatest range of tibial rotation is available when the knee is flexed 90°.[2] Knee movements are described in Table 7-1.

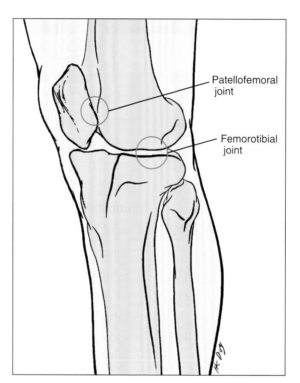

Patellofemoral joint

Femorotibial joint

Figure 7-1 Knee joint articulations, anterolateral view.

The patellofemoral articulation (Fig. 7-1), an incongruous joint, is also contained within the capsule of the knee joint. The patellar articular surface, divided by a vertical ridge, is flat or slightly convex mediolaterally and superoinferiorly[13] and articulates with the anterior surface of the femur, a surface that is divided by the intercondylar groove and is concave mediolaterally and convex superoinferiorly.[1] The "motion of the patella relative to the femur or femoral groove in knee flexion and extension" is referred to as patellar tracking.[14 (p. 241)] The gliding of the patella on the femur during knee flexion and extension is essential for normal motion at the knee. In full knee flexion, the patella slides distally and lies in the intercondylar notch.[13] In full knee extension, the patella slides proximally, and the lower portion of the patellar surface articulates with the anterior surface of the femur.[1] In addition to proximal–distal glide, the patella glides mediolaterally during knee joint movement.[15] At the beginning of knee flexion, the patella shifts slightly medial, and as knee flexion increases, the patella gradually shifts laterally.[14]

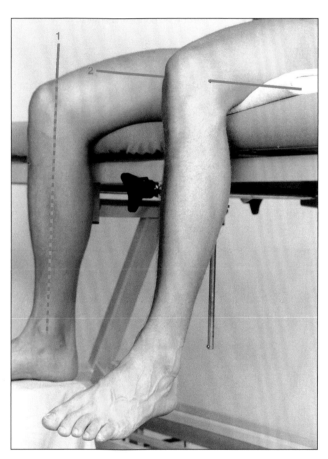

Figure 7-2 Knee joint axes: (*1*) tibial internal–external rotation; (*2*) flexion–extension.

TABLE 7-1   Joint Structure: Knee Movements

	Flexion	Extension	Internal Rotation	External Rotation
Articulation[1,3]	Femorotibial Patellofemoral	Femorotibial Patellofemoral	Femorotibial	Femorotibial
Plane	Sagittal	Sagittal	Horizontal	Horizontal
Axis	Frontal	Frontal	Longitudinal	Longitudinal
Normal limiting factors[2–6],* (see Fig. 7-3A and B)	Tension in the rectus femoris (with the hip in extension); tension in the vasti muscles; soft tissue apposition of the posterior aspects of the calf and thigh or the heel and buttock	Tension in parts of both cruciate ligaments, the medial and lateral collateral ligaments, the posterior aspect of the capsule, and the oblique popliteal ligament	Tension in the cruciate ligaments	Tension in the collateral ligaments
Normal end feel[4,7]	Firm/soft	Firm	Firm	Firm
Normal AROM[8],† (AROM[9])	0°–135° (0°–140°–145°)	135°–0° (0°)	40°[11] to 58°[12] total active range at 90° knee flexion	
Capsular pattern[7,10]	Tibiofemoral joint: flexion, extension			

*Note: There is a paucity of definitive research that identifies the normal limiting factors (NLF) of joint motion. The NLF and end feels listed here are based on knowledge of anatomy, clinical experience, and available references.

†AROM, active range of motion.

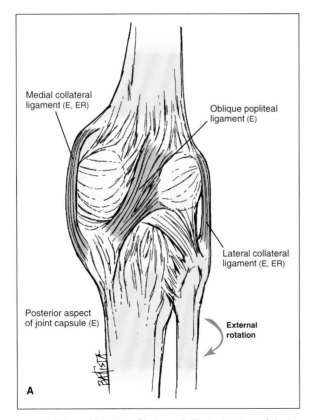

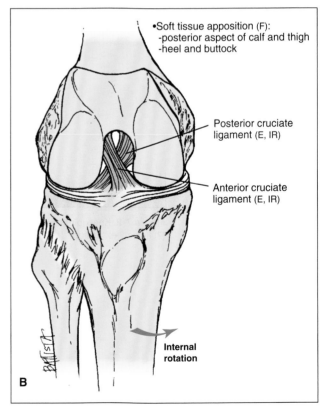

Figure 7-3 Normal Limiting Factors. A. Posterior view of the knee showing noncontractile structures that normally limit motion. **B.** Anterior view of the knee showing noncontractile structures that normally limit motion. Motion limited by structure is identified in brackets, using the following abbreviations: E, extension; ER, external rotation; IR, internal rotation. Muscles normally limiting motion are not illustrated.

ANATOMICAL LANDMARKS (FIGS. 7-4 AND 7-5)

Anatomical landmarks are described and illustrated below. Anatomical landmarks numbered 1, 2, 7, and 8 are used to assess knee ROM and/or to align the goniometer axis and arms, or position the OB goniometer to measure ROM at the knee.

Structure	Location
1. Greater trochanter	The superior border of the greater trochanter can be found with the tip of the thumb placed on the iliac crest at the midline and the tip of the third finger placed distally on the lateral aspect of the thigh.
2. Patella	Large triangular sesamoid bone on the anterior aspect of the knee. The base is proximal and the apex distal.
3. Ligamentum patellae	Extends from the apex of the patella to the tibial tuberosity tendon (patellar ligament or patellar tendon). As the patient attempts to extend the knee, the edges of the tendon are palpable.
4. Tibial tuberosity	Bony prominence at the proximal end of the anterior border of the tibia and the insertion of the ligamentum patellae.
5. Tibial plateaus	The upper edges of the medial and lateral tibial plateaus are located in the soft tissue depressions on either side of the ligamentum patellae. Follow the plateaus medially and laterally to ascertain the knee joint line.
6. Head of the fibula	A round bony prominence on the lateral aspect of the leg on a level with the tibial tuberosity.
7. Lateral malleolus	The prominent distal end of the fibula on the lateral aspect of the ankle.
8. Lateral epicondyle of the femur	Small bony prominence on the lateral condyle of the femur.

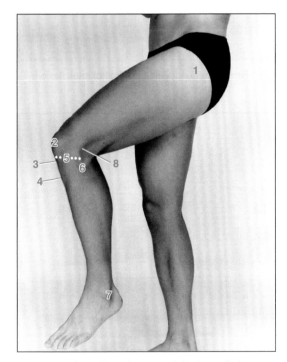

Figure 7-4 Anterolateral aspect of the lower limb.

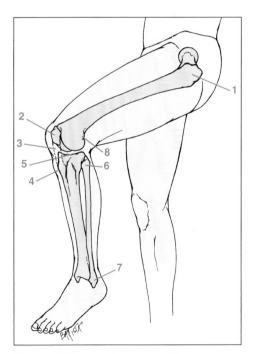

Figure 7-5 Bony anatomy, anterolateral aspect of the lower limb.

RANGE OF MOTION ASSESSMENT AND MEASUREMENT

 Practice Makes Perfect

To aid you in practicing the skills covered in this section, or for a handy review, use the Summary & Evaluation Forms found at

http://thepoint.lww.com/ClarksonJM2e.

Knee Flexion–Extension

AROM Assessment

Substitute Movement. Hip flexion.

PROM Assessment

Forms
7-1, 7-2

Start Position. The patient is supine with the hip and knee in the anatomical position (Fig. 7-6). A towel is placed under the distal thigh.

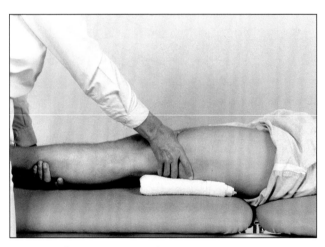

Figure 7-6 Start position: knee flexion and extension or hyperextension.

Stabilization. The pelvis is stabilized by the weight of the patient's body. The therapist stabilizes the femur.

Therapist's Distal Hand Placement. The therapist grasps the distal tibia and fibula.

End Positions. The therapist moves the lower leg to flex the hip and knee to the limit of knee flexion (Fig. 7-7).

The therapist extends the knee, to the limit of knee extension/hyperextension (Fig. 7-8).

End Feels. *Flexion*—firm/soft; *extension/hyperextension*—firm.

Joint Glides. *Flexion*—the concave tibial condyles glide posteriorly on the fixed convex femoral condyles. *Extension*—the concave tibial condyles glide anteriorly on the fixed convex femoral condyles.

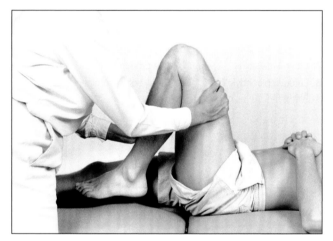

Figure 7-7 Firm or soft end feel at the limit of knee flexion.

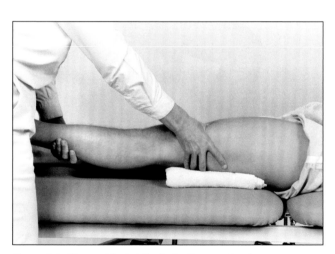

Figure 7-8 Firm end feel at the limit of knee extension or hyperextension.

Measurement: Universal Goniometer

Start Position. The patient is supine. The hip is in the anatomical position and the knee is in extension (0°) (Fig. 7-9). A towel is placed under the distal thigh.

Stabilization. The pelvis is stabilized by the weight of the patient's body. The therapist stabilizes the femur.

Goniometer Axis. The axis is placed over the lateral epicondyle of the femur (Fig. 7-10).

Stationary Arm. Parallel to the longitudinal axis of the femur, pointing toward the greater trochanter

Movable Arm. Parallel to the longitudinal axis of the fibula, pointing toward the lateral malleolus

End Position. From the start position of **knee extension (0°)**, the hip and knee are flexed (Fig. 7-11). The heel is moved toward the buttock to the limit of **knee flexion (135°)**.

Hyperextension. The femur is stabilized, and the lower leg is moved in an anterior direction beyond 0° of extension (Fig. 7-12). **Knee hyperextension from 0° to 10° may be present**.

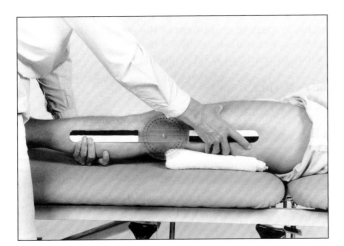

Figure 7-9 Start position: goniometer placement for knee flexion and extension/hyperextension.

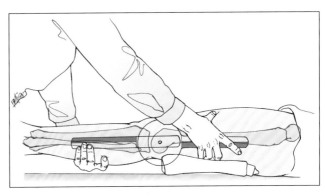

Figure 7-10 Goniometer placement for knee flexion and extension.

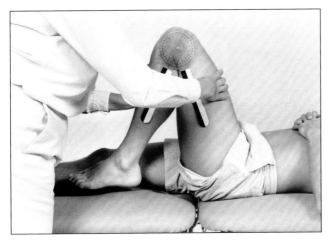

Figure 7-11 Knee flexion.

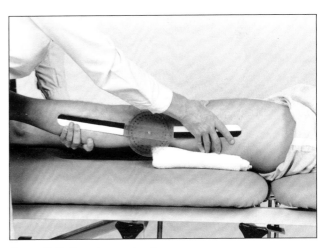

Figure 7-12 Knee hyperextension.

Patellar Mobility—Distal Glide

PROM Assessment

Form 7-3

Start Position. The patient is supine; a roll supports the knee joint in slight flexion (Fig. 7-13).

Stabilization. The femur rests on the plinth.

Procedure.[16] The heel of one hand is against the base of the patella, with the forearm lying along the thigh. The other hand is placed on top, and both hands move the patella in a distal direction to the end of the movement. Movement of the patella in a posterior direction compresses the patella against the femur and should be avoided. The therapist records whether the movement is full or restricted. The patella moves vertically a total of 8 cm from full flexion to full extension of the knee.[17]

End Feel. Firm.

Patellar Mobility—Mediolateral Glide

PROM Assessment

Form 7-4

Start Position. The patient is supine; a roll supports the knee joint in slight flexion (Fig. 7-14).

Stabilization. The therapist stabilizes the femur and tibia.

Procedure. The palmar aspects of the thumbs are placed on the lateral border of the patella. The pads of the index fingers are placed on the medial border of the patella. The thumbs move the patella medially, and the index fingers move the patella laterally in a side-to-side motion. With the knee in extension, passive movement of the **patella should average 9.6 mm medially and 5.4 mm laterally.**[18] Excessive, normal, or restricted ROM is recorded.

End Feel. Firm.

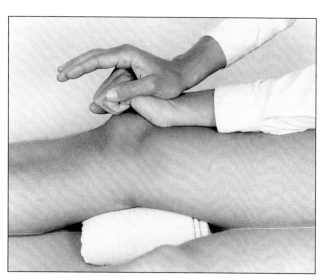

Figure 7-13 Distal glide of the patella.

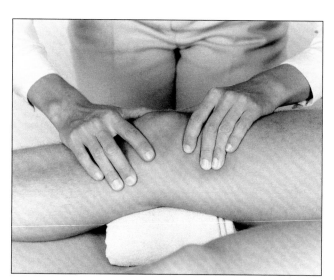

Figure 7-14 Mediolateral glide of the patella.

Tibial Rotation

Tibial rotation is an essential component of normal ROM at the knee. Assessment of total rotation ROM is more reliable than assessment of internal and external tibial rotation because of the difficulty of defining the zero start position for the individual movements.[19] The greatest range of tibial rotation is available when the knee is flexed 90°.[13]

AROM Assessment

Substitute Movement. Tibial internal rotation—hip internal rotation, ankle dorsiflexion/plantarflexion, subtalar joint inversion, forefoot adduction. Tibial external rotation—hip external rotation, ankle dorsiflexion/plantarflexion, subtalar joint eversion, forefoot abduction.

PROM Assessment

Form
7-5

Start Position. The patient is sitting with the knee in 90° flexion and the tibia in full internal rotation (Fig. 7-15A). A pad is placed under the distal thigh to maintain the thigh in a horizontal position.

Stabilization. The therapist stabilizes the femur.

Procedure. From full internal rotation, the therapist rotates the tibia externally through the full available ROM (Fig. 7-16A). The total range of tibial rotation is observed (average total active range, about 40° in women[11] and 58° in men[12]) and recorded as excessive, normal, or restricted.

End Feels. *Internal rotation—firm; external rotation—firm.*

Joint Spin. The proximal concave surface of the tibia spins on the convex condyles of the fixed femur. This spin occurs in conjunction with roll and glide of the articular surface during flexion and extension at the knee joint.

Measurement: OB Goniometer

Start Position. The patient is sitting with the knee in 90° flexion and the tibia in full internal rotation (Fig. 7-15A). A pad is placed under the distal thigh to maintain the thigh in a horizontal position. In the start position, the fluid-filled container of the goniometer is rotated until the 0° arrow lines up directly underneath the compass needle (Fig. 7-15B).

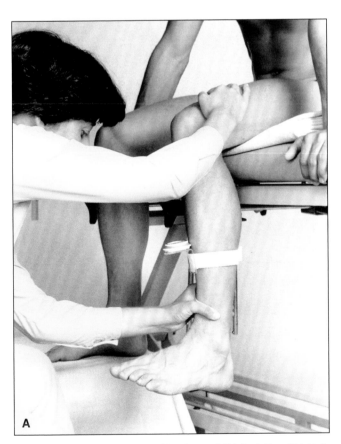

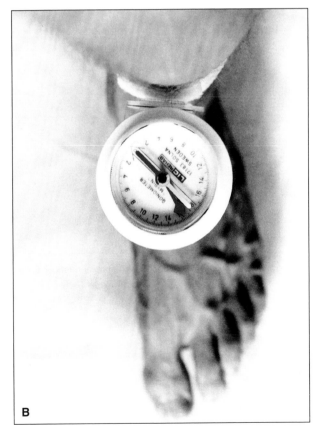

Figure 7-15 A and B. Start position for total tibial rotation: tibial internal rotation.

Goniometer Placement. The strap is placed around the leg distal to the gastrocnemius muscle, and the dial is placed on the right-angle extension plate on the anterior aspect of the leg.

Stabilization. The therapist stabilizes the femur.

End Position. From full internal rotation, the therapist rotates the tibia externally through the full available PROM (see Fig. 7-16A). The number of degrees the compass needle moves away from the 0° arrow on the compass dial is recorded as the **total range of tibial rotation** (see Fig. 7-16B) **(average total active range, about 40° in women[11] and 58° in men[12]).**

It is difficult to establish definitive normal values for active and passive total tibial rotation ROM from the literature. However, a study by Almquist and colleagues[20] used the "Rottometer" to evaluate the total tibial rotation PROM of 60 men and 60 women ranging in age from 15 to greater than 60 years, with normal knees. The total tibial rotation PROM was evaluated at three different knee flexion positions (i.e., 30°, 60°, and 90°), and the tibia was passively rotated using three different torques (i.e., 6 Nm, 9 Nm, and the examiner's determination of end feel). The researchers found no significant differences in total tibial rotation PROM between the subject's right and left knees at any of the knee flexion angles or applied torques (including the examiner's stopping of movement based on end feel). Based on these findings, the patient's contralateral normal knee, if available, may be used to define the patient's normal tibial rotation PROM.

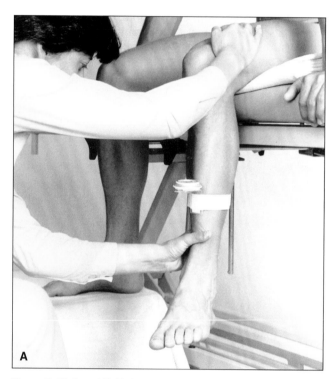

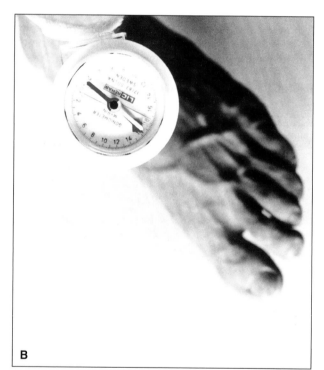

Figure 7-16 A and B. End position for total tibial rotation: tibial external rotation.

CHAPTER 7

MUSCLE LENGTH ASSESSMENT AND MEASUREMENT

Practice Makes Perfect

To aid you in practicing the skills covered in this section, or for a handy review, use the Summary & Evaluation Forms found at

http://thepoint.lww.com/ClarksonJM2e.

Hamstrings (Semitendinosus, Semimembranosus, Biceps Femoris)

Origins[1]	Insertions[1]
Semitendinosus	
Inferomedial impression on the superior aspect of the ischial tuberosity.	Proximal part of the medial surface of the tibia.
Semimembranosus	
Superolateral aspect of the ischial tuberosity.	Tubercle on the posterior aspect of the medial tibial condyle.
Biceps Femoris	
a. Long head: inferomedial impression of the superior aspect of the ischial tuberosity; lower portion of the sacrotuberous ligament. b. Short head: lateral lip of the linea aspera and lateral supracondylar line.	Head of the fibula; slip to the lateral condyle of the tibia; slip to the lateral collateral ligament.

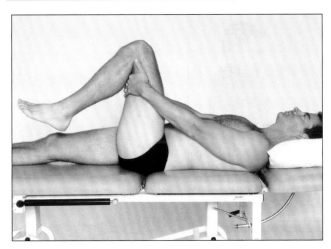

Figure 7-17 PKE: hamstrings length.

Passive Knee Extension (PKE) Supine[21]

Form 7-6

Start Position. The patient is supine (Fig. 7-17). The hip is flexed to 90°. The patient supports the thigh in this position by placing both hands around the distal thigh. If the patient cannot hold this position, the therapist stabilizes the thigh. The knee is flexed, and the ankle is relaxed in plantarflexion.

Stabilization. The patient or the therapist stabilizes the femur to maintain the hip in 90° flexion. Posterior tilt of the pelvis is avoided through use of a precise start position, observation of pelvic motion, and, if necessary, use of a strap placed over the anterior aspect of the distal thigh on the nontest side (see Fig. 6-41).

Goniometer Placement. The goniometer is placed the same as for knee flexion (Fig. 7-18). Should the therapist stabilize the thigh, a second therapist may be required to assist with the alignment and reading of the universal goniometer.

End Position. While maintaining the hip in 90° flexion, the knee is extended to the limit of motion so that the hamstring muscles are put on full stretch (Fig. 7-18). The ankle is relaxed in plantarflexion during the test.

The angle of knee flexion is used to indicate the hamstring muscle length. If the knee cannot be extended beyond 20° knee flexion, according to some sources,[22,23] this indicates hamstring tightness. However, Youdas and colleagues[24] performed the PKE test with 214 men and women, aged 20 to 79 years, and reported mean knee flexion PROM of 28° for women and 39° for men.

End Feel. Hamstrings on stretch—firm.

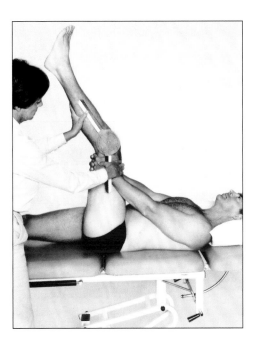

Figure 7-18 End position: universal goniometer measurement of knee flexion for hamstrings length.

Alternate Position—Sitting

Form
7-7

Start Position. The patient is sitting, grasps the edge of the plinth, and has the nontest foot supported on a stool (Fig. 7-19). A pad is placed under the distal thigh to maintain the thigh in a horizontal position. The ankle on the test side is relaxed in plantarflexion.

Stabilization. The therapist stabilizes the femur. The patient grasps the edge of the plinth and is instructed to maintain the upright sitting position.

Goniometer Placement. The goniometer is placed the same as for knee flexion–extension (Fig. 7-20).

End Position. The therapist extends the knee to the limit of motion so that hamstrings are put on full stretch (Fig. 7-20). The ankle is relaxed in plantarflexion throughout the test movement to prevent gastrocnemius muscle tightness from limiting knee ROM.

End Feel. Hamstrings on stretch—firm.

Substitute Movement. The patient leans back to posteriorly tilt the pelvis, extending the hip joint to place the hamstrings on slack, and thus allow increased knee extension (Fig. 7-21).

Alternate Position—Passive Straight Leg Raise (PSLR)

The PSLR technique used to evaluate hamstring muscle length is described in Chapter 6, page 189. Note: the PKE and PSLR tests should not be used interchangeably when assessing hamstring muscle length.[23]

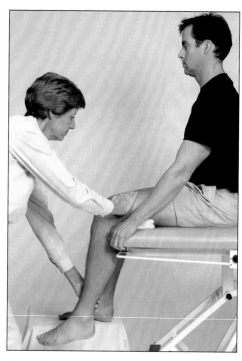

Figure 7-19 Start position: length of hamstrings.

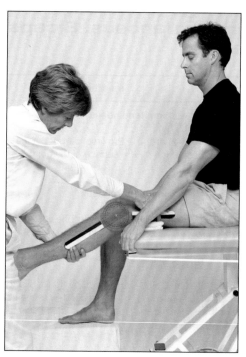

Figure 7-20 Goniometer measurement: length of hamstrings.

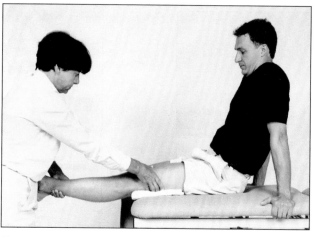

Figure 7-21 Substitute movement: backward lean during hamstrings length test.

Rectus Femoris

Origins[1]	Insertion[1]
Rectus Femoris	
a. Straight head: anterior inferior iliac spine.	Base of the patella, via the quadriceps tendon into the tibial tuberosity.
b. Reflected head: groove above the acetabulum and the capsule of the hip joint.	

Form 7-8

Start Position. The patient is prone. To position the pelvis in a posterior tilt, the nontest leg is over the side of the plinth with the hip flexed and the foot on the floor (Fig. 7-22). This positioning of the nontest leg has been shown to effectively tilt the pelvis posteriorly, and thus increase hip extension of the test leg to better ensure maximum stretch of the rectus femoris muscle.[25] The test leg is in the anatomical position with the knee in extension (0°). A towel may be placed under the thigh to eliminate pressure on the patella.

Stabilization. The patient's prone position with the nontest leg over the side of the plinth with the hip flexed and the foot on the floor stabilizes the pelvis. A strap may also be placed over the buttocks to stabilize the pelvis. The therapist stabilizes the femur.

Goniometer Placement. The goniometer is placed the same as for knee flexion–extension.

End Position. The lower leg is moved in a posterior direction so that the heel approximates the buttock to the limit of knee flexion. Decreased length of the rectus femoris restricts the range of knee flexion when the patient is prone (Fig. 7-23).

End Feel. Rectus femoris on stretch—firm.

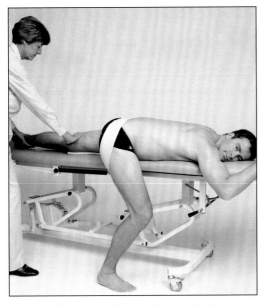

Figure 7-22 Start position: length of rectus femoris.

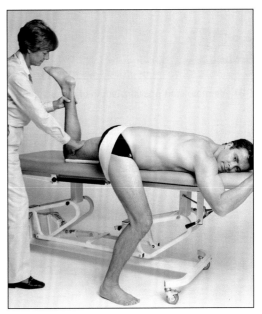

Figure 7-23 End position: length of rectus femoris.

CHAPTER 7

Alternate Position—Ely Test

Form 7-9

Start Position. The patient is prone. A towel may be placed under the thigh to eliminate pressure on the patella. The leg is in the anatomical position with the knee in extension (0°) (Fig. 7-24).

Stabilization. The patient's prone position stabilizes the pelvis. A strap may also be placed over the buttocks to stabilize the pelvis. The therapist observes the pelvis to ensure there is no tilting. The therapist stabilizes the femur.

Goniometer Placement. The goniometer is placed the same as for knee flexion–extension.

End Position. The lower leg is moved in a posterior direction so the heel approximates the buttock to the limit of knee flexion. Decreased length of the rectus femoris restricts the range of knee flexion when the patient is prone (Fig. 7-25).

End Feel. Rectus femoris on stretch—firm.

Substitute Movement. The patient anteriorly tilts the pelvis and flexes the hip to place the rectus femoris on slack and thus allows increased knee flexion (Fig. 7-26).

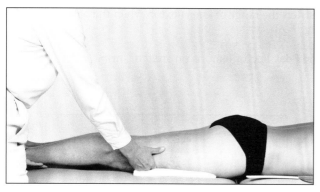

Figure 7-24 Alternate start position: length of rectus femoris.

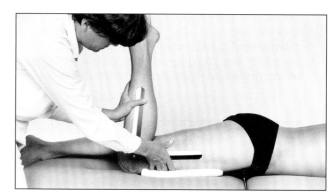

Figure 7-25 Goniometer measurement: length of rectus femoris.

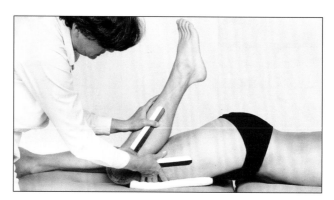

Figure 7-26 Substitute movement: anterior pelvic tilt and hip flexion placing rectus femoris on slack.

Alternate Position—Thomas Test Position

Start Position. The patient sits at the end of the plinth with the edge of the plinth at midthigh level. From this position, the patient is assisted into supine. Using both hands, the patient holds the hip of the nontest leg in flexion so that the sacrum and lumbar spine are flat on the plinth. Care should be taken to avoid flexion of the lumbar spine due to excessive hip flexion ROM. With the hip abducted, the hip is extended to the limit of motion[26] (Fig. 7-27).

Stabilization. The patient's supine position and holding of the nontest hip in flexion stabilize the pelvis and lumbar spine. The therapist observes the anterior superior iliac spine (ASIS) to ensure there is no pelvic tilting. The therapist stabilizes the femur.

Goniometer Placement. The goniometer is placed the same as for knee flexion–extension (Fig. 7-29).

End Position. The knee is flexed to the limit of motion to assess shortness of the rectus femoris (Figs. 7-28 and 7-29). If the rectus femoris is shortened, knee flexion PROM will be restricted proportional to the decrease in muscle length. Knee flexion of less than 80° indicates the degree of muscle shortening.[27]

End Feel. Rectus femoris on stretch—firm.

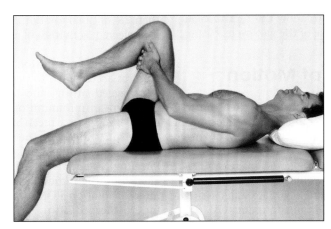

Figure 7-27 Alternate start position: length of rectus femoris.

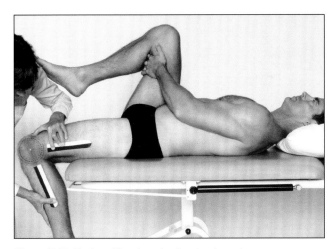

Figure 7-28 End position: length of rectus femoris.

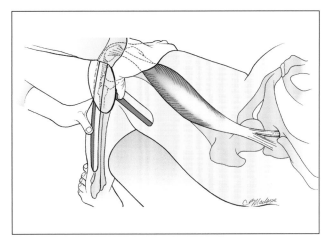

Figure 7-29 Alternate goniometer measurement: length of rectus femoris.

FUNCTIONAL APPLICATION

Joint Function

The knee joint functions to support the body weight and to shorten or lengthen the lower limb.[2] Knee flexion with the foot planted lowers the body closer to the ground, while knee extension raises the body.[28] With the foot off the ground, foot orientation in space is provided[2] by flexing or extending the knee or rotating the tibia. The rotational mobility of the knee joint makes twisting movements of the body possible when the foot is planted on the ground.[28] In walking, the knee joint acts as a shock absorber, decreases the vertical displacement of the body, and, through knee flexion, shortens the lower limb to allow the toes to clear the ground during the swing phase of the gait cycle.[29,30]

Functional Range of Motion

The normal AROM at the knee is from 0° of extension to 135° of flexion. Full extension is required for normal function, but many daily activities require less than 135° of knee flexion. Rowe and colleagues[31] suggest 0° to at least 110° of knee flexion would be an appropriate target for rehabilitation. A target of 110° knee flexion would enable one to walk, sit in and stand up from a chair, and negotiate stairs. Using the bath would require greater ROM of approximately 135° flexion to be performed in a normal manner.

The knee must be fully extended to stand erect (Fig. 7-30). Full or near-full knee extension is required to reach a height (Fig. 7-31) or to contact a distant object or surface with the foot, such as depressing the brake pedal of a car or going downstairs (Fig. 7-32). When dressing, the knee is extended to put on a pair of trousers (Fig. 7-33) or shorts. The fully extended position of the knee usually occurs in asymmetrical postures, for example, prolonged standing when one leg is used to support most of the body weight or when powerful thrusting motions[1] such as jumping are performed.

Daily activities involving ranges of knee motion up to an average of 117° of flexion include lifting an object off the floor (Fig. 7-34), sitting down in a chair (Fig. 7-35), descending and ascending stairs (Figs. 7-32 and 7-36), and tying a shoelace[33] or pulling on a sock (Fig. 7-37). Many of the daily functions previously mentioned require on average less than 25° of tibial rotation.[33] The knee flexion ROM required for selected activities of daily living (ADL) is shown in Table 7-2.

Far greater knee flexion ROM is utilized by non-Western cultures accustomed to performing ADL such as squatting, cross-legged sitting, and kneeling[35,36] (Table 7-3). A range with a mean minimum of 135° knee flexion when sitting cross-legged[36] to a mean maximum of about 157° flexion when squatting with the heels up[35] is required for these ADL. Positions (i.e., squatting, cross-legged sitting, and kneeling) essential for ADL in Asian and Eastern cultures all require high knee flexion ROM accompanied by tibial internal rotation ROM up to an average maximum of 33° for cross-legged sitting.[35] To achieve the knee flexion ROM required to squat and kneel, the hip is flexed placing the

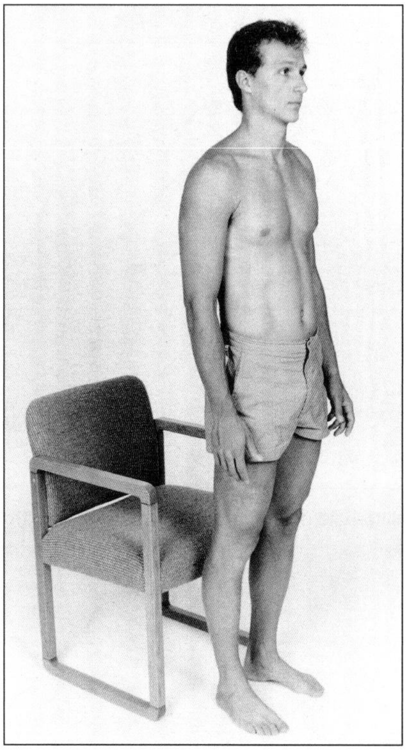

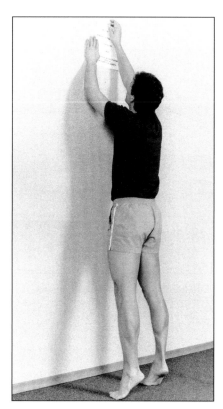

Figure 7-30 Full knee extension is required to stand erect.

Figure 7-31 To reach a height, full or near-full knee extension is required.

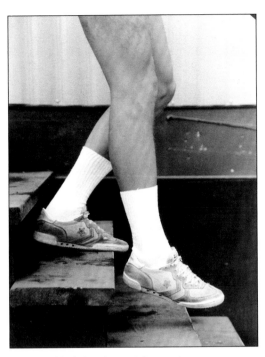

Figure 7-32 Going down stairs requires an average of 86° to 107° of knee flexion, and full or near-full knee extension.[32]

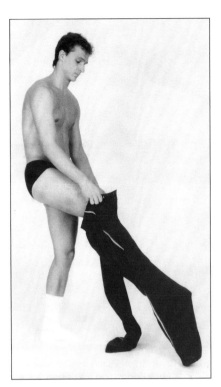

Figure 7-33 The knee is in extension to put on a pair of trousers.

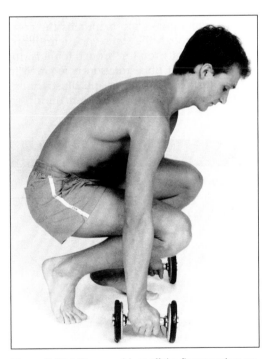

Figure 7-34 Lifting an object off the floor requires an average of 117° of knee flexion.[33]

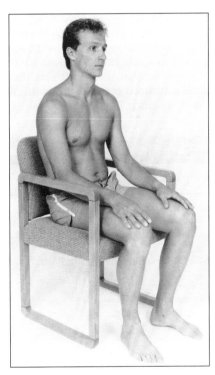

Figure 7-35 To sit down in a chair requires an average of 93° of knee flexion.[33]

rectus femoris on slack, and body weight assists in passively flexing the knee joint.

Livingston and coworkers[32] evaluated the knee flexion ROM required to ascend and descend three stairs of different dimensions. Depending on the stair dimensions and subject height, the maximum knee flexion ROM required ranged between averages of 83° and 105° to ascend and 86° and 107° to descend the stairs. Minimum knee flexion ROM averages of between 1° or 2° and 15° were required to ascend or descend stairs. It appears that changes of ROM at the knee joint, rather than the hip and ankle, are used to adjust to different stair dimensions.[32]

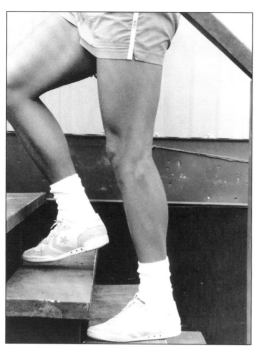

Figure 7-36 Climbing stairs requires an average of 83° to 105° of knee flexion and full or near-full knee extension.[32]

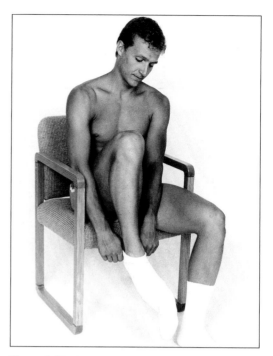

Figure 7-37 Knee range within the arc of 0° to 117° of flexion.

Gait

Walking requires an ROM from about 0° of knee extension as the leg advances forward to make initial contact with the ground (Fig. 7-38), to a maximum of about 60° of knee flexion at initial swing so that the foot clears the ground as the extremity is advanced forward (from the Rancho Los Amigos gait analysis forms, as cited in the work of Levangie

and Norkin [2]). The tibia rotates internally on the femur at the end of the swing phase and maintains the position of internal rotation through the stance phase until preswing, when the tibia externally rotates through to midswing.[38] An average of about 13° of tibial rotation is required for normal gait.[39] For further description and illustrations of the positions and motions at the knee joint during gait, see Appendix D.

TABLE 7-2 **Knee Flexion ROM Average Values Required for ADL**	
Activity	**Knee Flexion**
Taking a bath[31]	135°
Tying shoe: sitting and bringing the foot up from the floor*	106°
Sitting: without touching the chair with the hands*	93°

Lifting object from floor*
    Bending at hips to reach down
    Back straight, bending knees
	
	71°
	117°

Stairs†
    Ascending
    Descending
	
	83°–105°
	86°–107°

Walking‡	60°
Fast-paced running[34] (faster than 7.5-minute mile)	103°

*Knee flexion ROM for 30 subjects were measured from the subject's normal stance position and not anatomical zero position.[33]

†Knee flexion ROM for 15 subjects during ascent and descent of three stairs of different dimensions. Maximum knee flexion ROM requirements varied depending on the stair dimensions and subject height.[32]

‡Data from the Rancho Los Amigos gait analysis forms as cited in Levangie and Norkin.[2]

TABLE 7-3 **Positions Essential for ADL in Asian and Eastern Cultures: Average Knee Flexion ROM Values Required**

Activity	Knee Flexion
Sitting cross-legged	135°[36] to 150°[35]
Kneeling with:	
ankles plantarflexed	144°[35]
ankles dorsiflexed	140°[37] to 155°[35]
Squatting[35] with:	
heels down	154°
heels up	157°

Pink and colleagues[34] investigated and described the ROM requirement at the knee for slow-paced running (slower than an 8-minute mile) and fast-paced running (faster than a 7.5-minute mile). Fast-paced running required a range of knee joint motion from an average of 11° flexion at terminal swing to an average 103° maximum knee flexion near the end of middle swing. Slower-paced running required less flexion throughout most of the swing phase compared to fast-paced running.

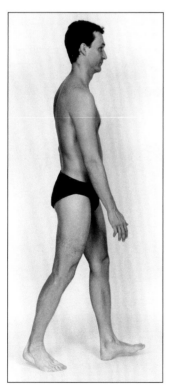

Figure 7-38 Full knee extension is required for normal gait.

References

1. Standring S, ed. *Gray's Anatomy: The Anatomical Basis of Clinical Practice.* 39th ed. London, UK: Elsevier Churchill Livingstone; 2001.
2. Levangie PK, Norkin CC. *Joint Structure and Function. A Comprehensive Analysis.* 3rd ed. Philadelphia, PA: FA Davis; 2001.
3. Kapandji IA. *The Physiology of the Joints. Vol. 2. The Lower Limb.* 6th ed. New York, NY: Churchill Livingstone Elsevier; 2011.
4. Norkin CC, White DJ. *Measurement of Joint Motion: A Guide to Goniometry.* 4th ed. Philadelphia, PA: FA Davis Company; 2009.
5. Daniels L, Worthingham C. *Muscle Testing: Techniques of Manual Examination.* 5th ed. Philadelphia, PA: WB Saunders; 1986.
6. Woodburne RT. *Essentials of Human Anatomy.* 5th ed. London: Oxford University Press; 1973.
7. Magee DJ. *Orthopedic Physical Assessment.* 5th ed. St. Louis, MO: Saunders Elsevier; 2008.
8. American Academy of Orthopaedic Surgeons. *Joint Motion: Method of Measuring and Recording.* Chicago, IL: AAOS; 1965.
9. Berryman Reese N, Bandy WD. *Joint Range of Motion and Muscle Length Testing.* 2nd ed. St. Louis, MO: Saunders Elsevier; 2010.
10. Cyriax J. *Textbook of Orthopaedic Medicine. Vol. 1. Diagnosis of Soft Tissue Lesions.* 8th ed. London, UK: Bailliere Tindall; 1982.
11. Mossberg KA, Smith LK. Axial rotation of the knee in women. *J Orthop Sports Phys Ther.* 1983;4(4):236-240.
12. Osternig LR, Bates BT, James SL. Patterns of tibial rotary torque in knees of healthy subjects. *Med Sci Sports Exerc.* 1980;12:195-199.
13. Levangie PK, Norkin CC. *Joint Structure and Function. A Comprehensive Analysis.* 4th ed. Philadelphia, PA: FA Davis; 2005.
14. Katchburian MV, Bull AMJ, Shih Y-F, Heatley FW, Amis AA. Measurement of patellar tracking: assessment and analysis of the literature. *Clin Orthop Relat Res.* 2003;412:241-259.
15. Heegaard J, Leyvraz P-F, Van Kampen A, Rakotomanana L, Rubin PJ, Blankevoort L. Influence of soft structures on patellar three-dimensional tracking. *Clin Orthop Relat Res.* 1994;299:235-243.
16. Kaltenborn FM. *Mobilization of the Extremity Joints: Examination and Basic Treatment Techniques.* 3rd ed. Oslo, Norway: Olaf Norlis Bokhandel; 1985.
17. Soderberg GL. *Kinesiology: Application to Pathological Motion.* 2nd ed. Baltimore, MD: Williams & Wilkins; 1997.

18. Skalley TC, Terry GC, Teitge RA. The quantitative measurement of normal passive medial and lateral patellar motion limits. *Am J Sports Med*. 1993;21:728-732.

19. Zarins B, Rowe CR, Harris BA, Watkins MP. Rotational motion of the knee. *Am J Sports Med*. 1983;11:152-156.

20. Almquist PO, Ekdahl C, Isberg P-E, Fridén T. Knee rotation in healthy individuals related to age and gender. *J Orthop Res*. 2013;31(1):23-28. doi: 10.1002/jor.22184.

21. Holt KS. *Assessment of Cerebral Palsy. I. Muscle Function, Locomotion and Hand Function*. London: Lloyd-Luke Medical Books; 1965.

22. Palmer ML, Epler ME. *Clinical Assessment Procedures in Physical Therapy*. Philadelphia, PA: JB Lippincott; 1990.

23. Davis DS, Quinn RO, Whiteman CT, Williams JD, Young CR. Concurrent validity of four clinical tests used to measure hamstring flexibility. *J Strength Cond Res*. 2008;22(2):583-588.

24. Youdas JW, Krause DA, Hollman JH, Harmsen WS, Laskowski E. The influence of gender and age on hamstring muscle length in healthy adults. *J Orthop Sports Phys Ther*. 2005; 35:246-252.

25. Hamberg J, Bjorklund M, Nordgren B, Sahistedt B. Stretchability of the rectus femoris muscle: investigation of validity and intra-tester reliability of two methods including x-ray analysis of pelvic tilt. *Arch Phys Med Rehabil*. 1993;74:263-270.

26. Van Dillen LR, McDonnell MK, Fleming DA, Sahrmann SA. Effect of knee and hip position on hip extension range of motion in individuals with and without low back pain. *J Orthop Sports Phys Ther*. 2000;30:307-316.

27. Kendall FP, McCreary EK, Provance PG, Rodgers MM, Romani WA. *Muscles Testing and Function*. 5th ed. Baltimore, MD: Williams & Wilkins; 2005.

28. Smith LK, Weiss EL, Lehmkuhl LD. *Brunnstrom's Clinical Kinesiology*. 5th ed. Philadelphia, PA: FA Davis; 1996.

29. Edelstein JE. Biomechanics of normal ambulation. *J Can Physiother Assoc*. 1965;17:174-185.

30. Inman VT, Ralston HJ, Todd F. *Human Walking*. Baltimore, MD: Williams & Wilkins; 1981.

31. Rowe PJ, Myles CM, Walker C, Nutton R. Knee joint kinematics in gait and other functional activities measured using flexible electrogoniometry: how much knee motion is sufficient for normal daily life? *Gait Posture*. 2000;12:143-155.

32. Livingston LA, Stevenson JM, Olney SJ. Stairclimbing kinematics on stairs of differing dimensions. *Arch Phys Med Rehabil*. 1991;72:398-402.

33. Laubenthal KN, Smidt GL, Kettelkamp DB. A quantitative analysis of knee motion during activities of daily living. *Phys Ther*. 1972;52:34-42.

34. Pink M, Perry J, Houglum PA, Devine DJ. Lower extremity range of motion in the recreational sport runner. *Am J Sports Med*. 1994;22:541-549.

35. Hemmerich A, Brown H, Smith S, Marthandam SSK, Wyss UP. Hip, knee, and ankle kinematics of high range of motion activities of daily living. *J Orthop Res*. 2006;24:770-781.

36. Kapoor A, Mishra SK, Kewangan SK, Mody BS. Range of movements of lower limb joints in cross-legged sitting posture. *J Arthroplasty*. 2008;23:451-453.

37. Zhou H, Wang D, Liu T, Zeng X, Wang C. Kinematics of hip, knee, ankle of the young and elderly Chinese people during kneeling activity. *J Zhejiang Univ Sci B*. 2012;13(10):831-838.

38. Mann RA, Hagy JL. The popliteus muscle. *J Bone Joint Surg Am*. 1977;59:924-927.

39. Kettelkamp DB, Johnson RJ, Smidt GL, Chao EYS, Walker M. An electrogoniometric study of knee motion in normal gait. *J Bone Joint Surg Am*. 1970;52:775-790.

EXERCISES AND QUESTIONS

See the Answer Guide in Appendix E for suggested answers to the following exercises and questions.

1. PALPATION

A. Identify the anatomical reference points a therapist would use to align the universal goniometer axis and stationary and moveable arms when measuring the following ROM or muscle length at the knee.

   i.   Knee flexion–extension:

   Goniometer axis _____

   Stationary arm _____

   Moveable arm _____

   ii. Hamstrings or rectus femoris:

   Goniometer axis _____

   Stationary arm _____

   Moveable arm _____

   iii. Whether measuring knee flexion or extension ROM or muscle length at the knee for hamstrings or rectus femoris, the alignment of the goniometer is the same. True or false?

B. i.   Palpate the anatomical reference points used to align the goniometer when measuring knee flexion–extension ROM on a skeleton and on a partner.

   ii. Palpate the following anatomical structures on a skeleton and on a partner.

Borders of the patella	Tibial tuberosity
Ligamentum patellae	Head of the fibula

2. ASSESSMENT PROCESS

List the 10 main components of the assessment process performed by the therapist to assess the knee joint.

3. ASSESSMENT OF AROM AT THE KNEE ARTICULATIONS

A. Identify and describe the shape of the articular components that make up the femorotibial and patellofemoral articulations.

B. Demonstrate, define, and identify the axis and plane of movement for knee flexion and knee extension.

C. **Tibial Rotation**

   i.   The purpose of the following exercise is to demonstrate the presence of **active** internal and external rotation of the tibia.

   - Have a partner sit with the knees flexed 90° and the feet flat on the floor.
   - Using your index finger, palpate your partner's tibial tuberosity.
   - Instruct your partner to raise the right forefoot off the floor and move the toes inward toward the midline of the body while pivoting on the heel to position the tibia in full internal rotation.
   - Now instruct your partner to move the toes outward while pivoting on the heel to position the tibia in full external rotation.
   - Observe and feel the tibial tuberosity move externally under your index finger as this motion is performed.
   - From the position of full external rotation, have your partner internally rotate the tibia.
   - Observe and feel the tibial tuberosity move as your partner slowly repeats the tibial rotation ROM.

ii. The purpose of this exercise is to demonstrate the **automatic** external and internal rotation of the tibia, that occurs at the end of knee extension and at the beginning of knee flexion, respectively. This automatic rotation of the tibia is necessary for normal knee motion.

- Have your partner sit with the knee flexed 90° and the foot flat on the floor.
- Using your index finger, palpate your partner's tibial tuberosity.
- Instruct your partner to slowly extend the knee fully (to 0°). In a normal knee, you should observe and feel the tibial tuberosity move in a lateral direction (i.e., external rotation of the tibia) under your finger as the knee approaches full extension.
- Instruct your partner to move from the position of full extension to 90° flexion.
- Observe and feel the tibial tuberosity move in a medial direction (i.e., internal rotation of the tibia) under your finger at the beginning of the knee flexion motion.
- Have your partner repeat the above movements to observe and feel the tuberosity move under your finger.

4. ASSESSMENT AND MEASUREMENT OF PROM AT THE KNEE

For each of the movements listed below, demonstrate the assessment and measurement of PROM on a partner and answer the questions that follow. Record your findings on the ROM Recording Form on page 227 (i.e., record excessive, normal, or restricted tibial rotation and patellar mobility). Have a third partner evaluate your performance using the appropriate Practical Summary and Evaluation Forms in Appendix B.

Knee Flexion

i.   What normal end feel(s) would be expected when assessing knee flexion?
ii. What end feel for knee flexion did you identify on your partner?
iii. Identify the normal limiting factor(s) that result in a normal end feel for knee flexion.
iv. If knee flexion ROM is assessed with the patient in prone lying, what muscle(s) would be stretched at the hip that could restrict knee flexion ROM?

Knee Extension

i.   If knee extension ROM is assessed with the patient in sitting, what muscles could be stretched at the hip that could restrict knee extension ROM?
ii. If a patient presents with decreased knee extension PROM, what glide of the tibia would be decreased? Explain the reason for the glide being decreased in the direction indicated.

Tibial Rotation

i.   What normal end feels would be expected when assessing tibial internal rotation and tibial external rotation?
ii. What end feel for external tibial rotation did you identify on your partner?
iii. Identify the normal limiting factor(s) that create the normal end feels for tibial internal and external rotation.

Patellar Mobility

i.   Identify the patellar glides a therapist assesses to determine patellar mobility.
ii. What is the magnitude of the normal vertical displacement of the patella from full flexion to full extension of the knee?
iii. With the knee in extension, what is the normal PROM for medial and lateral movement of the patella?

ROM RECORDING FORM

Patient's Name _____   Age _____

Diagnosis _____   Date of Onset _____

Therapist Name _____   AROM or PROM _____

Therapist Signature _____   Measurement Instrument _____

Left Side					Right Side			
	*		*	Date of Measurement	*		*	
				Knee				
				Flexion (0–135°)				
				Tibial rotation				
				Patellar mobility – Distal glide				
				Patellar mobility – Medial-lateral glide				
				Hypermobility: Comments:				

5. MUSCLE LENGTH ASSESSMENT AND MEASUREMENT

For the hamstrings and the rectus femoris, demonstrate the assessment and measurement of muscle length on a partner. Have a third partner evaluate your performance using the appropriate Practical Summary and Evaluation Form in Appendix E.

Rectus Femoris
  i.   The therapist stabilizes the femur and the _____ for all tests used to evaluate rectus femoris length.
 ii.   Identify the means used to stabilize the pelvis when using the following start positions to assess rectus femoris muscle length:
    a.   Supine
    b.   Prone (two test positions)

6. FUNCTIONAL ROM AT THE KNEE

A. Have a partner perform or simulate the following functional activities. Use a universal goniometer to measure the maximum knee flexion ROM required to complete each activity.
  i.   Lifting a light object from the floor, bending the knees with the back straight
 ii.   Sitting in a chair
iii.   Tying a shoe: sitting and bringing the foot up from the floor
 iv.   Climbing stairs
  v.   Going down stairs

B. Walking requires a ROM from about _____° of knee extension as the leg advances forward to make _____ with the ground to a maximum of about _____° of knee flexion at _____ so that the foot _____ the ground as the extremity is advanced forward.

C. In general terms, tibial rotation occurs in ADL that require _____.

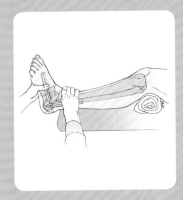

Ankle and Foot

8

ARTICULATIONS AND MOVEMENTS

Articulations of the ankle and foot are illustrated in Figure 8-1. The articulations at which range of motion (ROM) is commonly measured are the talocrural (ankle) joint, the subtalar joint, and the metatarsophalangeal (MTP) and interphalangeal (IP) joints of the great toe. The movements of these joints are described in Tables 8-1 and 8-2.

The ankle joint is classified as a hinge joint. The proximal concave articulating surface of the joint, commonly referred to as the ankle mortise, is formed by the medial aspect of the lateral malleolus, the distal tibia, and the lateral aspect of the medial malleolus. This concave surface is mated with the convex surface of the body of the talus. The primary movements at the ankle, dorsiflexion, and plantarflexion, occur around an oblique frontal axis in an oblique sagittal plane (Fig. 8-2). With the ankle in plantarflexion, the narrower posterior aspect of the body of the talus lies within the mortise and allows additional motion to occur at the joint. This movement is slight and includes side-to-side gliding, rotation, and abduction and adduction.[2]

The subtalar joint consists of two separate articulations between the talus and calcaneus that are separated by the tarsal canal. Posterior to the tarsal canal, the concave surface on the inferior aspect of the talus articulates with the convex posterior facet on the superior surface of the calcaneus. Anterior to the canal, the convex head of the talus articulates with the concave middle and anterior facets on the superior surface of the calcaneus. The subtalar joint axis runs posteroanteriorly, obliquely upward from the transverse plane and medial to the sagittal plane (Fig. 8-3). Owing to the obliqueness of the joint axis and the opposite shapes of the surfaces of the two

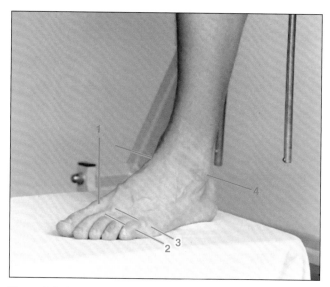

Figure 8-2 Ankle and foot axes: (*1*) metatarsophalangeal (MTP) joint abduction–adduction; (*2*) interphalangeal (IP) joint flexion–extension; (*3*) MTP joint flexion–extension; (*4*) talocrural joint dorsiflexion–plantarflexion.

joints (i.e., talar surfaces: posteriorly concave, anteriorly convex; calcaneal surfaces: posteriorly convex, anteriorly concave) that make up the subtalar joint, movement at the subtalar joint occurs in three planes and is identified as supination and pronation. In non–weight-bearing (NWB) conditions, when the subtalar joint is supinated, the calcaneus inverts in the frontal plane around a sagittal axis, adducts in the transverse plane around a vertical axis, and plantarflexes in the sagittal plane around a frontal axis.[5] Pronation includes calcaneal eversion, abduction, and dorsiflexion. In the clinical setting, it is not possible to directly measure triplanar subtalar ROM. "By convention, single-axis calcaneal inversion and eversion is considered representative of triplanar motion of the subtalar joint."[11 (p. 430)] Therefore, the more easily observed movements of inversion and eversion[5] are assessed and measured in the clinical setting to indicate subtalar joint ROM.

Movement at the transverse tarsal (i.e., talocalcaneo-navicular and calcaneocuboid articulations), intertarsal,

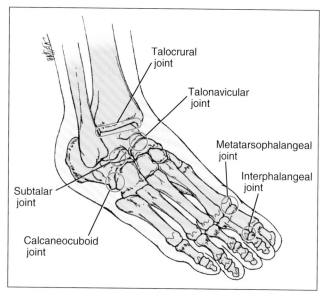

Figure 8-1 Ankle and foot articulations.

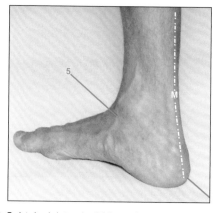

Figure 8-3 Subtalar joint axis: (*5*) inversion–eversion (*M*, midline of leg and heel).

TABLE 8-1 Joint Structure: Ankle and Foot Movements

	Plantarflexion	Dorsiflexion	Inversion	Eversion
Articulation[1,2]	Talocrural	Talocrural	Subtalar	Subtalar
Plane	Oblique sagittal	Oblique sagittal	Oblique frontal	Oblique frontal
Axis	Oblique frontal	Oblique frontal	Oblique sagittal	Oblique sagittal
Normal limiting factors[1-6,*] **(see Fig. 8-4A and B)**	Tension in the anterior joint capsule, anterior portion of the deltoid, anterior talofibular ligaments, and the ankle dorsiflexors; contact between the talus and the tibia	Tension in the posterior joint capsule, the deltoid, calcaneofibular and posterior talofibular ligaments, and the soleus; contact between the talus and the tibia	Tension in the lateral collateral ligament, ankle evertors, lateral talocalcaneal ligaments, cervical ligament, and the lateral joint capsule	Contact between the talus and calcaneus; tension in the medial joint capsule, medial collateral ligaments, medial talocalcaneal ligament, tibialis posterior, flexor hallucis longus, and flexor digitorum longus
Normal end feel[3,7]	Firm/hard	Firm/hard	Firm	Hard/firm
Normal AROM[8,†] **(AROM**[9]**)**	0°–50° (0°–40° to 50°)	0°–20° (0–15° to 20°)	0°–5°: forefoot 0°–35° (0°–30° to 35°)	0°–5°: forefoot 0°–15° (0°–20°)
Capsular pattern[7,10]	Talocrural joint: plantarflexion, dorsiflexion Subtalar joint: varus (i.e., inversion), valgus (i.e., eversion)			

*Note: There is a paucity of definitive research that identifies the normal limiting factors (NLFs) of joint motion. The NLFs and end feels listed here are based on knowledge of anatomy, clinical experience, and available references.
†AROM, active range of motion.

tarsometatarsal, and intermetatarsal joints (Fig. 8-1) is essential for normal ankle and foot function. These joints function to accommodate motions between the hindfoot and forefoot to either raise or flatten the arch of the foot, and thus enable the foot to conform to the supporting surface.

In the clinical setting, it is not possible to directly measure movements at these joints.

The MTP and IP joints of the toes make up the distal articulations of the foot (Fig. 8-1). The MTP joints are ellipsoidal joints,[2] each formed proximally by the

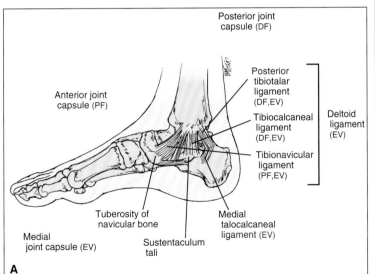
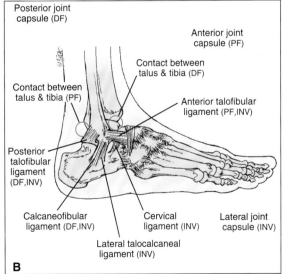

Figure 8-4 Normal Limiting Factors. A. Medial view of the ankle and foot showing noncontractile structures that normally limit motion at the ankle and subtalar joints. **B.** Lateral view of the ankle and foot showing noncontractile structures that normally limit motion at the ankle and subtalar joints. Motion limited by structures is identified in brackets, using the following abbreviations: *DF*, dorsiflexion; *PF*, plantarflexion; *INV*, inversion; *EV*, eversion. Muscles normally limiting motion are not illustrated.

TABLE 8-2 Joint Structure: Toe Movements

	Flexion	Extension	Abduction	Adduction
Articulation[1,2]	Metatarsophalangeal (MTP), proximal interphalangeal (PIP), distal interphalangeal (DIP) (second to fifth toes)	MTP PIP DIP	MTP	MTP
Plane	Sagittal	Sagittal	Transverse	Transverse
Axis	Frontal	Frontal	Vertical	Vertical
Normal limiting factors[3,4,6,*] (see Fig. 8-5)	MTP: tension in the dorsal joint capsule, extensor muscles, collateral ligaments PIP: soft tissue apposition between the plantar aspects of the phalanges; tension in the dorsal joint capsule, collateral ligaments DIP: tension in the dorsal joint capsule, collateral ligaments, and oblique retinacular ligaments	MTP: tension in the plantar joint capsule, plantar ligament, flexor muscles PIP: tension in the plantar joint capsule, plantar ligament DIP: tension in the plantar joint capsule, plantar ligament	MTP: tension in the medial joint capsule, collateral ligaments, adductor muscles, fascia and skin of the web spaces, and the plantar interosseous muscles	MTP: contact between the toes
Normal end feel[3,7]	MTP firm PIP soft/firm DIP firm	MTP firm PIP firm DIP firm	Firm	Soft
Normal AROM[8]	Great toe MTP 0°–45° IP 0°–90° Toes 2–5 MTP 0°–40° PIP 0°–35° DIP 0°–60°	Great toe MTP 0°–70° IP 0° Toes 2–5 MTP 0°–40° IP 0°		
Capsular pattern[7,10]	First MTP joint: extension, flexion Second to fifth MTP joints: variable, tend to fix in extension with the IP joints in flexion			

*Note: There is a paucity of definitive research that identifies the normal limiting factors (NLFs) of joint motion. The NLFs and end feels listed here are based on knowledge of anatomy, clinical experience, and available references.

convex head of the metatarsal articulating with the concave base of the adjacent proximal phalanx. The movements at the MTP articulations include flexion, extension, abduction, and adduction. Flexion and extension movements occur in the sagittal plane around a frontal axis, and the movements of abduction/adduction occur in the transverse plane around a vertical axis (Fig. 8-2). The IP joints are classified as hinge joints, formed by the convex head of the proximal phalanx articulating with the concave base of the adjacent distal phalanx. The IP joints allow flexion and extension movements of the toes.

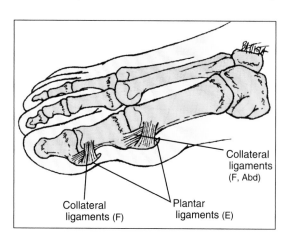

Collateral ligaments (F, Abd)

Collateral ligaments (F)

Plantar ligaments (E)

Figure 8-5 Normal Limiting Factors. Anteromedial view of the foot showing noncontractile structures that normally limit motion at the MTP and IP joints (medial collateral ligaments not shown). Motion limited by structures is identified in brackets, using the following abbreviations: F, flexion; E, extension; Abd, abduction. Muscles normally limiting motion are not illustrated.

ANATOMICAL LANDMARKS (FIGS. 8-6 THROUGH 8-8)

Anatomical landmarks are described and illustrated below. Anatomical landmarks numbered 1, 2, 4, 5, 8, 9, and 10 are used to assess ankle and foot ROM and/or to align the goniometer axis and arms, or position the OB goniometer to measure ROM at the ankle and foot.

Structure	Location
1. Head of the fibula	Round bony prominence on the lateral aspect of the leg level with the tibial tuberosity
2. Anterior border of the tibia	Subcutaneous bony ridge along the anterior aspect of the leg
3. Achilles tendon	Prominent ridge on the posterior aspect of the ankle; tendon edges are palpable proximal to the posterior aspect of the calcaneus
4. Medial malleolus	Prominent distal end of the tibia on the medial aspect of the ankle
5. Lateral malleolus	Prominent distal end of the fibula on the lateral aspect of the ankle
6. Tuberosity of the navicular bone	About 2.5 cm inferior and anterior to the medial malleolus
7. Base of the fifth metatarsal bone	Small bony prominence at the midpoint of the lateral border of the foot
8. Head of the first metatarsal	Round bony prominence at the medial aspect of the ball of the foot, at the base of the great toe
9. Calcaneus	Posterior aspect of the heel
10. Tibial tuberosity	Bony prominence at the proximal end of the anterior border of the tibia and the insertion of the ligamentum patellae (see anatomical landmark number 4 in Figs. 7-4 and 7-5)

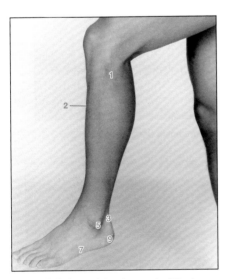

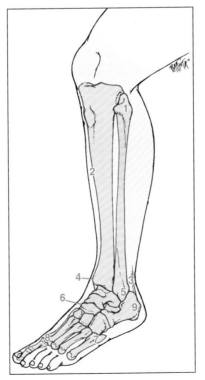

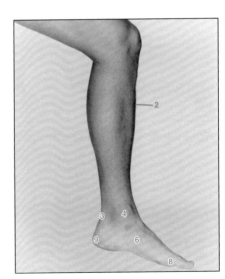

Figure 8-6 Anterolateral aspect of the leg and foot.

Figure 8-7 Bony anatomy, anterolateral aspect of the leg and foot.

Figure 8-8 Medial aspect of the leg and foot.

RANGE OF MOTION ASSESSMENT AND MEASUREMENT

Practice Makes Perfect

To aid you in practicing the skills covered in this section, or for a handy review, use the Summary & Evaluation Forms found at

http://thepoint.lww.com/ClarksonJM2e.

Ankle Dorsiflexion and Plantarflexion

AROM Assessment

Substitute Movement. *Dorsiflexion*—Knee extension, toe extension. *Plantarflexion*—Knee flexion, toe flexion.

PROM Assessment

Ankle Dorsiflexion

Start Position. The patient is supine. A roll is placed under the knee to position the knee in 20° to 30° flexion and place the gastrocnemius on slack (Fig. 8-9A). Research conducted by Baumbach and colleagues[12] supports positioning of the knee in at least 20° flexion to fully eliminate the restraining effect of the gastrocnemius muscle on ankle dorsiflexion ROM. The ankle is in the anatomical or neutral position with the foot perpendicular to the lower leg (see Fig. 8-9B).

Stabilization. The therapist stabilizes the tibia and fibula.

Therapist's Distal Hand Placement. The therapist grasps the posterior aspect of the calcaneus and places the forearm against the plantar aspect of the forefoot (Fig. 8-10).

End Position. The therapist applies traction to the calcaneus and using the forearm moves the dorsal aspect of the foot toward the anterior aspect of the lower leg to the limit of ankle dorsiflexion (Fig. 8-10).

End Feel. Dorsiflexion—firm/hard

Joint Glide. Dorsiflexion—convex body of the talus glides posteriorly on the fixed concave ankle mortise.

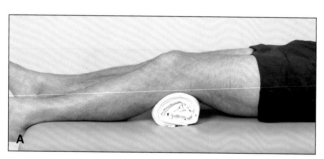
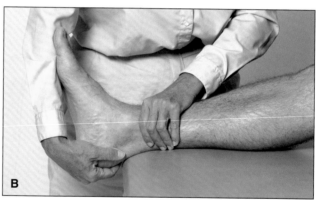

Figure 8-9 **A.** Position of knee in 20° to 30° flexion for assessment of ankle dorsiflexion. **B.** Start position: ankle dorsiflexion.

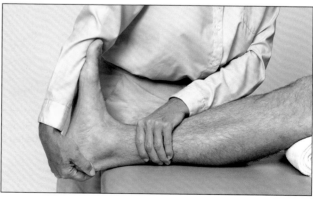

Figure 8-10 Firm or hard end feel at the limit of ankle dorsiflexion.

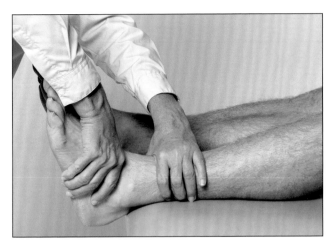

Figure 8-11 Start position for ankle plantarflexion.

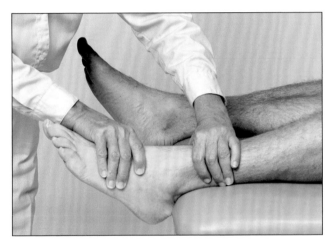

Figure 8-12 Firm or hard end feel at the limit of ankle plantarflexion.

Ankle Plantarflexion

Form 8-2

Start Position. The patient is supine. A roll is placed under the knee to maintain 20° to 30° knee flexion, and the ankle is in the neutral position (Fig. 8-11).

Stabilization. The therapist stabilizes the tibia and fibula.

Therapist's Distal Hand Placement. The therapist grasps the dorsum of the foot with the radial border of the index finger over the anterior aspects of the talus and calcaneus.

End Position. The therapist moves the talus and calcaneus in a downward direction to the limit of ankle plantarflexion (Fig. 8-12).

End Feel. Plantarflexion—firm/hard

Joint Glide. Plantarflexion—convex body of the talus glides anteriorly on the fixed concave ankle mortise.

Measurement: Universal Goniometer

Ankle Dorsiflexion and Plantarflexion

Start Position. The patient is supine with a roll placed under the knee to maintain 20° to 30° knee flexion and place the gastrocnemius on slack (see Fig. 8-9A). The ankle is in the anatomical position 0° (Fig. 8-13). Alternatively, the patient may be sitting with the knee flexed to 90° and the ankle in anatomical position (Fig. 8-14).

Stabilization. The therapist stabilizes the tibia and fibula.

Goniometer Axis. The axis is placed inferior to the lateral malleolus (Fig. 8-15). This measurement may also be obtained by placing the axis inferior to the medial malleolus (not shown).

Stationary Arm. Parallel to the longitudinal axis of the fibula, pointing toward the head of the fibula.

Movable Arm. Parallel to the sole of the heel (see reference line Fig. 8-15), to eliminate forefoot movement from the measurement. In the start position described, the goniometer will indicate 90°. This is recorded as 0°. For example, if the goniometer reads 90° at the start position for ankle dorsiflexion and 80° at the end position, the ankle dorsiflexion PROM would be 10°.

End Positions. Dorsiflexion (20°) (Fig. 8-16): The ankle is flexed with the dorsal aspect of the foot approximating the anterior aspect of the lower leg. **Plantarflexion (50°)** (Fig. 8-17): The ankle is extended to the limit of motion.

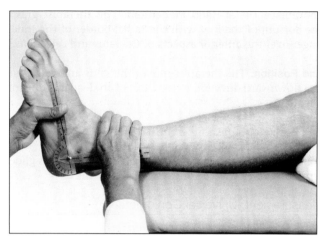

Figure 8-13 Start position for ankle dorsiflexion and plantarflexion.

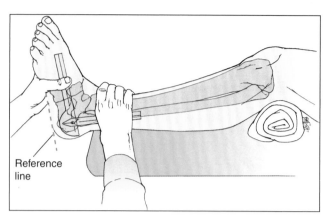

Reference line

Figure 8-15 Goniometer alignment for ankle dorsiflexion and plantarflexion.

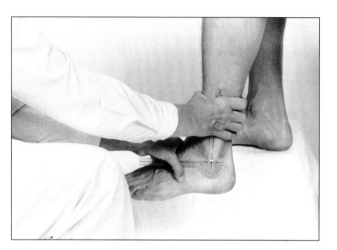

Figure 8-14 Alternate start position for ankle dorsiflexion and plantarflexion.

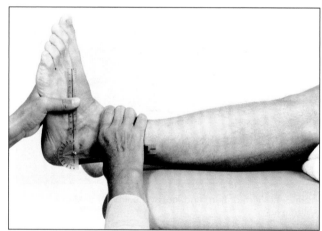

Figure 8-16 Dorsiflexion.

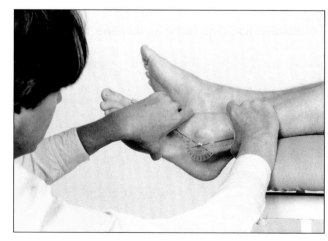

Figure 8-17 Plantarflexion.

Alternate Measurement

This test may be contraindicated for patients with poor standing balance or generalized or specific lower extremity weakness.

Measures of ankle dorsiflexion passive ROM (PROM) are significantly greater when assessed in weight-bearing (WB) than in non–weight-bearing (NWB) positions; therefore, these assessment techniques should not be used interchangeably.[13,14] When possible, ankle dorsiflexion PROM should be measured in standing to evaluate the patient's ability to perform activities of daily living (ADL) normally performed in WB.[13]

Start Position. The patient is standing erect (Fig. 8-18). The nontest foot is off the ground or only lightly touching the ground to assist with balance (Fig. 8-19).

Stabilization. The patient uses the parallel bars or other stable structure for balance. The foot on the test side is stabilized by the patient's body weight.

End Position. The patient is instructed to maintain the foot on the test side flat on the floor, with the toes pointing forward, and to flex the knee as far as possible (Fig. 8-19). *Note:* If the soleus muscle is shortened, the patient will feel a muscle stretch over the posterior aspect of the calf and ankle dorsiflexion ROM will be restricted proportional to the decrease in muscle length.

Measurement: Universal Goniometer

The therapist measures and records the available ankle dorsiflexion PROM. The goniometer is placed as described for measuring ankle dorsiflexion ROM (see Fig. 8-15). Ankle dorsiflexion PROM measured in weight-bearing (WB) is greater than in NWB positions. If dorsiflexion is measured in WB, this is noted when recording the ROM.

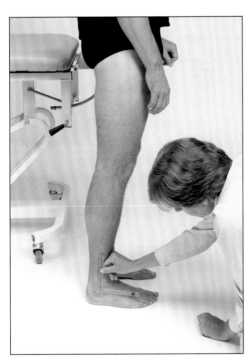

Figure 8-18 Alternate start position for ankle dorsiflexion.

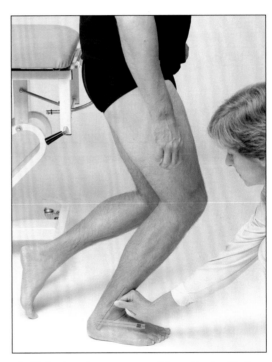

Figure 8-19 Goniometer measurement for ankle dorsiflexion.

Measurement: OB Goniometer

Goniometer Placement. The strap is placed around the lower leg proximal to the ankle. The dial is placed on the lateral aspect of the lower leg (Fig. 8-20). With the patient in the start position, the inclination needle is aligned with the 0° arrow of the fluid-filled container. At the end position, the number of degrees the inclination needle moves away from the 0° arrow on the inclinometer dial is recorded as the ankle dorsiflexion PROM (Fig. 8-21). (Alternatively, a standard inclinometer can be placed on the anterior border of the tibia to measure ankle dorsiflexion in standing [not shown].)

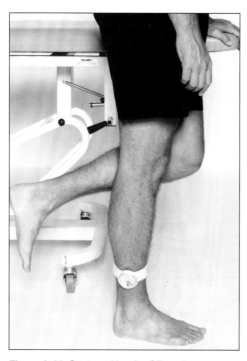

Figure 8-20 Start position for OB goniometer measurement of ankle dorsiflexion.

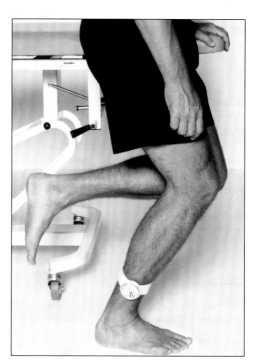

Figure 8-21 End position for ankle dorsiflexion.

Subtalar Inversion and Eversion

AROM Assessment

Substitute Movement. Inversion—hip external rotation. Eversion—hip internal rotation.

Measurement: Universal Goniometer

Form
8-3

Start Position. The patient is supine (Fig. 8-22). A roll is placed under the knee to maintain slight flexion. The ankle is in the neutral position. A piece of paper, adhered to a flat surface, is placed under the heel. A flat-surfaced object (plexiglass or book) is placed against the full sole of the foot. A line is drawn along the plexiglass or book as shown in Figure 8-22.

Stabilization. The therapist stabilizes the tibia and fibula.

End Positions. The foot is placed in inversion to the limit of motion (Fig. 8-23). The plexiglass is again positioned against the full sole of the foot in this position, and a line is again drawn along the plexiglass (Fig. 8-24). The process is repeated at the limit of eversion AROM (Figs. 8-25 and 8-26).

Goniometer Axis and Arms. The goniometer is placed on the line graphics to obtain a measure of the arc of movement (Figs. 8-27 and 8-28).

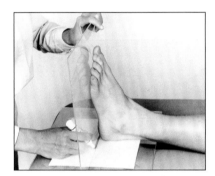

Figure 8-22 Start position for foot inversion and eversion AROM.

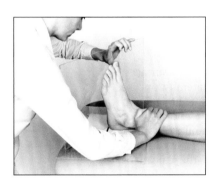

Figure 8-23 Placement of the foot in inversion.

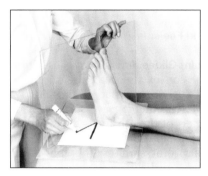

Figure 8-24 Inversion.

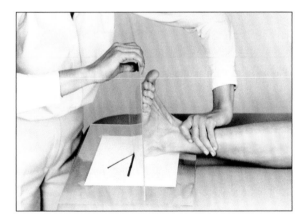

Figure 8-25 Placement of the foot in eversion.

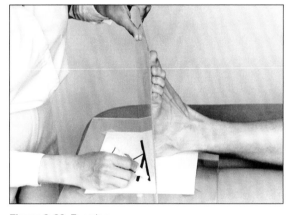

Figure 8-26 Eversion.

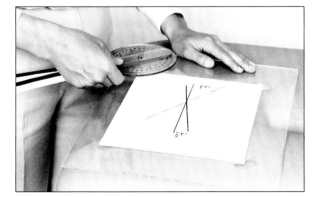

Figure 8-27 Completed measurements of inversion and eversion AROM.

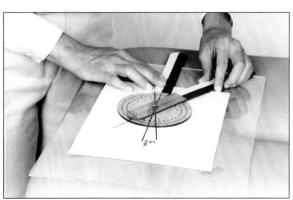

Figure 8-28 Goniometer placement for measurement of inversion AROM.

PROM Assessment

Start Position. The patient is supine. The ankle is in the neutral position (Fig. 8-29).

Forms 8-4, 8-5

Stabilization. The therapist stabilizes the talus immediately anterior and inferior to the medial and lateral malleoli. Current research[11] appears to support positioning the ankle in dorsiflexion to assist in stabilizing the talus, as the wider anterior aspect of the body of the talus is wedged within the mortise.

Therapist's Distal Hand Placement. The therapist grasps the posterior aspect and sides of the calcaneus.

End Positions. The therapist moves the calcaneus inward to the limit of inversion (Fig. 8-30) and outward to the limit of eversion (Fig. 8-31).

End Feels. *Inversion*—firm; *eversion*—hard/firm.

Joint Glides. *Inversion*—(1) posterior subtalar joint surfaces: the convex surface of the calcaneus glides laterally on the fixed concave surface of the talus; (2) anterior subtalar joint surfaces: the concave surfaces of the middle and anterior facets of the calcaneus glide medially on the fixed convex surface of the head of the talus. *Eversion*—(1) posterior subtalar joint surfaces: the convex surface of the calcaneus glides medially on the fixed concave surface of the talus; (2) anterior subtalar joint surfaces: the concave surfaces of the middle and anterior facets of the calcaneus glide laterally on the fixed convex surface of the head of the talus.

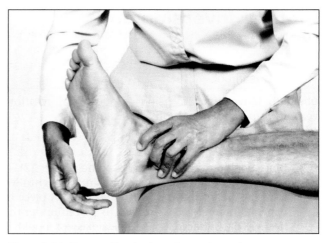

Figure 8-29 Start position for inversion and eversion.

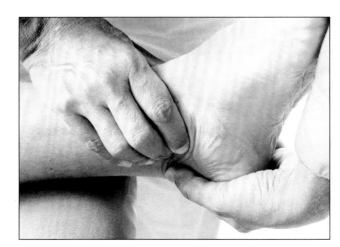

Figure 8-30 Firm end feel at the limit of inversion.

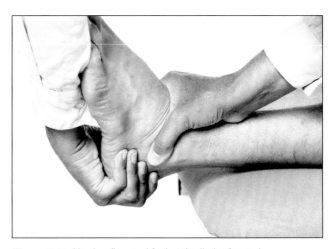

Figure 8-31 Hard or firm end feel at the limit of eversion.

Measurement: Universal Goniometer

Start Position. The patient lies prone with the feet off the end of the plinth and the ankle in the neutral position. For alignment of the goniometer, the therapist marks the skin over the midlines of the superior aspect of the calcaneus posteriorly and the inferior aspect of the heel pad posteriorly (Fig. 8-32A).

Stabilization. The therapist stabilizes the tibia and fibula.

Goniometer Axis. The axis is placed over the mark placed at the midline of the superior aspect of the calcaneus (Figs. 8-32B and 8-33).

Stationary Arm. Parallel to the longitudinal axis of the lower leg

Movable Arm. Lies along the midline of the posterior aspect of the calcaneus. Use the mark on the heel pad posteriorly to assist in maintaining alignment of the movable arm.

End Positions. The calcaneus is passively inverted (Fig. 8-34) and then passively everted (Fig. 8-35) to the limit of **inversion (5°)** and to the limit of **eversion (5°)**, respectively.

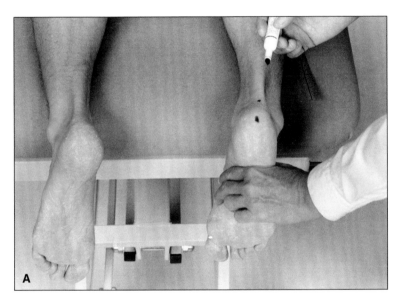
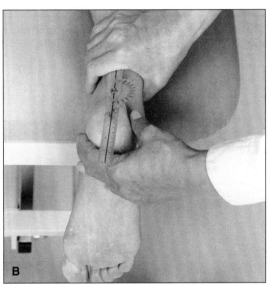

A   **B**

Figure 8-32 **A.** Subtalar inversion and eversion. Points marked for alignment of goniometer. **B.** Goniometer alignment for subtalar joint inversion and eversion.

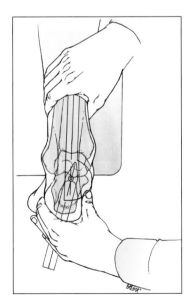

Figure 8-33 Goniometer placement for inversion and eversion. Shown with the subtalar joint in eversion.

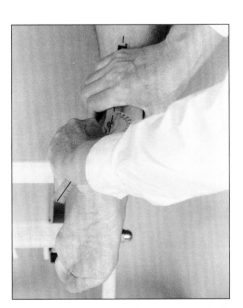

Figure 8-34 End position for measurement of right subtalar joint inversion.

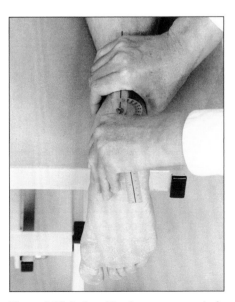

Figure 8-35 End position for measurement of right subtalar joint eversion.

CHAPTER 8

Ankle and Foot Supination/ Pronation: Inversion/Eversion Components

The inversion and eversion components of ankle and foot supination and pronation occur mainly at the subtalar and transverse tarsal (i.e., talocalcaneonavicular and calcaneo-cuboid) joints.

Ankle and Foot Supination: Inversion Component

AROM Assessment

Substitute Movement. Tibial internal rotation, knee flexion, hip external rotation, hip abduction.

PROM Assessment

Form
8-6

Start Position. The patient is sitting with the ankle and foot in anatomical position (Fig. 8-36).

Stabilization. The therapist stabilizes the tibia and fibula.

Therapist's Distal Hand Placement. The therapist grasps the lateral aspect of the forefoot.

End Position. The ankle and foot are inverted (Fig. 8-37).

End Feel. Ankle and foot are inverted—firm.

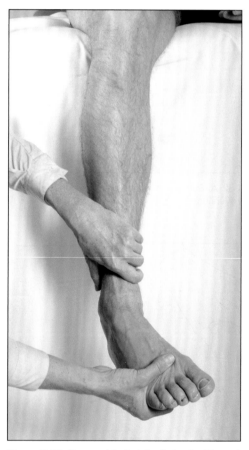

Figure 8-36 Start position: ankle and foot supination: inversion component.

Figure 8-37 Firm end feel at the limit of ankle and foot supination: inversion component.

Measurement: Universal Goniometer

Start Position. The patient is sitting with the ankle and foot in anatomical position.

Stabilization. The therapist stabilizes the tibia and fibula.

Goniometer Axis. The axis is placed anterior to the talocrural (ankle) joint midway between the medial and lateral malleoli (Fig. 8-38).

Stationary Arm. Parallel to the midline of the tibia, pointing toward the tibial tuberosity

Movable Arm. Parallel to the midline of the second metatarsal

End Position. Ankle and foot supination: inversion component (Fig. 8-39)

Ankle and Foot Pronation: Eversion Component

AROM Assessment

Substitute Movement. Tibial external rotation, knee extension, hip internal rotation, hip adduction

PROM Assessment

Form 8-7

Start Position. The patient is sitting with the ankle and foot in anatomical position (Fig. 8-40).

Stabilization. The therapist stabilizes the tibia and fibula.

Therapist's Distal Hand Placement. The therapist grasps the medial aspect of the forefoot.

End Position. The ankle and foot are everted (Fig. 8-41).

End Feel. Ankle and foot eversion—firm/hard.

Measurement: Universal Goniometer

Start Position. The patient is sitting with the ankle and foot in anatomical position.

Stabilization. The therapist stabilizes the tibia and fibula.

Goniometer Axis. The axis is placed anterior to the talocrural (ankle) joint midway between the medial and lateral malleoli (Fig. 8-42).

Stationary Arm. Parallel to the midline of the tibia, pointing toward the tibial tuberosity.

Movable Arm. Parallel to the midline of the second metatarsal.

End Position. Ankle and foot pronation: eversion component (Fig. 8-43).

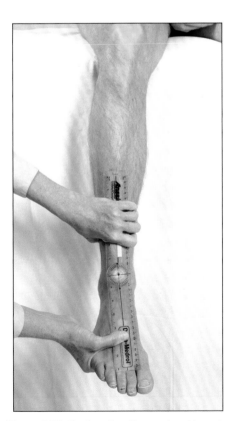

Figure 8-38 Goniometer alignment: ankle and foot supination: inversion component.

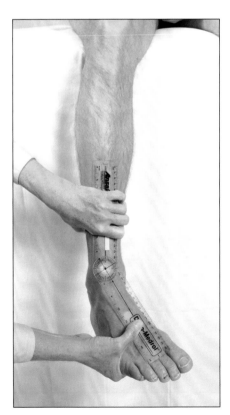

Figure 8-39 End position for measurement: ankle and foot supination: inversion component.

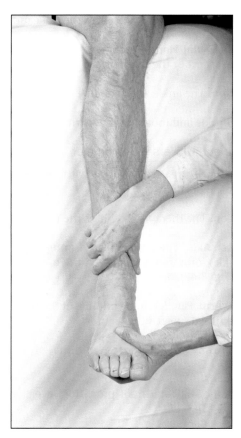

Figure 8-40 Start position: ankle and foot pronation: eversion component.

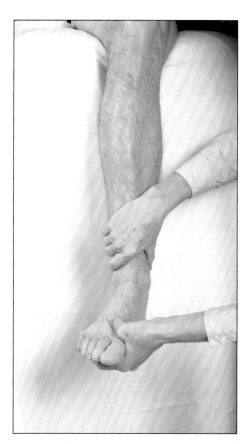

Figure 8-41 Firm or hard end feel at the limit of ankle and foot pronation: eversion component.

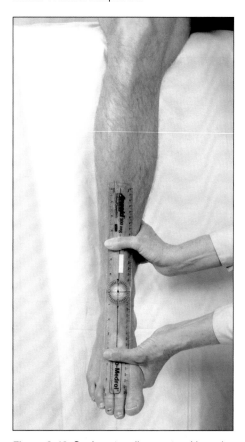

Figure 8-42 Goniometer alignment: ankle and foot pronation: eversion component.

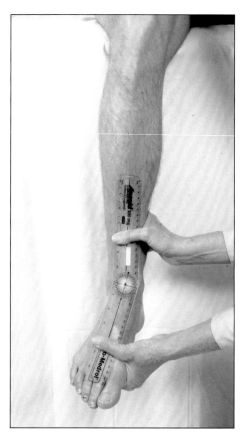

Figure 8-43 End position for measurement: ankle and foot pronation: eversion component.

MTP Joint Flexion and Extension of the Great Toe

AROM Assessment

Substitute Movement. *MTP flexion:* Ankle plantarflexion. *MTP extension:* Ankle dorsiflexion

PROM Assessment

Forms
8-8, 8-9

Start Position. The patient is supine. The ankle and toes are in the neutral position (Fig. 8-44).

Stabilization. The therapist stabilizes the first metatarsal.

Therapist's Distal Hand Placement. The therapist grasps the proximal phalanx.

End Positions. The therapist moves the proximal phalanx of the great toe to the limit of MTP joint flexion (Fig. 8-45) and MTP joint extension (Fig. 8-46).

End Feels. *MTP joint flexion*—firm; *MTP joint extension*—firm.

Joint Glides. *MTP joint flexion*—the concave base of the proximal phalanx glides in a plantar direction on the fixed convex head of the adjacent metatarsal. *MTP joint extension*—the concave base of the proximal phalanx glides in a dorsal direction on the fixed convex head of the adjacent metatarsal.

Measurement: Universal Goniometer

Start Position. The patient is supine or sitting. The ankle and toes are in the neutral position (Fig. 8-47).

Stabilization. The therapist stabilizes the first metatarsal.

Goniometer Axis. For MTP joint flexion, the axis is placed over the dorsum of the MTP joint (Fig. 8-47). For MTP joint extension, the goniometer axis is placed over the plantar aspect of the MTP joint (not shown). Alternatively, the axis can be placed over the MTP joint axis on the medial aspect of the great toe (Figs. 8-49 and 8-50).

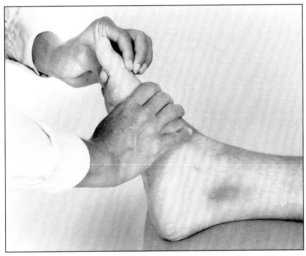

Figure 8-44 Start position for MTP joint flexion and extension.

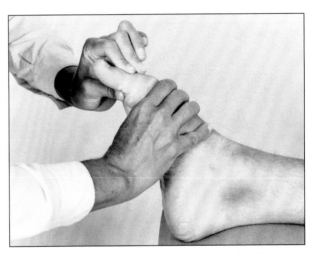

Figure 8-45 Firm end feel at the limit of MTP joint flexion of the great toe.

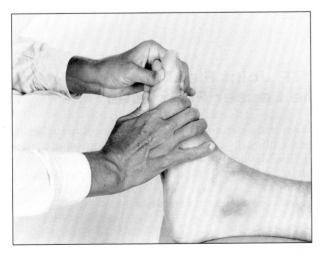

Figure 8-46 Firm end feel at the limit of MTP joint extension of the great toe.

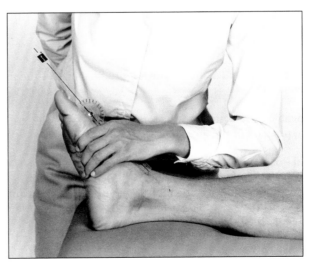

Figure 8-47 Start position for MTP joint flexion.

CHAPTER 8

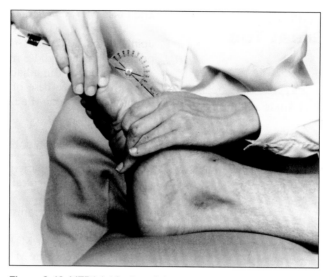

Figure 8-48 MTP joint flexion of the great toe.

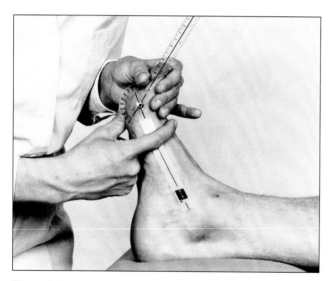

Figure 8-49 MTP joint extension of the great toe.

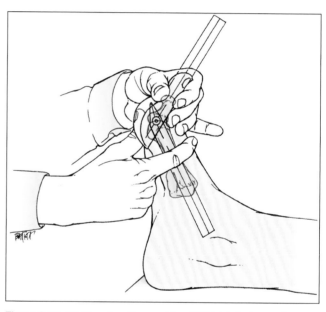

Figure 8-50 Goniometer alignment for MTP joint flexion and extension.

Stationary Arm. Parallel to the longitudinal axis of the first metatarsal

Movable Arm. Parallel to the longitudinal axis of the proximal phalanx of the great toe.

End Positions. The MTP joint is flexed to the limit of **MTP joint flexion (45° for the great toe)** (Fig. 8-48). The MTP joint of the toe being measured is extended to the limit of **MTP joint extension (70° for the great toe)** (Figs. 8-49 and 8-50).

MTP Joint Flexion/Extension of the Lesser Four Toes

Flexion and extension at the MTP joints of the lesser four toes are normally not measured using a universal goniometer. The MTP joints of the lesser four toes are flexed to the limit of **MTP joint flexion (40°)** and extended to the limit of **MTP joint extension (40°)**. The ROM is observed and recorded as either full or decreased.

MTP Joint Abduction and Adduction of the Great Toe

PROM Assessment (MTP Joint Abduction)

Forms
8-10, 8-11

Start Position. The patient is supine. The ankle and great toe are in the neutral position.

Stabilization. The therapist stabilizes the first metatarsal.

Therapist's Distal Hand Placement. The therapist grasps the proximal phalanx of the great toe.

End Position. The therapist moves the proximal phalanx to the limit of MTP joint abduction (Fig. 8-51).

End Feel. MTP joint abduction—firm.

Joint Glide. MTP joint abduction—the concave base of the proximal phalanx glides laterally (relative to the midline of the foot that passes through the second toe) on the fixed convex head of the first metatarsal.

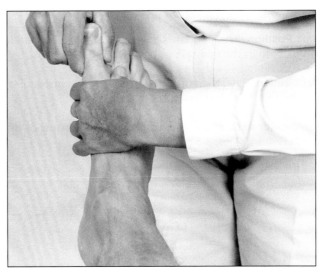

Figure 8-51 Firm end feel at the limit of MTP joint abduction.

Measurement: Universal Goniometer

Start Position. The patient is supine or sitting. The ankle and toes are in the neutral position (Fig. 8-52).

Stabilization. The therapist stabilizes the first metatarsal and the foot proximal to the MTP joint.

Goniometer Axis. The axis is placed on the dorsum of the first MTP joint (Figs. 8-52 and 8-53).

Stationary Arm. Parallel to the longitudinal axis of the first metatarsal

Movable Arm. Parallel to the longitudinal axis of the proximal phalanx of the great toe

End Positions. The MTP joint is abducted to the limit of motion (Fig. 8-54) and adducted to the limit of motion (Fig. 8-55).

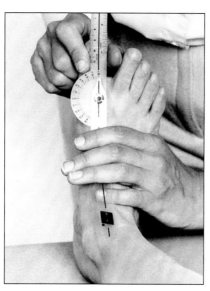

Figure 8-52 Start position for MTP joint abduction and adduction.

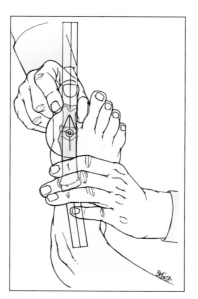

Figure 8-53 Start position and goniometer alignment for MTP joint abduction and adduction.

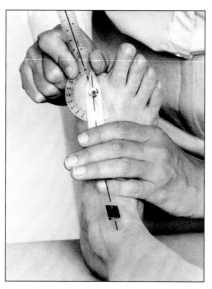

Figure 8-54 MTP joint abduction.

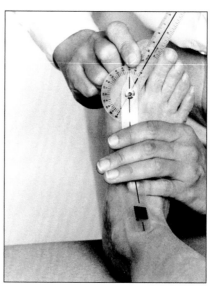

Figure 8-55 MTP joint adduction.

IP Joint Flexion/Extension of the Great Toe

AROM Assessment

Substitute Movement. *IP joint flexion:* MTP joint flexion, ankle plantarflexion; *IP joint extension:* MTP joint extension, ankle dorsiflexion

PROM Assessment

Forms
8-12, 8-13

Start Position. The patient is supine. The ankle and great toe are in the neutral position.

Stabilization. The therapist stabilizes the proximal phalanx of the great toe.

Therapist's Distal Hand Placement. The therapist grasps the distal phalanx of the great toe.

End Positions. The therapist moves the distal phalanx to the limit of IP joint flexion (Fig. 8-56) and IP joint extension (Fig. 8-57).

End Feels. *IP joint flexion*—soft/firm; *IP joint extension*—firm.

Joint Glides. *IP joint flexion*—the concave base of the distal phalanx of the great toe glides in a plantar direction on the fixed convex head of the proximal phalanx of the great toe. *IP joint extension*—the concave base of the distal phalanx of the great toe glides in a dorsal direction on the fixed convex head of the proximal phalanx of the great toe.

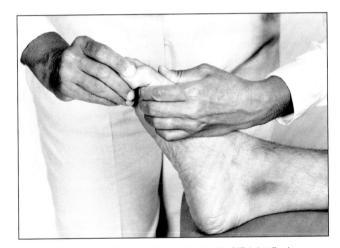

Figure 8-56 Soft or firm end feel at the limit of IP joint flexion.

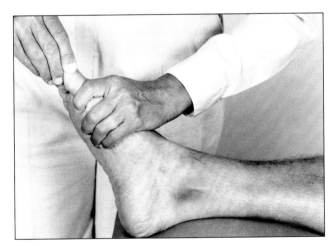

Figure 8-57 Firm end feel at the limit of IP joint extension.

CHAPTER 8

Measurement: Universal Goniometer

Start Position. The patient is supine or sitting. The ankle and toes are in the neutral position (Fig. 8-58).

Stabilization. The therapist stabilizes the proximal phalanx.

Goniometer Axis. The axis is placed over the dorsal aspect of the IP joint for flexion (Fig. 8-58) and the plantar aspect of the IP joint for extension (not shown).

Stationary Arm. Parallel to the longitudinal axis of the proximal phalanx

Movable Arm. Parallel to the longitudinal axis of the distal phalanx

End Positions. The IP joint is flexed to the limit of **IP joint flexion (90° for the great toe)** (Fig. 8-59). The IP joint is extended to the limit of **IP joint extension (0° for the great toe)** (not shown).

MTP and IP Joint Flexion/Extension of the Lesser Four Toes

The lesser four toes are flexed and extended as a group, and the ROM is observed and recorded as either full or decreased.

Flexion and extension at the MTP and IP joints of the lesser four toes are normally not measured using a universal goniometer. However, if used, the goniometer is placed according to the same principles used for measuring finger MTP and IP joint flexion and extension ROM.

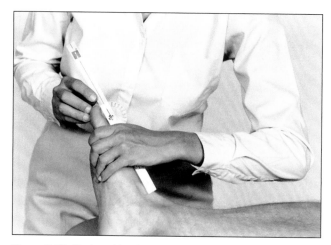

Figure 8-58 Start position for great toe IP joint flexion.

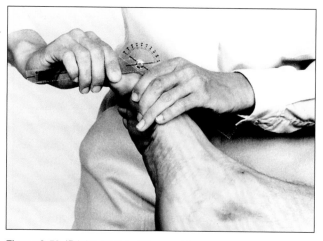

Figure 8-59 IP joint flexion of the great toe.

MUSCLE LENGTH ASSESSMENT AND MEASUREMENT

 Practice Makes Perfect

To aid you in practicing the skills covered in this section, or for a handy review, use the Summary & Evaluation Forms found at

http://thepoint.lww.com/ClarksonJM2e.

Gastrocnemius

Origins[2]	Insertion[2]
Gastrocnemius	
a. Medial head: proximal and posterior aspect of the medial condyle of the femur posterior to the adductor tubercle.	Via the Achilles tendon into the calcaneus.
b. Lateral head: lateral and posterior aspect of the lateral condyle of the femur; lower part of the supracondylar line.	

Start Position. The patient is standing erect with the lower extremity in the anatomical position. The patient is positioned facing a stable plinth or wall.

Form 8-14

End Position. The patient places the nontest leg ahead of the test leg and leans forward to place the hands on the plinth or wall (Fig. 8-60). The patient is instructed to maintain the foot on the test side flat on the floor, with the toes pointing forward, and to keep the knee in full extension as the leg moves over the foot. As the patient leans closer toward the supporting surface, the leg moves over the foot to the limit of ankle dorsiflexion and the gastrocnemius is placed on full stretch. Research[15] supports the use of ankle dorsiflexion PROM as an indicator of Achilles tendon length.

Measurement: Universal Goniometer

If the gastrocnemius is shortened, ankle dorsiflexion ROM will be restricted proportional to the decrease in muscle length. The therapist measures and records the available ankle dorsiflexion PROM.

Universal Goniometer Placement. The goniometer is placed as described for measuring ankle dorsiflexion ROM (Figs. 8-61 and 8-62).

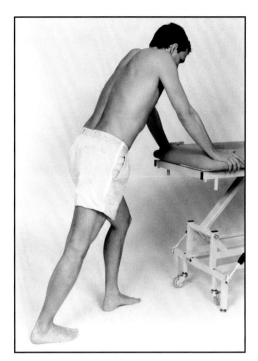

Figure 8-60 End position for measurement of the length of gastrocnemius.

Measurement: OB Goniometer

The strap is placed around the lower leg proximal to the ankle (Fig. 8-63). The dial is placed on the lateral aspect of the lower leg. With the patient in the start position, the inclination needle is aligned with the 0° arrow of the fluid-filled container. At the end position, the number of degrees the inclination needle moves away from the 0° arrow on the inclinometer dial is recorded to represent the length of the gastrocnemius muscle.

Note: If the contralateral (i.e., nontest) leg is not placed ahead of the test leg, ensure the heel of the nontest leg is raised slightly off the floor. This position ensures a true test for gastrocnemius tightness on the test side because the amount of forward lean the patient achieves will not be limited by contralateral gastrocnemius tightness, if present.

Alternate Test

Start Position. The patient is supine. The leg is in the anatomical position with the knee in extension (0°) (Fig. 8-64).

Stabilization. The therapist stabilizes the lower leg.

End Position. The foot is moved to the limit of ankle dorsiflexion (Fig. 8-65).

Assessment and Measurement. If the gastrocnemius muscle is shortened, ankle dorsiflexion ROM will be restricted proportional to the decrease in muscle length. The therapist either observes the available PROM or uses a universal goniometer to measure and record the available ankle dorsiflexion PROM. A second therapist is required to measure the PROM when using a goniometer.

End Feel. Gastrocnemius on stretch—firm.

CHAPTER 8

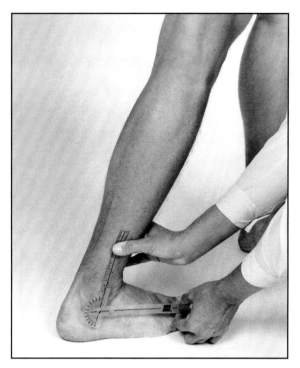

Figure 8-61 Goniometer measurement for length of gastrocnemius.

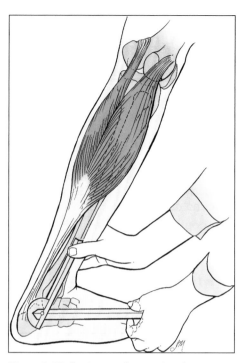

Figure 8-62 Gastrocnemius on stretch.

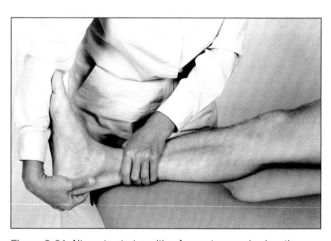

Figure 8-64 Alternate start position for gastrocnemius length.

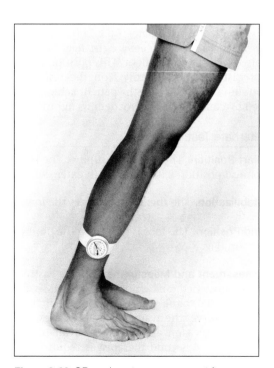

Figure 8-63 OB goniometer measurement for gastrocnemius muscle length.

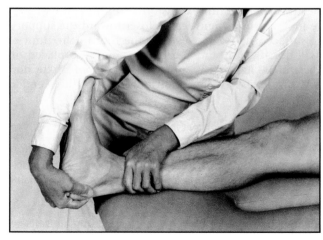

Figure 8-65 Gastrocnemius on stretch.

FUNCTIONAL APPLICATION

Joint Function

The foot functions as a flexible base to accommodate rough terrain[16] and functions as a rigid lever during terminal stance of the walking pattern.[5] In transmitting forces between the ground and the leg, the foot absorbs shock.[16] With the foot planted, the ankle and foot elevate the body, and when off the ground, the foot is used to manipulate machinery.[16] When weight is taken through the foot, the MTP joints allow movement of the rigid foot over the toes.[5]

Functional Range of Motion (Table 8-3)

Ankle Dorsiflexion and Plantarflexion

The normal AROM of the ankle joint is 20° dorsiflexion and 50° plantarflexion. However, ankle dorsiflexion ROM measured in WB (e.g., on stairs, when rising from sitting, squatting, and kneeling) is greater than in NWB positions.

The full range of ankle dorsiflexion is necessary to descend stairs (Fig. 8-66). Rising from sitting (Fig. 8-67) also requires significant ankle dorsiflexion ROM (i.e., an average of 28°[17]). Ankle dorsiflexion ROM is utilized by non-Western

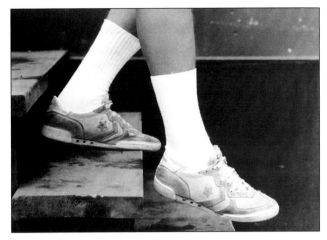

Figure 8-66 Full range of ankle dorsiflexion is required to descend stairs.

cultures accustomed to performing ADL such as kneeling and squatting.[21,23]

Full ankle plantarflexion may be required when climbing, jumping, or reaching high objects (Fig. 8-68). Less than the full range of ankle plantarflexion may be used to perform activities such as depressing the accelerator of a motor vehicle (Fig. 8-69) or the foot pedals of a piano, and wearing high-heeled shoes. Cross-legged sitting, a position essential in ADL used by Asian and Eastern cultures, requires less than full ankle plantarflexion ROM of about 26°[21] to 29°[22].

Livingston, Stevenson, and Olney[18] found that maximum ankle dorsiflexion ROM requirements to ascend and

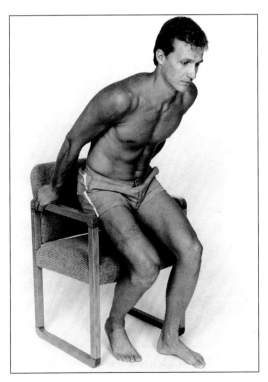

Figure 8-67 Ankle dorsiflexion is required to rise from sitting.

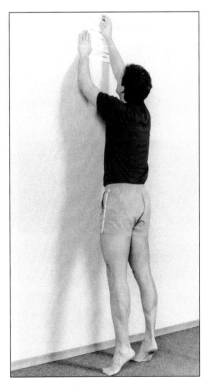

Figure 8-68 Toe extension, ankle plantarflexion, and contraction of the ankle plantarflexors.

TABLE 8-3 Ankle and Great Toe ROM Required for Selected ADL[5,17–23]

Activity	Ankle Dorsiflexion	Ankle Plantarflexion	Great Toe MTP Extension
Rising from sitting[17]*	28°		
Ascending stairs[18]†	14–27°	23°–30°	
Descending stairs[18]†	21°–36°	24°–31°	
Walking	10°[5]‡	20°[5]‡	90°[19]
Running[20]§	17°	32°	
Sitting cross-legged		26°[21]–29°[22]	
Kneeling with ankles dorsiflexed	37°[23]**–40°[21]		
Squatting with heels down	39°[21]		

*Average of young and elderly average values from original source.[17]
†Ankle dorsiflexion and plantarflexion ROM values for 15 subjects during ascent and descent of three stairs of different dimensions. Maximum ankle dorsiflexion and plantarflexion requirements varied depending on the stair dimensions and subject height.[18]
‡Data from the Rancho Los Amigos gait analysis forms as cited in the work of Levangie and Norkin[5].
§There were no differences in average ankle ROM at fast-paced (faster than a 7.5-minute mile) and slow-paced (slower than an 8-minute mile) running.[20]
**Average of young and old mean values from original source.[23]

descend stairs ranged between averages of 14° and 27° to ascend and 21° and 36° to descend stairs. The average maximum ankle plantarflexion ROM requirements ranged from 23° to 30° to ascend and 24° to 31° to descend stairs.[18]

Movements of the Foot

The AROM of the subtalar joint is 5° each for inversion and eversion without forefoot movement. The ranges of inversion and eversion may be augmented by forefoot movement of 35° and 15°, respectively. The subtalar, transverse tarsal joints, and joints of the forefoot must be fully mobile to allow the foot to accommodate to varying degrees of rough terrain (Fig. 8-70). With the foot across the opposite thigh, inversion is required to inspect the foot.

In standing, the MTP joints are in at least 25° extension due to the downward slope of the metatarsals.[2] Ranges approximating the full 90° of extension of the MTP joint of the great toe are required for many ADL.[19] Extension of the great toe and lesser four toes is essential for activities such as rising onto the toes to reach high objects (see Fig. 8-68) and squatting (Fig. 8-71). For most ADL, only a few degrees of flexion are required at the great toe.[19] There appears to be

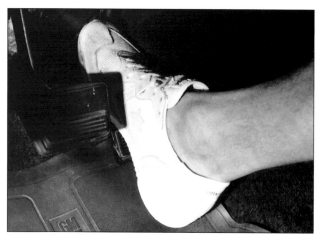

Figure 8-69 Ankle plantarflexion is used to depress the accelerator of a motor vehicle.

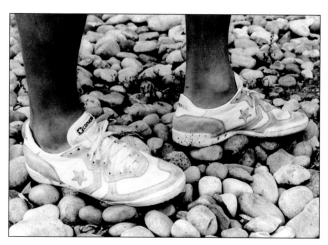

Figure 8-70 The mobile joints of the ankle and foot accommodate rough terrain.

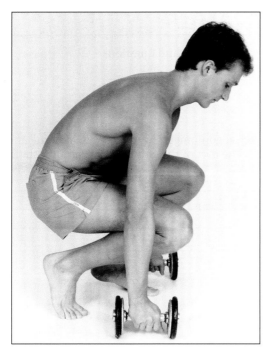

Figure 8-71 Extension of the toes is essential for squatting.

no significant function that can be attributed to abduction and adduction at the MTP joints.[5]

Gait

Normal walking (see Appendix D) requires a maximum of 10° of ankle dorsiflexion at midstance to terminal stance as the tibia advances over the fixed foot and a maximum of 20° of plantarflexion at the end of preswing (from the Rancho Los Amigos gait analysis forms as cited in the work of Levangie and Norkin[5]). At the MTP joint of the great toe, almost 90° of extension is required at preswing.[19] Extension of the lesser four toes is also required.[19] Extension of the toes stretches the plantar aponeurosis, resulting in significant longitudinal arch support.[24]

Running requires a range of ankle joint motion from an average of 17° dorsiflexion at midstance to an average 32° maximum ankle plantarflexion at early swing.[20] Ankle ROM was the same when fast-paced running was compared to slow-paced running.[20]

References

1. Kapandji IA. *The Physiology of the Joints. Vol. 2. The Lower Limb.* 6th ed. New York, NY: Churchill Livingstone Elsevier; 2011.
2. Soames RW. Skeletal system. Salmon S, ed. Muscle. In: *Gray's Anatomy.* 38th ed. New York, NY: Churchill Livingstone; 1995.
3. Norkin CC, White DJ. *Measurement of Joint Motion: A Guide to Goniometry.* 4th ed. Philadelphia, PA: FA Davis; 2009.
4. Daniels L, Worthingham C. *Muscle Testing: Techniques of Manual Examination.* 5th ed. Philadelphia, PA: WB Saunders; 1986.
5. Levangie PK, Norkin CC. *Joint Structure & Function: A Comprehensive Analysis.* 3rd ed. Philadelphia, PA: FA Davis; 2001.
6. Woodburne RT. *Essentials of Human Anatomy.* 5th ed. London, UK: Oxford University Press; 1973.
7. Magee DJ. *Orthopedic Physical Assessment.* 5th ed. St. Louis, MO: Saunders Elsevier; 2008.
8. American Academy of Orthopaedic Surgeons. *Joint Motion: Method of Measuring and Recording.* Chicago, IL: AAOS; 1965.
9. Berryman Reese N, Bandy WD. *Joint Range of Motion and Muscle Length Testing.* 2nd ed. St. Louis, MO: Saunders Elsevier; 2010.
10. Cyriax J. *Textbook of Orthopaedic Medicine. Vol. 1. Diagnosis of Soft Tissue Lesions.* 8th ed. London, UK: Bailliere Tindall; 1982.
11. Taylor Major KF, Bojescul Captain JA, Howard RS, Mizel MS, McHale KA. Measurement of isolated subtalar range of motion: a cadaver study. *Foot Ankle Int.* 2001;22:426-432.
12. Baumbach SF, Brumann M, Binder, J Mutschler W, Regauer M, Polzer H. The influence of knee position on ankle dorsiflexion—a biometric study. *BMC Musculoskelet Disord.* 2014;15:246-252.
13. Whitting JW, Steele JR, McGhee DE, Munro BJ: Passive dorsiflexion stiffness is poorly correlated with passive dorsiflexion range of motion. *J Sci Med Sport.* 2013;16:157-161.
14. Kang M, Oh J: Relationship between weightbearing ankle dorsiflexion passive range of motion and ankle kinematics during gait. *J Am Podiatr Med Assoc.* 2017;107(1):39-45.
15. Costa ML, Logan K, Heylings D, Donell ST, Tucker K. The effects of Achilles tendon lengthening on ankle dorsiflexion: a cadaver study. *Foot Ankle Int.* 2006;27(6):414-417.
16. Smith LK, Weiss EL, Lehmkuhl LD. *Brunnstrom's Clinical Kinesiology.* 5th ed. Philadelphia, PA: FA Davis; 1996.
17. Ikeda ER, Schenkman ML, Riley PO, Hodge WA. Influence of age on dynamics of rising from a chair. *Phys Ther.* 1991;71:473-481.
18. Livingston LA, Stevenson JM, Olney SJ. Stairclimbing kinematics on stairs of differing dimensions. *Arch Phys Med Rehabil.* 1991;72:398-402.
19. Sammarco GJ, Hockenbury RT. Biomechanics of the foot and ankle. In: Nordin M, Frankel VH eds. *Basic Biomechanics of the Musculoskeletal System.* 3rd ed. Philadelphia, PA: Lippincott Williams & Wilkins; 2001.
20. Pink M, Perry J, Houglum PA, Devine DJ. Lower extremity range of motion in the recreational sport runner. *Am J Sports Med.* 1994;22:541-549.
21. Hemmerich A, Brown H, Smith S, Marthandam SSK, Wyss UP. Hip, knee, and ankle kinematics of high range of motion activities of daily living. *J Orthop Res.* 2006;24:770-781.
22. Kapoor A, Mishra SK, Kewangan SK, Mody BS. Range of movements of lower limb joints in cross-legged sitting posture. *J Arthroplasty.* 2008;23:451-453.
23. Zhou H, Wang D, Liu T, Zeng X, Wang C. Kinematics of hip, knee, ankle of the young and elderly Chinese people during kneeling activity. *J Zhejiang Univ Sci B.* 2012;13(10):831-838.
24. Thordarson DB, Schmotzer H, Chon J, Peters J. Dynamic support of the human longitudinal arch. *Clin Orthop Relat Res.* 1995;316:165-172.

EXERCISES AND QUESTIONS

See the Answer Guide in Appendix E for suggested answers to the following exercises and questions.

1. PALPATION

A. When the following anatomical structures are used to align the universal goniometer to measure ROM at the ankle or foot: (a) identify the ROM that would be measured and (b) identify the part of the goniometer (i.e., axis, stationary arm, or moveable arm) aligned with the anatomical structure.

   i. Proximal phalanx of the great toe. _____

   ii. Mark placed at the midline of the posterior superior aspect of the calcaneus. _____

   iii. Head of the fibula. _____

B. On a skeleton and on a partner, palpate the following anatomical structures.

First MTP joint line	Tip of the lateral malleolus
Posterior surface of the calcaneus	Head of the first metatarsal
Head of the fibula	

2. ASSESSMENT PROCESS

Identify whether the following statements are true or false:

   i. AROM is assessed prior to assessing PROM at a joint.

   ii. End feels are determined when assessing PROM at a joint.

   iii. The presence or absence of pain is noted when assessing AROM and PROM at a joint.

   iv. The therapist always measures all PROM through goniometry when assessing a joint.

3. ASSESSMENT OF AROM AT THE ANKLE AND FOOT

For the ankle joint, subtalar joint, and IP joints:

   i. List the AROM a therapist would assess.

   ii. For each AROM listed in (i) above, identify the axis and plane of movement.

   iii. Assume the start position for the assessment and measurement of the AROM and demonstrate the full available AROM at the joint.

4. ASSESSMENT AND MEASUREMENT OF PROM AT THE ANKLE AND FOOT

For each of the movements listed below, demonstrate the assessment and measurement of PROM on a partner and answer the questions that follow. Have a third partner evaluate your performance using the appropriate Practice Makes Perfect Summary and Evaluation Form at http://thepoint.lww.com/ClarksonJM2e.
Record your findings on the ROM Recording Form on page 258.

Ankle Dorsiflexion

   i. What normal end feel(s) would be expected when assessing ankle dorsiflexion? Identify the end feel for ankle dorsiflexion on your partner.

   ii. What position is the knee placed in when assessing ankle dorsiflexion ROM? Explain why the knee is placed in this position.

   iii. Identify and describe the shape of the articular components that make up the ankle joint.

Ankle Plantarflexion

   i. Have your partner assume the start position for assessment of ankle dorsiflexion/plantarflexion. Have your partner perform full ankle dorsiflexion and plantarflexion, and observe the contour of the lateral border of the foot. What part of the lateral border of the foot is mobile and what part is immobile? Using the universal goniometer to measure ankle joint dorsiflexion/plantarflexion, to what part of the lateral border of the foot would the therapist align the moveable arm of the goniometer to avoid an erroneous measurement due to substitute motion?

    ii. Identify the direction of glide of the talus during ankle plantarflexion.

    iii. Identify the normal limiting factors that create the normal end feel(s) for ankle plantarflexion. What normal end feel(s) is/are produced by these normal limiting factors?

Subtalar Inversion

If a patient presented with decreased subtalar joint inversion PROM:

    i. Identify the glide of the posterior facet of the calcaneus that would be limited.

    ii. Identify the glide of the anterior and middle facets of the calcaneus that would be limited.

    iii. Explain the reason for the glides being decreased in the direction(s) indicated in (i) and (ii).

Great Toe MTP Joint Extension

    i. When assessing great toe MTP joint extension PROM, you note decreased PROM and a firm end feel. Would the firm end feel be considered a normal finding? Explain.

    ii. If a patient has decreased great toe MTP joint extension PROM, what glide of the base of the proximal phalanx of the great toe would be decreased? Explain the reason for the glide being decreased in the direction indicated.

    iii. Identify the pattern of movement restriction at the first MTP joint in the presence of a capsular pattern.

5. MUSCLE LENGTH ASSESSMENT AND MEASUREMENT

Gastrocnemius

    i. Identify the origin and insertion of the gastrocnemius muscle.

    ii. What movements of the lower extremity would move the origin and insertion of the gastrocnemius muscle farther apart and thus place the gastrocnemius muscle on stretch?

    iii. Demonstrate the assessment and measurement of gastrocnemius muscle length on a partner. Have a third partner evaluate your performance using the appropriate Practice Makes Perfect Summary and Evaluation Form at http://thepoint.lww.com/ClarksonJM2e.

    iv. If the gastrocnemius muscle is shortened, what end feel would the therapist note at the limit of ankle PROM when assessing gastrocnemius muscle length?

6. FUNCTIONAL ROM AT THE ANKLE AND FOOT

A. Normal walking requires a maximum of ____° ankle dorsiflexion at midstance to terminal stance as the tibia advances over the fixed foot and a maximum of ___° plantarflexion at the end of preswing.

B. For each movement listed below, identify three daily activities that require the specified movement, and demonstrate each activity:

    i. ankle dorsiflexion

    ii. ankle plantarflexion

    iii. toe extension

C. Have a partner perform the following activities and, using a universal goniometer, determine the maximum ankle dorsiflexion ROM required to perform each activity in a normal manner.

    i. Rise from sitting on a standard-height chair

    ii. Descend a standard-height step

ROM RECORDING FORM

Patient's Name _____   Age _____

Diagnosis _____   Date of Onset _____

Therapist Name _____   AROM or PROM _____

Therapist Signature _____   Measurement Instrument _____

Left Side   **Right Side**

	*		*	Date of Measurement	*		*	
				Ankle				
				Dorsiflexion (0–20°)				
				Plantarflexion (0–50°)				
				Inversion (0–35°)				
				Eversion (0–15°)				
				Hypermobility:				
				Comments:				
				Toes				
				MTP great toe flexion (0–45°)				
				extension (0–70°)				
				abduction				
				MTP digit 2 flexion (0–40°)				
				extension (0–40°)				
				MTP digit 3 flexion (0–40°)				
				extension (0–40°)				
				MTP digit 4 flexion (0–40°)				
				extension (0–40°)				
				MTP digit 5 flexion (0–40°)				
				extension (0–40°)				
				IP great toe flexion (0–90°)				
				PIP digit 2 flexion (0–35°)				
				PIP digit 3 flexion (0–35°)				
				PIP digit 4 flexion (0–35°)				
				PIP digit 5 flexion (0–35°)				
				Hypermobility:				
				Comments:				

Summary of Limitation:

Additional Comments:

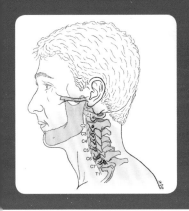

Head, Neck, and Trunk

9

(Continued)

QUICK FIND *(continued)*

ARTICULATIONS AND MOVEMENTS: HEAD AND NECK

The articulations and joint axes of the temporomandibular joint (TMJ) and cervical spine are illustrated in Figures 9-1 to 9-3. The joint structure and movements of the TMJ and cervical spine are described below and summarized in Tables 9-1 and 9-2.

The Temporomandibular Joints

The TMJs, located on each side of the head just anterior to the ears, are individually described as condylar joints and together form a bicondylar articulation,[2] being linked via the mandible (lower jaw). The TMJs are evaluated together as a functional unit. The articular surfaces of the TMJ are incongruent mates, but an articular disc positioned between these surfaces promotes congruency and divides the TMJ into upper and lower compartments (Fig. 9-4C).

The upper compartment of each TMJ is formed superiorly by the concave mandibular fossa and the convex temporal articular eminence that lies anterior to the fossa. These bony surfaces together form the superior TMJ surface and articulate with the reciprocally shaped superior surface of the articular disc, which is anteroposteriorly concavoconvex. The inferior surface of the articular disc is concave and mated with the convex condyle of the mandible to form the lower compartment of the TMJ.

Simultaneous movement of the TMJs produces depression (to open the mouth), elevation (to close the mouth), protrusion, retraction, or lateral deviation of the mandible. Elevation and depression of the mandible occur in the sagittal plane with movement around a frontal axis (Fig. 9-2). On mouth opening, a two-part sequence of motion occurs within the lower compartment of each TMJ. First, the mandibular condyle rotates, and glides forward and downward on the articular disc. Second, because of the posterior attachment of the disc to the mandibular condyle, both structures move together anteriorly.[2] This motion results in the anterior gliding of the articular disc over the temporal joint surfaces within the upper compartment.[2] These motions are reversed with mouth closing.

When the lower jaw is protracted and retracted, the articular disc of each TMJ moves with the mandibular condyle[2] as the mandible moves in the transverse plane anteriorly and posteriorly, respectively. Movement within the upper compartment of each TMJ occurs between the articular disc and the temporal bone.[14]

Lateral deviation of the mandible includes rotation of the mandibular condyle in the mandibular fossa on the side toward which the deviation occurs and a gliding forward of the contralateral mandibular condyle over the mandibular fossa and temporal articular eminence.[2]

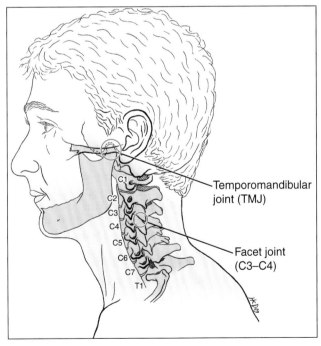

Figure 9-1 TMJ and cervical spine articulations.

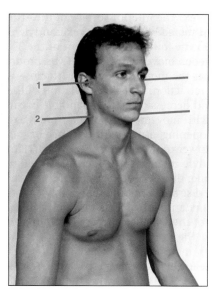

Figure 9-2 (*1*) TMJ axis: elevation–depression. (*2*) Cervical spine axis: flexion–extension.

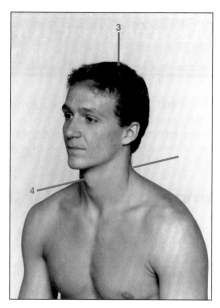

Figure 9-3 Cervical spine axes: (*3*) rotation; (*4*) lateral flexion.

The Neck: Cervical Spine

There are seven vertebrae that make up the cervical spine (Fig. 9-1). The third through seventh vertebrae (C3–C7) have a similar structure, and C1 and C2 each have a different structure.

The first cervical vertebra, also referred to as C1 or the atlas, articulates with the occiput of the skull via the atlanto-occipital joints (Figs. 9-1 and 9-5A). These joints are formed superiorly by the convex condyles of the occiput articulating with the concave superior articular facets of C1, which lie in the transverse plane and face superiorly and medially. The orientation of the facets determines the motion at the atlanto-occipital articulations. The main movements being flexion and extension, there is slight lateral flexion,[14] and no rotation.[15]

There are three atlantoaxial articulations between the atlas (C1) and the axis (C2) (Figs. 9-1 and 9-5). A pivot is formed[2] between the odontoid process (dens) of C2 as it articulates anteriorly with the concave posterior surface of the anterior arch of C1 and posteriorly with the cartilaginous posterior surface of the transverse ligament. The transverse ligament retains the odontoid process in place. There are two facet joints, one on each side between C1 and C2, which lie posterior to the transverse ligament in the transverse plane. Each of the inferior facets of C1 articulates with a superior facet of C2. The orientation of the facets results

in rotation being the primary motion at the atlantoaxial joints. Most of the rotation of the cervical spine occurs at the atlantoaxial joints.[15]

From C2 to C7, a vertebral segment consists of two vertebrae and the three articulations between these vertebrae. Anteriorly, the intervertebral disc is positioned between the adjacent vertebral bodies (Fig. 9-5B and C). Two facet joints are located posteriorly on each side of the vertebral segment. Each facet joint (Fig. 9-1) is formed by the inferior facet of the superior vertebra (oriented inferiorly and anteriorly) and the superior facet of the inferior vertebra (oriented superiorly and posteriorly). The surfaces of the facet joints lie at an angle of about 45° to the transverse plane. The orientation of the facets from C2 through C7 permits cervical spine flexion, extension, lateral flexion, and rotation.

When assessing cervical spine range of motion (ROM), the combined motions of the segments between the occiput and C7 are assessed and measured, since segmental motion cannot be measured clinically. Cervical spine movements include neck flexion and extension, which occur in the sagittal plane about a frontal axis (Fig. 9-2); lateral flexion, which occurs in the frontal plane around a sagittal axis (Fig. 9-3); and rotation, which occurs in the transverse plane around a vertical axis (Fig. 9-3). About 40% of cervical flexion and 60% of cervical rotation occur at the occiput/C1/C2 complex of the cervical spine.[16]

TABLE 9-1 Joint Structure: Jaw Movements

	Opening of the Mouth (Depression of the Mandible)	Closing of the Mouth (Occlusion)	Protrusion	Retrusion	Lateral Deviation
Articulation[1,2]	Temporomandibular (TM)	TM	TM	TM	TM
Plane	Sagittal	Sagittal	Horizontal	Horizontal	Horizontal
Axis	Frontal	Frontal			
Normal limiting factors[2,3]* (see Fig. 9-4)	Tension in the lateral/ temporomandibular ligament and the retrodiscal tissue	Occlusion or contact of the teeth	Tension in the lateral/ temporomandibular, sphenomandibular, and stylomandibular ligaments		Tension in the lateral/ temporomandibular ligament
Normal AROM† (ruler)	35–50 cm[4]	Contact of teeth	3–7 mm[5]	10–15 mm[4]	
Capsular pattern[4,6]	Limitation of mouth opening				

*There is a paucity of definitive research that identifies the normal limiting factors (NLF) of joint motion. The NLF and end feels listed here are based on knowledge of anatomy, clinical experience, and available references.

†AROM, active range of motion.

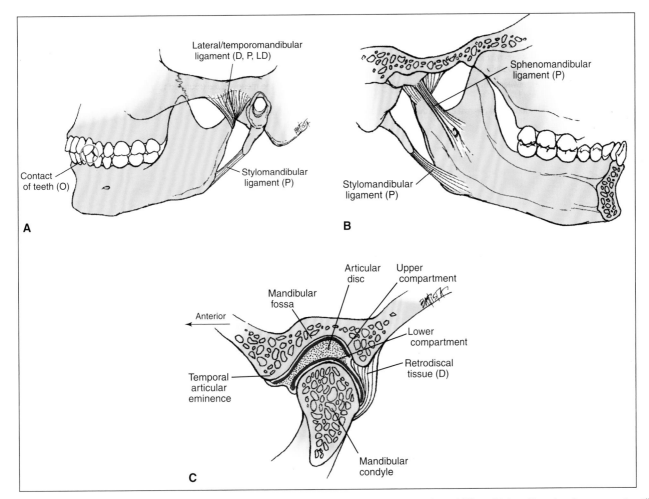

Figure 9-4 Normal Limiting Factors: TMJ. (A) Lateral view, **(B)** medial view (sagittal section), and **(C)** sagittal section showing noncontractile structures that normally limit motion. Motion limited by structures is identified in brackets, using the following abbreviations: *D*, depression of mandible; *O*, occlusion; *P*, protrusion; *LD*, lateral deviation.

CHAPTER 9

TABLE 9-2 Joint Structure: Cervical Spine Movements

	Flexion	Extension	Lateral Flexion	Rotation
Articulation[1,2]	Atlanto-occipital Atlantoaxial Intervertebral	Atlanto-occipital Atlantoaxial Intervertebral	Atlanto-occipital Intervertebral (with rotation)	Atlanto-occipital Atlantoaxial Intervertebral (with lateral flexion)
Plane	Sagittal	Sagittal	Frontal	Transverse
Axis	Frontal	Frontal	Sagittal	Vertical
Normal limiting factors[7,8*] (see Fig. 9-5)	Tension in the tectorial membrane, posterior atlantoaxial ligament, posterior longitudinal ligament, ligamentum nuchae, ligamentum flavum, posterior neck muscles, and posterior fibers of annulus; contact between anterior rim of foramen magnum of skull and dens (atlanto-occipital joint)	Tension in the anterior longitudinal ligament and anterior atlanto-axial neck muscles; anterior fibers of annulus; bony contact between the spinous processes	Tension in the alar ligament limits lateral flexion to the contralateral side; lateral fibers of annulus; uncinate processes	Tension in the alar ligament limits rotation to the ipsilateral side; tension in the annulus fibrosis
Normal AROM				
CROM[9†]	0°–45°	0°–65°	0°–35°	0°–60°
Tape Measure[10,11‡]	3 cm	20 cm	13 cm	11 cm
Inclinometer[12]	0°–50°	0°–60°	0°–45°	0°–80°
Universal Goniometer[13]	0°–45°	0°–45°	0°–45°	

*There is a paucity of definitive research that identifies the normal limiting factors (NLF) of joint motion. The NLF and end feels listed here are based on knowledge of anatomy, clinical experience, and available references.

†AROM for 337 healthy subjects between 11 and 97 years of age. Values represent the means of the mean values (rounded to the nearest 5°) from each age group as derived from the original source.[9]

‡Values represent the mean (rounded to the nearest cm) of the mean values derived from both studies.[10,11]

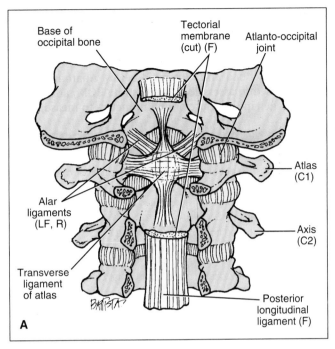

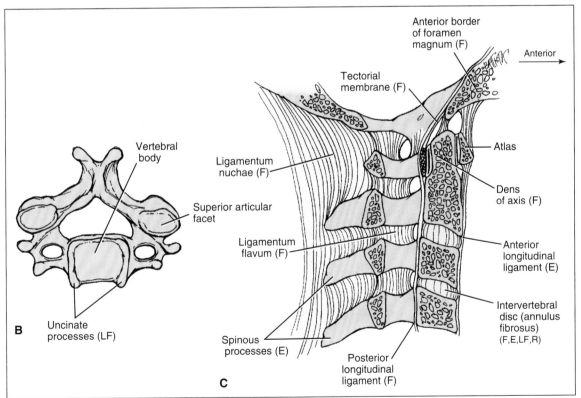

Figure 9-5 Normal Limiting Factors. (A) Posterior view (frontal section) of the occiput and upper cervical spine, **(B)** superior view of a cervical vertebra, and **(C)** sagittal section of the occiput and cervical spine (C1–C4) showing non-contractile structures that normally limit motion. Motion limited by structures is identified in brackets, using the following abbreviations: *F*, flexion; *E*, extension; *LF*, lateral flexion; *R*, rotation. Muscles normally limiting motion are not illustrated.

ANATOMICAL LANDMARKS: HEAD AND NECK (FIGS. 9-6 THROUGH 9-9)

Anatomical landmarks are described and illustrated below. Anatomical landmarks numbered 1, 7, and 8 through 13 are used to assess TMJ and C-spine ROM, and/or align the goniometer axis and arms, or position the tape measure or inclinometers to measure ROM at the C spine.

Structure	Location
1. Suprasternal (jugular) notch	The rounded depression at the superior border of the sternum and between the medial ends of each clavicle.
2. Thyroid cartilage	The most prominent laryngeal cartilage located at the level of the 4th and 5th cervical vertebrae; subcutaneous projection (Adam's apple).
3. Hyoid bone	A submandibular U-shaped bone located above the thyroid cartilage at the level of the 3rd cervical vertebra; the body is felt in the midline below the chin at the angle formed between the floor of the mouth and the front of the neck.
4. Angle of the mandible	The angle of the lower jaw located medially and distally to the earlobe.
5. Angle of the mouth	The lateral angle formed by the upper and lower lips.
6. Nasolabial fold	The fold of skin extending from the nose to the angle of the mouth.
7. Temporomandibular joint	The joint may be palpated anterior to the tragus of the external ear during opening and closing of the mouth.
8. Mastoid process	Bony prominence of the skull located behind the ear.
9. Acromion process	Lateral aspect of the spine of the scapula at the tip or point of the shoulder.
10. Spine of the scapula	The bony ridge running obliquely across the upper four-fifths of the scapula.
11. C7 spinous process	Often the most prominent spinous process at the base of the neck.
12. T1 spinous process	The next spinous process inferior to the C7 spinous process.
13. Lobule of the ear	The soft lowermost portion of the auricle of the ear.

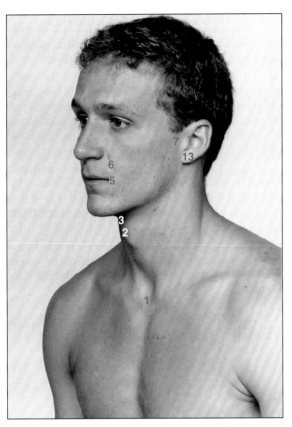

Figure 9-6 Anterolateral aspect of the head and neck.

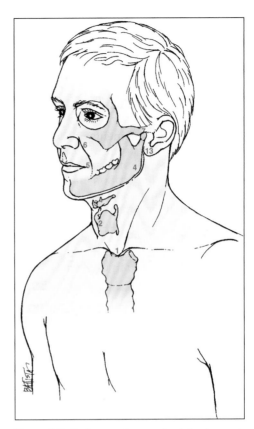

Figure 9-7 Surface anatomy, anterolateral aspect of the head and neck.

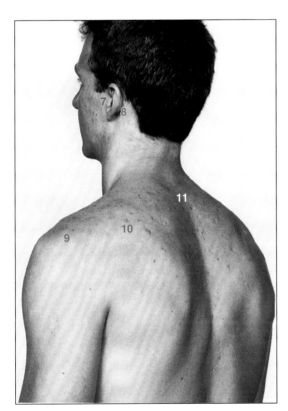

Figure 9-8 Posterolateral aspect of the head and neck.

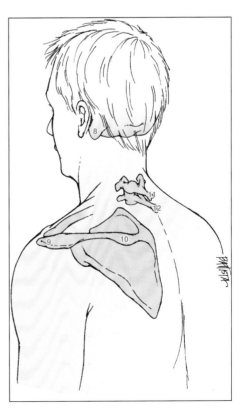

Figure 9-9 Bony anatomy, posterolateral aspect of the head and neck.

INSTRUMENTATION AND MEASUREMENT PROCEDURES: TMJ AND SPINE

Active ROM (AROM) measurements of the TMJs are made using a ruler or calipers. Instruments used to measure spinal AROM include the tape measure, standard inclinometer, the Cervical Range-of-Motion Instrument (CROM)[17] (Performance Attainment Associates, Roseville, MN), the Back Range-of-Motion Instrument (BROMII), and the universal goniometer. These instruments and the general principles for use of each instrument are described, with the exception of the universal goniometer and OB "Myrin" goniometer that are described in Chapter 1.

Tape Measure/Ruler/Calipers

A ruler or calipers are used to measure the AROM of the TMJs, and a tape measure is commonly used to measure AROM of the spine.

Measurement Procedure: Tape Measure/Ruler

A linear measurement of AROM is obtained using a tape measure and one of the following three methods:

Method 1 (Fig. 9-10): The patient moves to the end position for the motion being tested. Using a tape measure, the therapist measures the distance between two specified anatomical landmarks or a specified anatomical landmark and a stationary external surface, such as the plinth or floor to determine the ROM in centimeters.

Method 2 (Fig. 9-11): The distance between two specified vertebral levels is measured at the start position and at the end position for the ROM being measured. The difference between the two measures is the ROM in centimeters.

Method 3 (Fig. 9-12): The location of an anatomical landmark that moves with the test motion is marked on a stationary part of the body at the start and at the end of the ROM. The distance between the marks is the ROM for the movement.

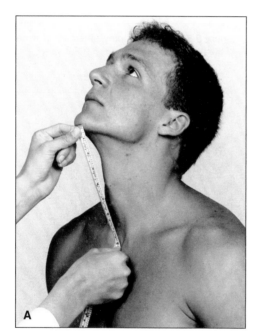

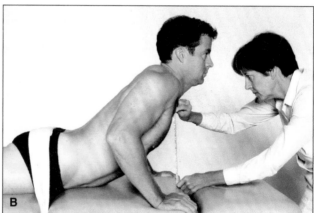

Figure 9-10 Tape measure method 1: the distance measured between **(A)** two anatomical landmarks, for example, neck extension AROM, or **(B)** an anatomical landmark and an external surface, for example, the plinth for thoracolumbar extension AROM.

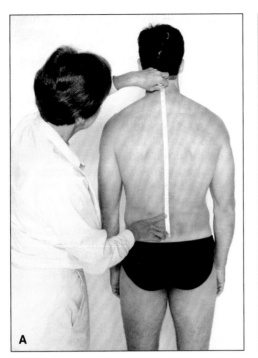
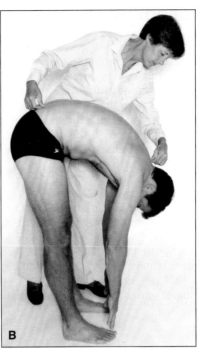

Figure 9-11 Tape measure method 2: for example, thoracolumbar flexion AROM—the difference between the distances measured between the two vertebral levels S2 and C7 at the **(A)** start position and **(B)** end position is the AROM for thoracolumbar flexion.

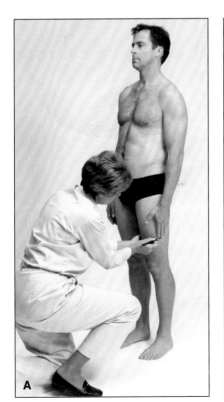
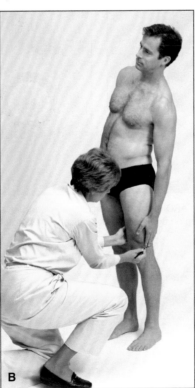
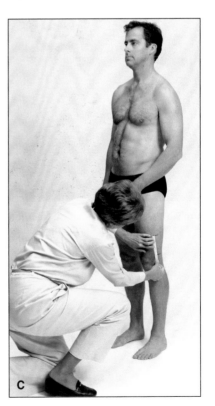

Figure 9-12 Tape measure method 3: for example, trunk lateral flexion AROM—the location of the tip of the third finger is marked on the thigh at the **(A)** start position, **(B)** end position, and **(C)** the distance between the marks is the AROM for trunk lateral flexion.

Standard Inclinometer

The standard inclinometer contains a gravity-dependent needle and a 360° protractor scale (Fig. 9-13). On some inclinometers, the protractor scale can be rotated so that the gravity inclination needle is zeroed at the start position for the measured motion. In this case, the final position of the inclination needle relative to the protractor scale provides the ROM or joint position in degrees. If the needle cannot be zeroed, the ROM will be recorded as the difference in degrees between the readings on the inclinometer at the start and end positions for the assessed motion.

The therapist normally holds the standard inclinometer in place over an anatomical landmark. The surface of the inclinometer placed in contact with the patient may consist of a fixed flat surface, fixed feet, or adjustable feet. Adjustable feet (see Fig. 1-30) facilitate placement of the inclinometer over curved body surfaces. The American Medical Association (AMA)[12] has advocated using the inclinometer to evaluate spinal ROM when evaluating permanent impairment of the spine. One or two standard inclinometers may be used to assess ROM.

Measurement Procedure: Standard Inclinometer

Single Inclinometry (Fig. 9-13). One inclinometer is normally used to assess the AROM when either the proximal or distal joint body segment is stabilized. With the patient in the start position, the inclinometer is positioned in relation to a specified anatomical landmark, normally located on the distal end of the moving joint segment. If possible, the protractor of the inclinometer is adjusted to 0° in the start position, or the reading on the inclinometer is noted. The patient is instructed to move through the AROM. At the end of the movement, the therapist reads the inclinometer. If the inclinometer was zeroed in the start position, the reading is the ROM in degrees. If the inclinometer was not zeroed at the start position, the difference between the reading on the inclinometer at the start and the end positions is recorded as the ROM.

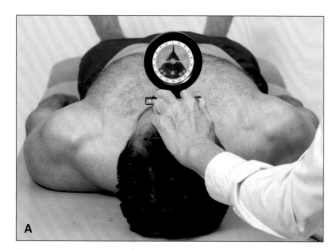
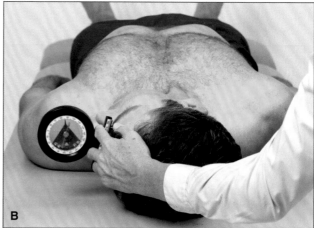

Figure 9-13 Single inclinometry. **A.** Neck rotation AROM start position: supine with trunk stabilized, single inclinometer aligned on forehead with dial zeroed. **B.** End position: reading on the inclinometer indicates neck rotation AROM.

Double Inclinometry (Fig. 9-14). When two standard inclinometers are used to assess AROM, the patient is in the start position with one inclinometer placed at a specified anatomical landmark at the inferior end of the spinal segments being measured. A second inclinometer is placed at a specified anatomical landmark at the superior end of the spinal segments being measured. The protractor of each inclinometer is either

i. adjusted to 0° in the start position by a second therapist, or

ii. the readings on the inclinometers are noted at the start position

The patient is instructed to move through the AROM.

At the end of the movement, the therapist reads each inclinometer.

If the inclinometers were zeroed in the start position, the difference between the two readings on the inclinometers at the end position is the AROM for the spinal movement being assessed.

If the inclinometers were not zeroed in the start position, the difference between the readings at the start and at the end position on each inclinometer provides the ROM at each inclinometer location. The difference between the ROM at each inclinometer location is recorded as the ROM for the assessed movement.

When measuring ROM, the therapist ensures that sources of error (described in Chapter 1) do not occur or are minimized, so that ROM measurements will be reliable and the patient's progress can be meaningfully monitored. Note that Mayer and colleagues[18] studied the sources of error with inclinometric measurement of spinal ROM and found that "training and practice was the most significant factor (eliminating the largest source of error) improving overall test performance"[18 (p. 1981)].

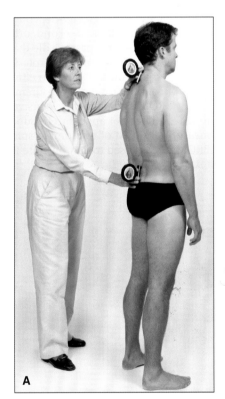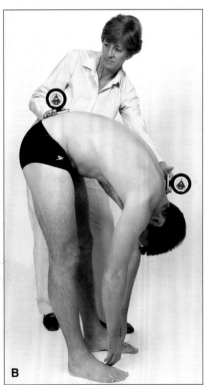

Figure 9-14 Double inclinometry. **A.** Thoracolumbar spine flexion AROM start position with inclinometers placed over S2 and C7 and zeroed. **B.** End position: the difference between the two inclinometer readings is the thoracolumbar flexion AROM.

CHAPTER 9

Cervical Range-of-Motion Instrument (CROM)

The CROM[17] (Fig. 9-15) is designed to measure cervical spine motion. It consists of a headpiece (i.e., frame that holds three inclinometers) and a magnetic yoke. The inclinometers are located on the front and side of the CROM; each contains an inclination needle that is influenced by the force of gravity. The third inclinometer, situated in the transverse plane, contains a compass needle that reacts to earth's magnetic field for measurement of cervical spine rotation.

Measurement Procedure: CROM

The CROM is positioned on the patient's head with the bridge of the frame placed comfortably on the nose and the occipital strap snug (Fig. 9-15). The magnetic yoke is used when measuring cervical spine rotation ROM and serves to eliminate substitute trunk motion from the cervical spine rotation measurement. The magnetic yoke is positioned over the shoulders with the arrow on the yoke pointing north (indicated by observing the position of the red needle on the compass inclinometer with the yoke greater than 4 ft away).

With the patient in the start position for movements in either the sagittal plane (i.e., flexion/extension) or the frontal plane (i.e., lateral flexion), the gravity inclinometer situated in the same plane as that of the motion to be measured should read 0°. With the patient in the start position for movement in the transverse plane (i.e., rotation), both gravity inclinometers should read 0° by adjusting the patient's head position. The compass inclinometer is then rotated to read 0°.

The patient moves through the AROM to be measured. At the end of the test movement, the therapist reads the appropriate gravity or compass inclinometer and records the angular AROM measurement for the cervical spine movement being assessed.

Back Range-of-Motion Instrument (BROMII)

The Back Range-of-Motion Instrument (BROMII)[19] (Performance Attainment Associates, Roseville, MN) is a relatively new tool designed to measure AROM of the lumbar spine. It consists of two units for the measurement of back ROM. First, a frame that contains a protractor scale is positioned over S1 and held in place using Velcro straps. An L-shaped extension arm slides into the frame, and this device is used to measure lumbar flexion and extension ROM. Second, a frame that holds two inclinometers is positioned horizontally over the T12 spinous process and held in place by the therapist during the measurement of lateral flexion and rotation. One inclinometer lies in the frontal plane with a gravity-dependent needle for measurement of lateral flexion; a second, oriented in the transverse plane, contains a compass needle that reacts to Earth's magnetic field for measurement of rotation. A magnetic yoke is positioned around the pelvis to eliminate substitute pelvic motion from the rotation measurement.

The BROMII is relatively expensive, and from the research to date, it does not appear to be superior to other means of measuring AROM of the lumbar spine. For this reason, the BROMII is not used to demonstrate ROM assessment in this text.

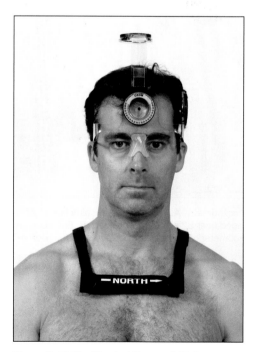

Figure 9-15 The Cervical Range-of-Motion Instrument (CROM).

ACTIVE RANGE OF MOTION ASSESSMENT AND MEASUREMENT: HEAD AND NECK

 ## Practice Makes Perfect

To aid you in practicing the skills covered in this section, or for a handy review, use the Summary & Evaluation Forms found at

http://thepoint.lww.com/ClarksonJM2e.

The use of the ruler and calipers to measure TMJ AROM is described and illustrated.

TMJ Movements

Start Position. The patient is sitting with the head, neck, and trunk in the anatomical position. The patient remains in this position throughout the test movements. It is important to maintain a standard position of the head and neck because the magnitude of mandibular opening is affected by head and neck position.[20,21] From the rest position (i.e., with the teeth not in contact), the patient performs elevation, depression, protrusion, or lateral deviation of the mandible.

Elevation of the Mandible

The patient elevates the lower jaw to a position where the **teeth are in contact at full elevation** (Fig. 9-16). The relative position of the mandibular teeth in relation to the maxillary teeth is observed.

Depression of the Mandible

 The patient is asked to open the mouth. On slow active opening of the mouth, the therapist observes for deviation of the mandible from the midline. In normal mouth opening, the mandible moves in a straight line. Deviation of the mandible to the left in the form of a C-type curve indicates hypomobility of the TMJ situated on the convex side of the C curve or hypermobility of the joint on the concave side of the curve.[4] Deviation in the shape of an S-type curve may indicate a muscular imbalance or displacement of the condyle.[4]

Functional ROM normally required for daily activity is determined by placing two or three flexed proximal interphalangeal joints between the upper and lower central incisors[4] (Fig. 9-17). The fingers represent a distance of about **25 to 35 mm.**[4]

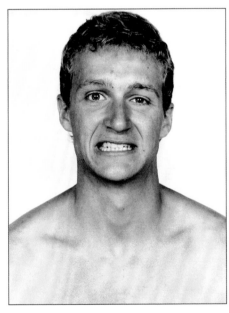
Figure 9-16 Occlusion of the teeth.

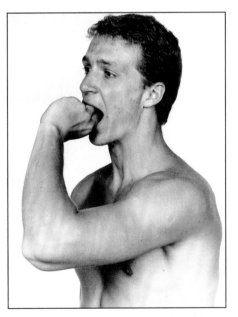
Figure 9-17 Functional ROM: opening of the mouth (depression of the mandible).

CHAPTER 9

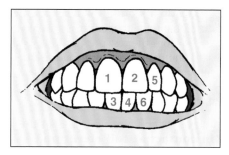

Figure 9-18 Teeth occluded. Maxillary central incisors (*1,2*). Mandibular central incisors (*3,4*). Lateral incisors (*5,6*).

Using a ruler and the edges of the upper and lower central incisors (Fig. 9-18) for reference, a measure of opening is obtained[22] for recording change (Fig. 9-19). Vernier calipers may also be used to measure the distance between the edges of the upper and lower central incisors to establish the range of mandibular depression (Fig. 9-20). **Normal depression of the mandible (mouth opening) is 35 to 50 mm.**[4]

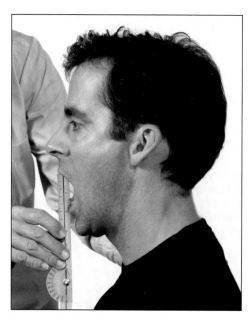

Figure 9-19 Mandibular depression measured with a ruler.

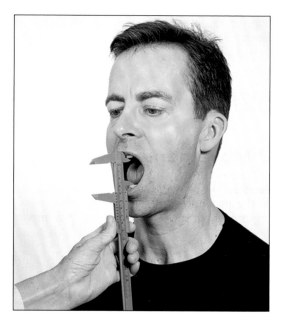

Figure 9-20 Vernier calipers measure mandibular depression.

Protrusion of the Mandible

Form 9-2

The patient protrudes the lower jaw (Fig. 9-21) to place the lower teeth beyond the upper teeth. A ruler measurement is obtained by measuring the distance between the upper and lower central incisors[22] (Fig. 9-21). From resting position, **normal protrusion is 3 to 7 mm.**[5]

Lateral Deviation of the Mandible

Form 9-3

The patient deviates the lower jaw to one side and then the other (Fig. 9-22). Lateral deviation of the mandible should be symmetrical. A measure is obtained for recording purposes by measuring the distance between two selected points that are level, one on the upper teeth and one on the lower teeth,[4] such as the space between the central incisors. **The normal range of lateral deviation is 10 to 15 mm.**[4]

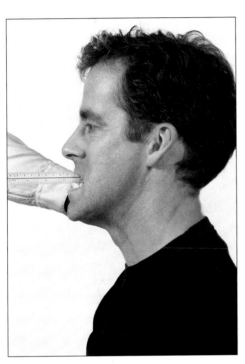

Figure 9-21 Ruler measurement of distance between the upper and lower central incisors, a measure of protrusion of the mandible.

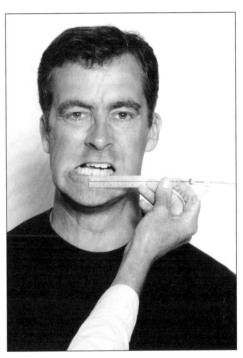

Figure 9-22 Lateral deviation of the mandible.

Neck Movements

Tests of head and neck movement are contraindicated in some instances. Contraindications include pathology that may result in spinal instability and pathology of the vertebral artery. In the absence of contraindications, cervical spine AROM may be assessed.

The measurement of cervical spine AROM is described and illustrated using the tape measure, inclinometer, CROM, and universal goniometer. When measuring cervical spine AROM, the start position (sitting) and the stabilization are the same for all neck movements regardless of the instrument used to measure the AROM, with one exception: the start position for active cervical spine rotation is supine when measured using an inclinometer.

Start Position. The patient is sitting in a chair with a back support. The feet are flat on the floor, and the arms are relaxed at the sides. The head and neck are in the anatomical (neutral zero) position (Fig. 9-23).

Stabilization. The back of the chair provides support for the thoracic and lumbar spines. The patient is instructed to avoid substitute movement and the therapist can stabilize the trunk.

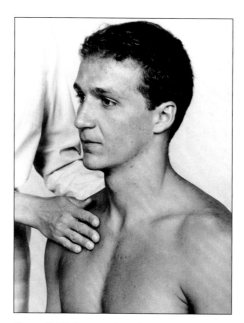

Figure 9-23 Start position for all movements of the neck with the exception of rotation when measured using the inclinometer.

Neck Flexion–Extension

End Positions. *Flexion*: The patient flexes the neck to the limit of the motion. *Extension*: The patient extends the neck to the limit of motion.

Substitute Movement. Mouth opening (for tape measurements), trunk flexion–extension.

Tape Measure Measurement

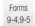
Forms
9-4,9-5

Flexion. The distance is measured between the tip of the chin and the suprasternal notch. A measure is taken in the flexed position (Fig. 9-24). The linear measure reflects the **neck flexion AROM (3 cm)**.

Extension. The same reference points are used. A measure is taken in the extended position (Fig. 9-25). The linear measure reflects the range of **neck extension AROM (20 cm)**.

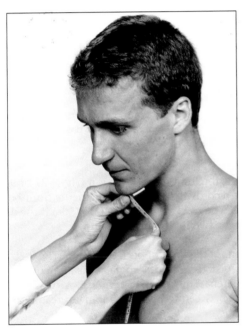

Figure 9-24 Neck flexion: limited AROM.

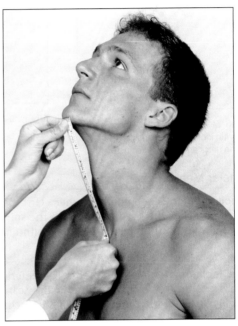

Figure 9-25 Neck extension: full AROM.

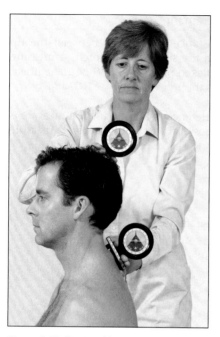

Figure 9-26 Start position: neck flexion and extension with inclinometers positioned on the vertex of the head and over the spine of T1.

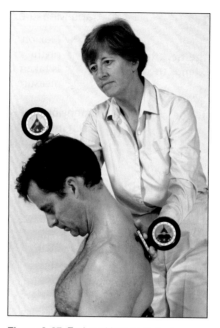

Figure 9-27 End position: neck flexion.

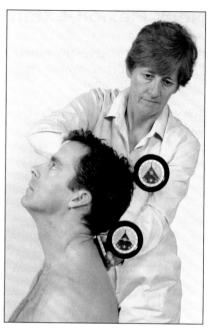

Figure 9-28 End position: neck extension.

Inclinometer Measurement

Forms 9-6,9-7

Inclinometer Placement. *Superior*: On the vertex (i.e., top[23]) of the head. *Inferior*: On the spine of T1. In the start position (Fig. 9-26), the inclinometers are zeroed.

Alternate Inclinometer Measurement. The inferior inclinometer is positioned over the spine of the scapula,[24] as shown in Figure 9-29, if the position of the inclinometer over T1 hinders neck extension ROM or a large neck extension ROM displaces the inclinometer.

Flexion. At the limit of neck flexion (Fig. 9-27 or 9-30), the therapist records the angle measurements from both inclinometers. The **neck flexion AROM (50°)** is the difference between the two inclinometer readings.

Extension. At the limit of neck extension (Fig. 9-28 or 9-31), the therapist records the angle measurements from both inclinometers. The **neck extension AROM (60°)** is the difference between the two inclinometer readings.

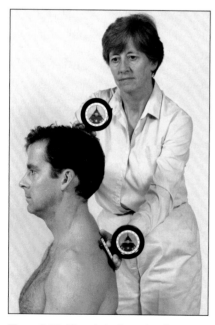

Figure 9-29 Alternate inclinometer placement, start position: neck flexion and extension with inclinometers positioned on the vertex of the head and over the spine of the scapula.

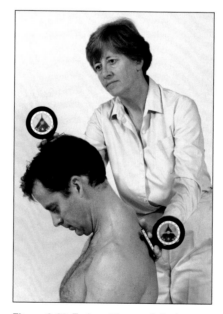

Figure 9-30 End position: neck flexion.

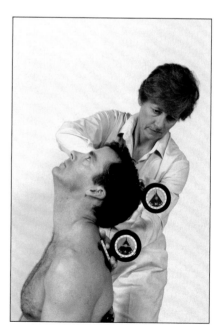

Figure 9-31 End position: neck extension.

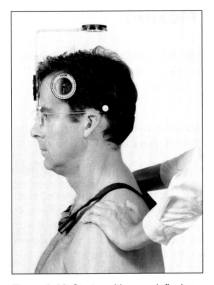

Figure 9-32 Start position: neck flexion and extension.

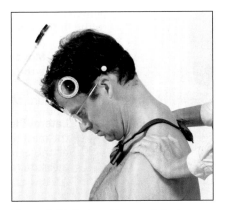

Figure 9-33 End position: neck flexion.

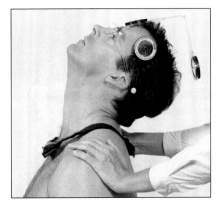

Figure 9-34 End position: neck extension.

CROM Measurement

By positioning the patient's head, the inclinometer on the lateral aspect of the CROM is zeroed in the start position (Fig. 9-32).

Forms 9-8,9-9

Flexion. The neck is flexed to the limit of motion, and the reading on the lateral inclinometer is the **neck flexion AROM (45°)** (Fig. 9-33).

Extension. The neck is extended to the limit of motion, and the reading on the lateral inclinometer is the **neck extension AROM (65°)** (Fig. 9-34).

Universal Goniometer Measurement

Goniometer Axis. Over the lobule of the ear (Fig. 9-35)

Stationary Arm. Perpendicular to the floor

Forms 9-10,9-11

Movable Arm. Lies parallel to the base of the nares. In the start position (Fig. 9-35), the goniometer will indicate 90°. This is recorded as 0°.

Flexion. The goniometer is realigned at the limit of neck flexion (Fig. 9-36). The number of degrees the movable arm lies away from the 90° position is recorded as the **neck flexion AROM (45°)**.

Extension. The goniometer is realigned at the limit of neck extension (Fig. 9-37). The number of degrees the movable arm lies away from the 90° position is recorded as the **neck extension AROM (45°)**.

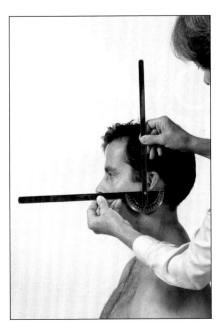

Figure 9-35 Start position: universal goniometer placement for neck flexion and extension.

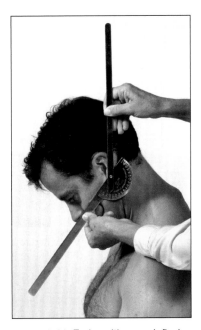

Figure 9-36 End position: neck flexion.

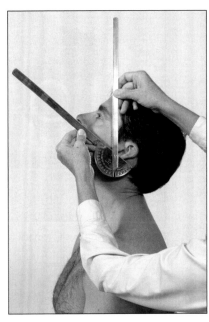

Figure 9-37 End position: neck extension.

CHAPTER 9

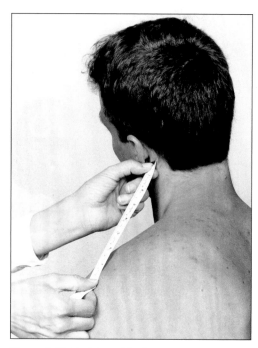

Figure 9-38 Neck lateral flexion.

Neck Lateral Flexion

End Positions. The patient flexes the neck to the left side (without rotation) to the limit of motion (Fig. 9-38). The patient flexes the neck to the right side (without rotation) to the limit of motion.

Substitute Movement. Elevation of the shoulder girdle to approximate the ear; ipsilateral trunk lateral flexion.

Tape Measure Measurement

Form 9-12

Lateral Flexion. The distance is measured between the mastoid process of the skull and the lateral aspect of the acromion process (see Fig. 9-38). The linear measure reflects the range of **neck lateral flexion AROM (13 cm)** to the side measured.

Inclinometer Measurement

Form 9-13

Inclinometer Placement. *Superior:* On the vertex (i.e., top) of the head. *Inferior:* On the spine of T1. In the start position (Fig. 9-39), the inclinometers are zeroed.

Lateral Flexion. At the limit of neck lateral flexion (Fig. 9-40), the therapist records the angle measurements from both inclinometers. The **neck lateral flexion AROM (45°)** is the difference between the two inclinometer readings.

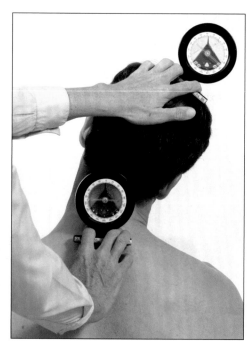

Figure 9-39 Start position: neck lateral flexion.

Figure 9-40 End position: neck lateral flexion.

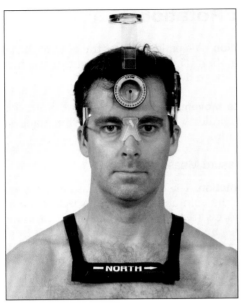

Figure 9-41 Start position: neck lateral flexion.

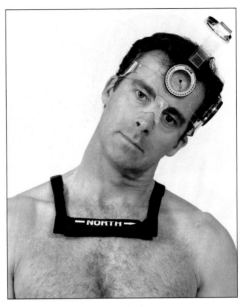

Figure 9-42 Neck lateral flexion.

CROM Measurement

By positioning the patient's head, the inclinometer on the anterior aspect of the CROM is zeroed in the start position (Fig. 9-41).

Form 9-14

Lateral Flexion. The neck is laterally flexed to the limit of motion, and the reading on the anterior inclinometer is the **neck lateral flexion AROM (35°)** to the side measured (Fig. 9-42).

Universal Goniometer Measurement

Goniometer Axis. Over the C7 spinous process (Fig. 9-43).

Form 9-15

Stationary Arm. Along the spine and perpendicular to the floor.

Movable Arm. Points toward the midpoint of the head. In the start position (Fig. 9-43), the goniometer will indicate 0°.

Lateral Flexion. The goniometer is realigned at the limit of neck lateral flexion (Fig. 9-44). The number of degrees the movable arm lies away from the 0° position is recorded as the **neck lateral flexion AROM (45°)** to the side measured.

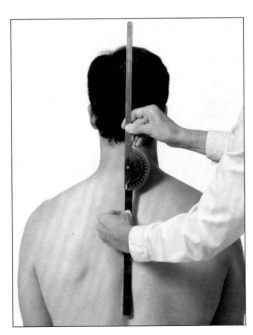

Figure 9-43 Start position: universal goniometer alignment neck lateral flexion.

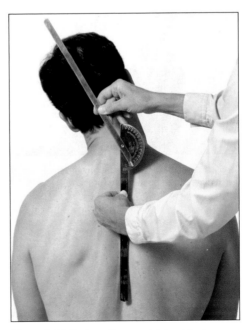

Figure 9-44 End position: neck lateral flexion.

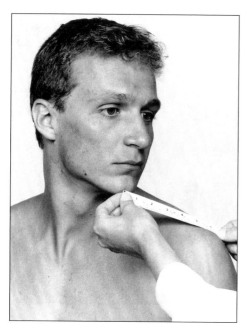

Figure 9-45 Neck rotation.

Neck Rotation

End Position. The patient rotates the head to the left to the limit of motion (Fig. 9-45). The patient rotates the head to the right side to the limit of motion.

Substitute Movement. Elevation and/or protrusion of the shoulder girdle to approximate the chin (tape measure); trunk rotation

Tape Measure Measurement

Form 9-16

Rotation. The distance is measured between the tip of the chin and the lateral aspect of the acromion process (see Fig. 9-45). The linear measure reflects the range of **neck rotation AROM (11 cm)** to the side measured.

Inclinometer Measurement

Form 9-17

Start Position. The patient is supine with the head and neck in anatomical position (Fig. 9-46).

Inclinometer Placement. In the midline at the base of the forehead. In the start position, the inclinometer is zeroed.

Rotation. At the limit of neck rotation (Fig. 9-47), the therapist records the inclinometer reading as the **neck rotation AROM (80°)** to the side measured.

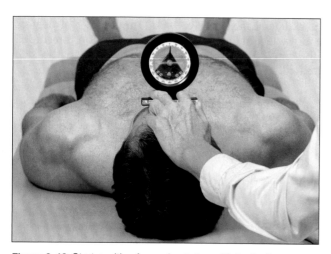

Figure 9-46 Start position for neck rotation with the inclinometer placed in the midline at the base of the forehead.

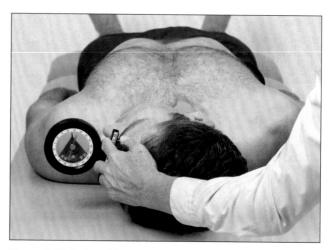

Figure 9-47 End position: neck rotation.

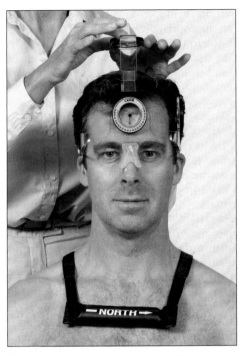

Figure 9-48 Start position: neck rotation.

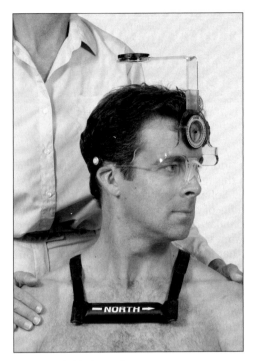

Figure 9-49 Neck rotation.

CROM Measurement

Form 9-18

The magnetic yoke is positioned over the shoulders with the arrow on the yoke pointing north. With the patient in the start position, both gravity inclinometers should read 0° (accomplished by adjusting the patient's head position). The compass inclinometer is then rotated to read 0° (Fig. 9-48).

Rotation. The neck is rotated to the limit of motion, and the reading on the compass inclinometer is the **neck rotation AROM (60°)** to the side measured (Fig. 9-49).

Universal Goniometer Measurement

Form 9-19

Goniometer Axis. Over the midpoint of the top of the head (Fig. 9-50).

Stationary Arm. Parallel to a line joining the two acromion processes.

Movable Arm. Aligned with the nose. In the start position (Fig. 9-50), the goniometer will indicate 90°. This is recorded as 0°.

Rotation. The goniometer is realigned at the limit of neck rotation (Fig. 9-51). The number of degrees the movable arm lies away from the 90° position is recorded as the neck rotation AROM.

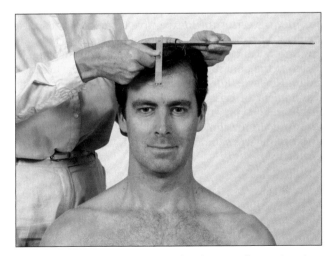

Figure 9-50 Start position: universal goniometer alignment neck rotation.

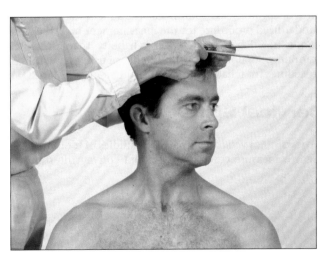

Figure 9-51 End position: neck rotation.

CHAPTER 9

VALIDITY AND RELIABILITY: MEASUREMENT OF THE TMJ AND CERVICAL SPINE AROM

TMJ

The ruler and calipers are the tools used to measure TMJ AROM in this text.

Walker, Bohannon, and Cameron[25] evaluated the construct *validity* of using a ruler to measure AROM of the TMJs for mandibular depression, lateral deviation, and protrusion. The measurement of mouth opening was the only measure that demonstrated construct validity for identifying TMJ pathology. Therefore, the authors concluded that mouth opening measured by a ruler might be a possible method for documenting and monitoring the status of patients with TMJ disorders.

Evaluating the intra- and intertester *reliability* of the ruler for measuring mouth opening AROM, researchers[21,25–28] found the ruler to be reliable. Dijkstra and coworkers[26] pointed out that mandibular length might influence how much the mouth can be opened. Therefore, when comparing different subjects with the same linear mouth opening, one cannot conclude similar TMJ mobility. However, using a ruler to measure the distance between the central incisors in maximal mouth opening is a reliable and accurate measure of TMJ mobility when evaluating progress in the same subject over time.

Al-Ani and Gray[28] evaluated intra-instrument reliability of the ruler and an Alma bite gauge for measuring mouth opening. The Alma bite gauge is a set of calipers with recesses on the arms for ease of positioning against the edges of the central incisors. These researchers found the Alma bit gauge to have better reliability and ease of use when compared to the ruler.

For measurements of lateral deviation and protrusion of the TMJs using the ruler, Walker, Bohannon, and Cameron[25] found acceptable intratester reliability and good-to-excellent intertester reliability, but Dworkin and colleagues[27] found less-than-desirable intertester reliability. Dworkin and colleagues[27] also found that examiners trained in the standardized procedure for the measurement of TMJ AROM demonstrated better intertester reliability than untrained examiners, supporting the importance of using standardized procedures for reliable clinical measurement of TMJ AROM.

Cervical Spine

Reviews[29–32] of *validity and reliability* studies of tools and tests used to measure cervical spine ROM convey the status of the research on this topic. This type of review, undertaken to select an appropriate measurement tool to assess ROM, is difficult due to the lack of optimized study designs, poor reporting in studies, lack of studies of some measurement methods, and studies having been conducted on a limited number of patient populations.[31]

Reviews by Williams and associates[31] and de Koning and colleagues[30] concluded that although more research is needed, the CROM and single inclinometer were the most valid and reliable instruments for use in assessing cervical spine ROM. Jordan,[29] in an earlier review of the literature on the reliability of tools used to measure cervical spine ROM in clinical settings, could give "no strong recommendation for any tool" but found the CROM to be the most reliable tool. He also noted the CROM shows promise but may not be the most practical tool in the clinical setting due to cost, portability, and specificity for use in measuring only cervical spine ROM. Jordan[29] suggested the tape measure might be the preferred clinical option as it is inexpensive, portable, and clinically acceptable, but he found the tape measure needs more support in the literature. Williams and associates[31] found visual estimation to be the least reliable and concurrently valid method, and along with de Koning and colleagues[30] recommended visual estimation not be used to measure cervical spine ROM.

A systematic review by Rondoni and associates[32] sought to compare the intra- and interrater reliability of measuring the cervical spine AROM of adults with nonspecific neck pain, using expensive technology-based devices versus inexpensive devices commonly used in the clinical setting. The commonly used inexpensive devices included the standard universal goniometer, universal inclinometer, gravity inclinometer, and the CROM. The expensive (i.e., costing more than 500 Euros) technology-based devices included the Cybex Electronic Digital Inclinometer 320 (EDI320), the Orthopedic Systems Incorporated Computerized Anatometry 6000 Spine Motion Analyzer (SMA), and the Flock-of-Birds electromagnetic tracking system.

Rondoni and associates[32] found there to be no significant difference in the inter and intrarater reliability of cervical spine AROM measures using the expensive technology-based devices versus the inexpensive commonly used measurement devices. The researchers[32] qualified the ability to draw strong conclusions from the review and meta-analysis, due to the poor methodological quality of the available studies. However, Rondoni and associates[32] concluded that measurement of cervical spine AROM can be carried out reliably and cost effectively, using inexpensive devices commonly used in the clinical setting, while expensive technology-based devices should be reserved for specific clinical or research use.

ARTICULATIONS AND MOVEMENTS: TRUNK

The Trunk: Thoracic and Lumbar Spines

The articulations and joint axes of the trunk are illustrated in Figures 9-52 to 9-54. The joint structure and movements of the trunk are described below and summarized in Table 9-3.

There are 12 vertebrae in the thoracic spine and 5 in the lumbar spine (Fig. 9-52). Vertebral segments are referred to when describing the articulations of the spine. A vertebral segment consists of two vertebrae and the three articulations between them (Fig. 9-55). Anteriorly, intervertebral discs are positioned between the adjacent vertebral bodies. However, it is the orientation of the facet joints, located posteriorly on each side of the vertebral segment that determines the predominant motions that occur between the vertebral segments. Each facet joint is formed by the inferior facet of the superior vertebra articulating with the superior facet of the inferior vertebra.

Although all segments of the thoracic and lumbar spines contribute to flexion, extension, lateral flexion, and rotation of the trunk, the regional contribution to these motions varies. The surfaces of the facets in the thoracic spine lie in the frontal plane, favoring the motions of lateral

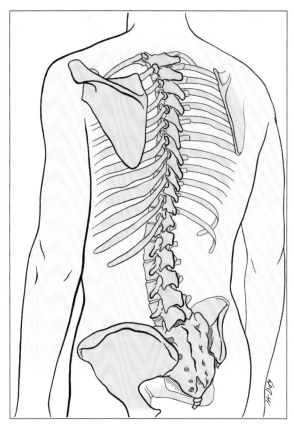

Figure 9-52 Trunk articulations.

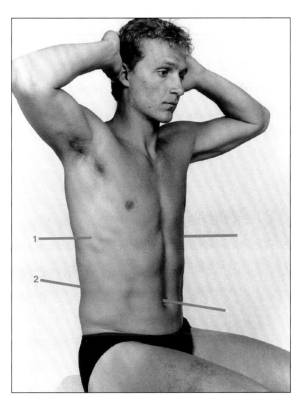

Figure 9-53 Trunk axes: (*1*) flexion–extension; (*2*) lateral flexion.

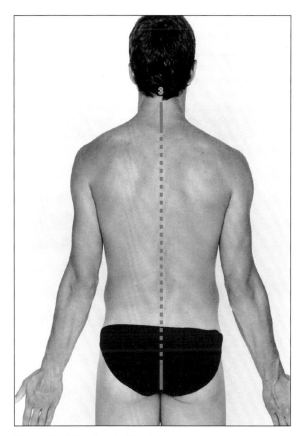

Figure 9-54 Trunk axis: (*3*) rotation.

TABLE 9-3　Joint Structure: Trunk Movements

	Flexion	Extension	Lateral Flexion	Rotation
Articulation[33]	Lumbar spine, thoracic spine (mainly T6–T12)	Lumbar spine, thoracic spine (mainly T6–T12)	Lumbar spine, thoracic spine	Thoracic spine, lumbosacral articulation
Plane	Sagittal	Sagittal	Frontal	Horizontal
Axis	Frontal	Frontal	Sagittal	Vertical
Normal limiting factors[8,9,34]* (see Fig. 9-55)	Tension in the posterior longitudinal, supraspinous, interspinous and intertransverse ligaments, the ligamentum flavum, facet joint capsules and spinal extensor muscles; compression of the intervertebral discs anteriorly and tension in the posterior fibers of the annulus; apposition of articular facets thoracic spine; rib cage	Tension in the anterior longitudinal ligament, abdominal muscles, facet joint capsules and the anterior fibers of the annulus; contact between adjacent spinous processes; apposition of articular facets thoracic spine	Contact between the iliac crest and thorax; tension in the contralateral trunk side flexors, intertransverse and iliolumbar ligaments and facet joint capsules; tension in the contralateral fibers of the annulus; apposition of articular facets lumbar spine	Tension in the costovertebral, supraspinous, interspinous, intertransverse, and iliolumbar ligaments and facet joint capsules, lumbar spine and annulus fibrosus of the intervertebral discs; tension in the ipsilateral external and contralateral internal abdominal oblique muscles; apposition of the articular facets lumbar spine
Normal AROM				
Tape measure	10 cm[5]† 6 cm[35]§		22 cm[36]‡	
Inclinometer[12] Universal goniometer[3]	0°–60+° L spine	0°–25° L spine	0°–25° L spine 0°–35°	0°–30° T spine
Capsular pattern	It is difficult to perform passive movements of the trunk due to its size and weight. It is difficult to determine the capsular pattern for the trunk.[6]			

*There is a paucity of definitive research that identifies the normal limiting factors (NLF) of joint motion. The NLF and end feels listed here are based on knowledge of anatomy, clinical experience, and available references.

†Measured between C7 and S1.

‡Measured between level of middle finger on thigh in anatomical position and at end of lateral flexion ROM. Value represents the mean of mean values from the original source[36] for right and left lateral flexion ROM of 39 healthy subjects.

§Measured between level of PSIS and 15 cm proximal. Value represents the rounded mean of mean values from the original source[35] for L-spine flexion ROM of 104 children 13 to 18 years of age.

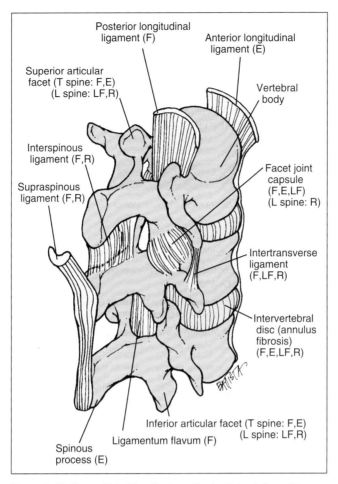

Posterior longitudinal ligament (F)

Anterior longitudinal ligament (E)

Superior articular facet (T spine: F,E) (L spine: LF,R)

Vertebral body

Interspinous ligament (F,R)

Facet joint capsule (F,E,LF) (L spine: R)

Supraspinous ligament (F,R)

Intertransverse ligament (F,LF,R)

Intervertebral disc (annulus fibrosis) (F,E,LF,R)

Inferior articular facet (T spine: F,E) (L spine: LF,R)

Ligamentum flavum (F)

Spinous process (E)

Figure 9-55 Normal Limiting Factors. Posterolateral view of the vertebral column to illustrate noncontractile structures that normally limit motion in the thoracic and lumbar spines. Motion limited by structures is identified in brackets, using the following abbreviations: *F*, flexion; *E*, extension; *LF*, lateral flexion; *R*, rotation. Muscles normally limiting motion are not illustrated.

flexion and rotation. The facet joint surfaces of the lumbar spine are oriented in the sagittal plane, favoring flexion and extension.

When assessing thoracic and lumbar spine ROM, the combined motions of the segments are assessed and measured since segmental motion cannot be measured clin- ically. Thoracic and lumbar spine movements include flex- ion and extension, which occur in the sagittal plane around a frontal axis (Fig. 9-53); lateral flexion, which occurs in the frontal plane around a sagittal axis (Fig. 9-53); and rotation, which occurs in the transverse plane around a vertical axis (Fig. 9-54).

ANATOMICAL LANDMARKS: TRUNK (FIGS. 9-56 THROUGH 9-59)

Anatomical landmarks are described and illustrated below. Anatomical landmarks numbered 1, 4, 5, 6, and 11 through 14 are used to assess T- and L-spine ROM, and/or align the goniometer axis and arms, or position the tape measure or inclinometers to measure ROM at the T and L spines. To measure chest expansion, the landmark numbered 2 is used to locate the xiphisternal joint and position the tape measure.

Structure	Location
1. Suprasternal (jugular) notch	The rounded depression at the superior border of the sternum, between the medial ends of each clavicle.
2. Xiphoid process	The lower end of the body of the sternum.
3. Anterior superior iliac spine (ASIS)	Round bony prominence at the anterior end of the iliac crest.
4. Iliac crest	Upper border of the ilium; a convex bony ridge, the top of which is level with the space between the spines of L4 and L5.
5. Posterior superior iliac spine (PSIS)	Round bony prominence at the posterior end of the iliac crest, felt subcutaneously at the dimples on the proximal aspect of the buttocks.
6. S2 spinous process	At the midpoint of a line drawn between each PSIS.
7. Inferior angle of the scapula	At the inferior aspect of the vertebral border of the scapula.
8. Spine of the scapula	The bony ridge running obliquely across the upper four-fifths of the scapula.
9. T7 spinous process	Midline of the body at the level of the inferior angle of the scapula with the body in the anatomical position.
10. T3 spinous process	With the body in the anatomical position, it is at the midpoint of a line drawn between the roots of the spines of each scapula.
11. C7 spinous process	Often the most prominent spinous process at the base of the neck.
12. T1 spinous process	The next spinous process inferior to the C7 spinous process.
13. Acromion process	Lateral aspect of the spine of the scapula at the tip or point of the shoulder.
14. Greater trochanter	With the tip of the thumb on the lateral aspect of the iliac crest, the tip of the third digit placed distally on the lateral aspect of the thigh locates the upper border of the greater trochanter.

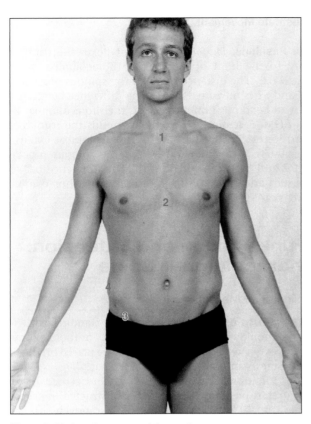

Figure 9-56 Anterior aspect of the trunk.

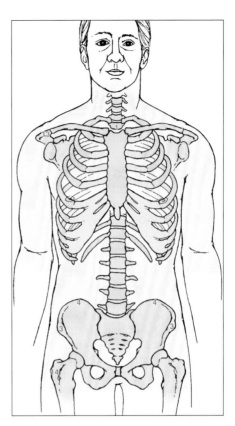

Figure 9-57 Bony anatomy, anterior aspect of the trunk.

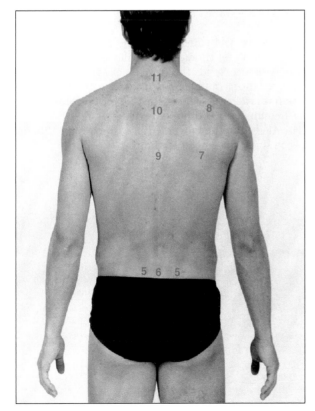

Figure 9-58 Posterior aspect of the trunk.

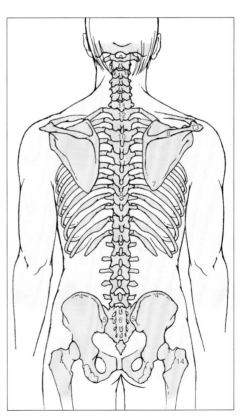

Figure 9-59 Bony anatomy, posterior aspect of the trunk.

ACTIVE RANGE OF MOTION ASSESSMENT AND MEASUREMENT: TRUNK

Practice Makes Perfect

To aid you in practicing the skills covered in this section, or for a handy review, use the Summary & Evaluation Forms found at

http://thepoint.lww.com/ClarksonJM2e.

The tape measure, universal goniometer, and standard inclinometer are the tools used to objectively measure spinal AROM as presented in this text. Description of the general principles of application for the tape measure, standard inclinometer, and BROMII can be found in the section "Instrumentation and Measurement Procedures: TMJ and Spine" at the beginning of this chapter. The measurement of spinal AROM is described and illustrated.

Trunk Flexion and Extension: Thoracolumbar Spine

Tape Measure Measurement

Forms
9-20,
9-21

Start Positions. *Flexion*: The patient is standing with feet shoulder width apart (Fig. 9-60). A tape measure is used to measure the distance between the spinous processes of C7 and S2. *Extension*: For thoracolumbar extension, the patient's hands are placed on the iliac crests and into the small of the back (Fig. 9-61). A tape measure is used to measure the distance between the spinous processes of C7 and S2. The patient is instructed to keep the knees straight when performing the test movements.

Substitute Movement. None.

End Positions. *Flexion*: The patient flexes the trunk forward to the limit of motion for thoracolumbar flexion (Fig. 9-62). The distance between the spinous processes of C7 and S2 is measured again. The difference between the start and end position measures is the thoracolumbar flexion ROM. *Extension*: The patient extends the trunk backward to the limit of motion for thoracolumbar extension (Fig. 9-63). The distance between the spinous processes of C7 and S2 is measured again. The difference between the start and end position measures is the thoracolumbar extension ROM.

Trunk Flexion and Extension: Thoracolumbar Spine

Inclinometer Measurement

Forms
9-22,
9-23

Start Positions. The patient is standing with feet shoulder width apart (Fig. 9-64). For thoracolumbar extension, the patient's hands are placed on the iliac crests and into the small of the back (Fig. 9-65). The inclinometers are positioned and zeroed in each start position. The patient is instructed to keep the knees straight when performing the test movements.

Substitute Movement. None.

Inclinometer Placement. *Superior*: On the spine of C7. *Inferior*: On the spine of S2.

End Positions. The patient flexes the trunk forward to the limit of motion for thoracolumbar flexion (Fig. 9-66).

The patient extends the trunk backward to the limit of motion for thoracolumbar extension (Fig. 9-67). At the end position for each movement, the therapist records the angle measurements from both inclinometers.

The AROM for the movement measured is the difference between the inclinometer readings.

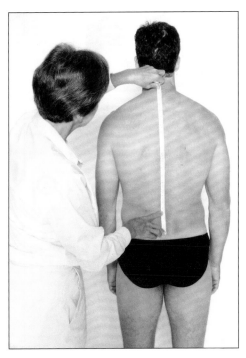

Figure 9-60 Start position: thoracolumbar spinal flexion. The distance is measured between the spinous processes of C7 and S2.

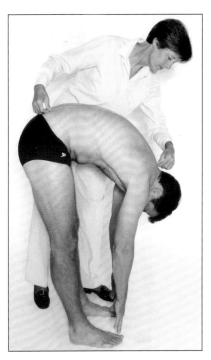

Figure 9-62 End position: thoracolumbar spinal flexion.

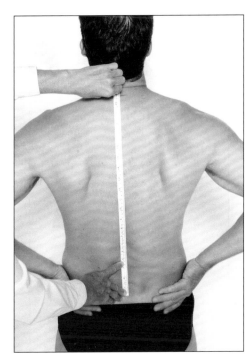

Figure 9-61 Start position for thoracolumbar extension.

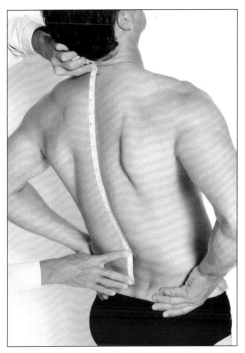

Figure 9-63 End position: thoracolumbar extension.

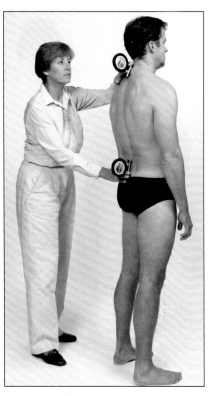

Figure 9-64 Start position: thoracolumbar flexion with inclinometer placement over the spines of C7 and S2.

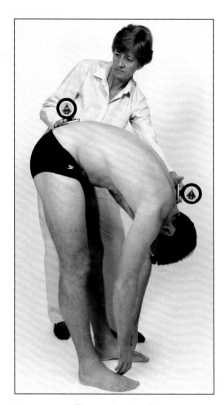

Figure 9-66 Thoracolumbar flexion.

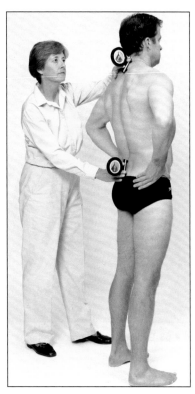

Figure 9-65 Start position: thoracolumbar extension.

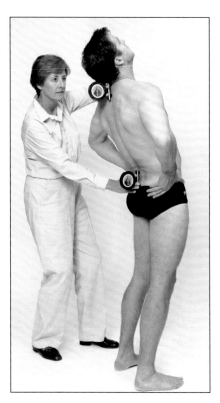

Figure 9-67 End position: thoracolumbar spine extension.

Trunk Extension: Thoracolumbar Spine

Tape Measure Measurement (Prone Press-Up)

Form
9-24

Start Position. The patient is prone (Fig. 9-68). The hands are positioned on the plinth at shoulder level.

Stabilization. A strap is placed over the pelvis.

Substitute Movement. Lifting the pelvis from the plinth.

End Position. The patient extends the elbows to raise the trunk and extends the thoracolumbar spine (Fig. 9-69). A tape measure is used to measure the perpendicular distance between the suprasternal notch and the plinth at the limit of motion. This method is unsuitable for patients who have upper extremity muscle weakness or who find the prone position uncomfortable. In these cases, spinal extension is assessed in standing using a tape measure.

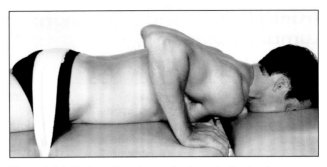

Figure 9-68 Start position: thoracolumbar spinal extension.

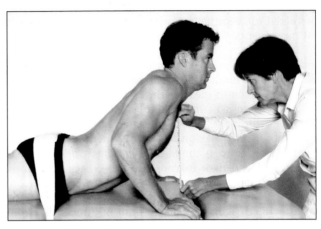

Figure 9-69 End position: thoracolumbar spinal extension.

Trunk Flexion and Extension: Lumbar Spine

Tape Measure Measurement

Start Positions. *Flexion*[35]: The patient is standing with feet shoulder width apart. A tape measure is used to measure a distance and mark a point 15 cm above the midpoint of the line connecting the PSISs (i.e., the spinous process of S2) with the patient in the start position (Fig. 9-70). *Extension*: For lumbar extension, the patient's hands are placed on the iliac crests and into the small of the back (Fig. 9-71). The patient is instructed to keep the knees straight when performing the test movements.

Forms
9-25,
9-26

End Positions. *Flexion*: The patient flexes the trunk forward to the limit of lumbar flexion motion (Fig. 9-72). A second measure is taken to measure the distance between the PSIS and the 15 cm skin mark at the limit of lumbar flexion ROM. The difference between the start and end measures is the lumbar spinal flexion ROM. This method of measurement is referred to as the *modified-modified Schöber method*. *Extension*: The patient extends the trunk backward to the limit of motion for lumbar extension (Fig. 9-73). A second measure is taken to measure the distance between the PSIS and the 15 cm skin mark at the limit of lumbar extension ROM. The difference between the start and end measures is the lumbar spinal extension ROM.

Trunk Flexion and Extension: Lumbar Spine

Inclinometer Measurement

Start Positions. *Flexion*: For lumbar flexion, the patient is standing with feet shoulder width apart (Fig. 9-74). *Extension*: For lumbar extension, the patient's hands are placed on the iliac crests and into the small of the back (Fig. 9-75).

Forms
9-27,
9-28

The inclinometers are positioned and zeroed in each start position. The patient is instructed to keep the knees straight when performing the test movements.

Inclinometer Placement. *Superior*: On a mark 15 cm above the spinous process of S2. *Inferior*: On the spine of S2.

End Positions. *Flexion*: The patient flexes the trunk forward to the limit of motion for lumbar flexion (Fig. 9-76). *Extension*: The patient extends the trunk backward to the limit of motion for lumbar extension (Fig. 9-77). At the end position for each movement, the therapist records the angle measurements from both inclinometers.

The AROM for lumbar spine flexion or extension is the difference between the inclinometer readings in the end position for the movement being measured.

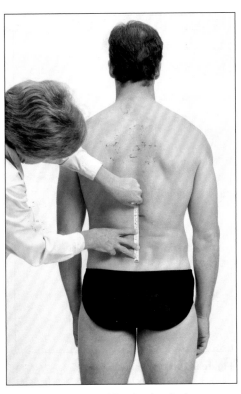

Figure 9-70 Start position: lumbar flexion, modified-modified Schöber method. The distance measured is between the spine of S2 and a point 15 cm above S2.

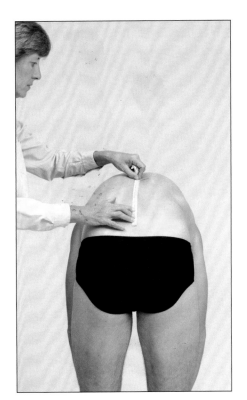

Figure 9-72 End position: lumbar flexion, modified-modified Schöber method.

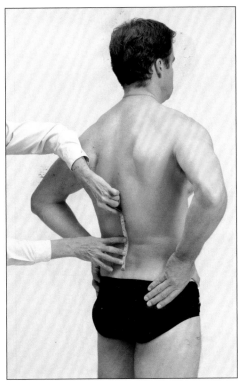

Figure 9-71 Start position: lumbar extension.

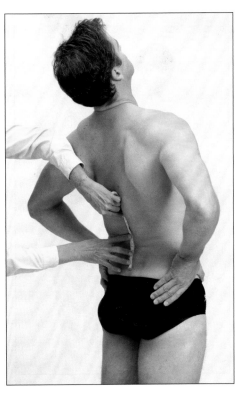

Figure 9-73 End position: lumbar extension.

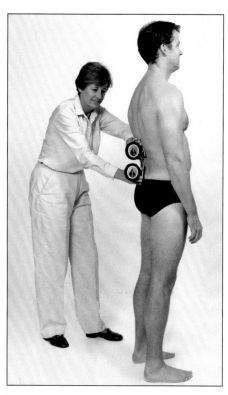

Figure 9-74 Start position: lumbar flexion with inclinometer placement over the spine of S2 and over a mark 15 cm above the spine of S2.

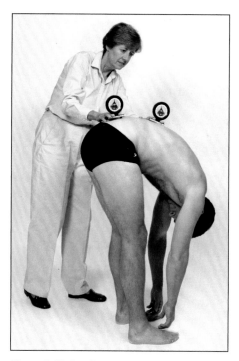

Figure 9-76 Lumbar spine flexion.

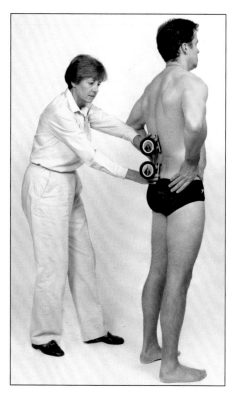

Figure 9-75 Start position: lumbar spine extension.

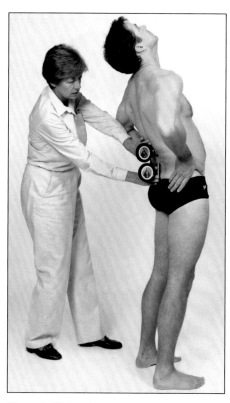

Figure 9-77 Lumbar spine extension.

Trunk Lateral Flexion

Tape Measure Measurement

Form
9-29

Start Position. The patient is standing with the feet shoulder width apart (Fig. 9-78). The patient is instructed to keep both feet flat on the floor when performing the test movements.

Stabilization. None.

Substitute Movement. Trunk flexion, trunk extension, ipsilateral hip and knee flexion, raising the contralateral or ipsilateral foot from the floor.

End Position. The patient laterally flexes the trunk to the limit of motion (Fig. 9-79). A tape measure is used to measure the distance between the tip of the third digit and the floor.

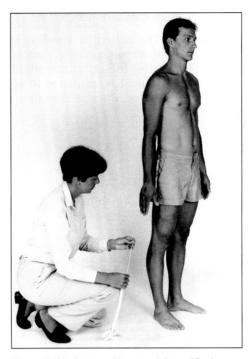

Figure 9-78 Start position: trunk lateral flexion.

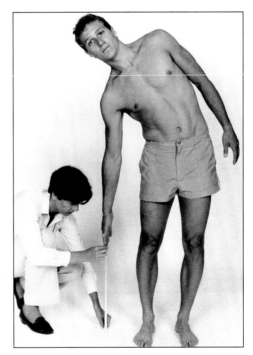

Figure 9-79 End position: trunk lateral flexion.

Alternate Tape Measure Measurement[36]

Form 9-30

Start Position. The patient is standing with the feet shoulder width apart. A mark is placed on the thigh at the level of the tip of the middle finger (Fig. 9-80). The patient is instructed to keep both feet flat on the floor when performing the test movements.

Stabilization. None.

End Position. The patient laterally flexes the trunk to the limit of motion. A second mark is placed on the thigh at the level of the tip of the middle finger (Fig. 9-81).

Measurement. A tape measure is used to measure the distance between the marks placed on the thigh at the level of the tip of the middle finger at the start position and at the end position (Fig. 9-82). The distance measured represents the lateral flexion ROM.

Inclinometer Measurement

Form 9-31

Start Position. The patient stands with feet shoulder width apart. The inclinometers are positioned and zeroed (Fig. 9-83). The patient is instructed to keep both feet flat on the floor when performing the test movements.

Inclinometer Placement. *Superior*: On the spine of T1. *Inferior*: On the spine of S2.

End Position. The patient laterally flexes the trunk to the limit of motion (Fig. 9-84). At the end position, the therapist records the angle measurements from both inclinometers. The AROM for lateral flexion is the difference between the inclinometer readings.

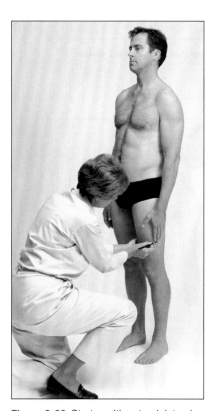

Figure 9-80 Start position: trunk lateral flexion.

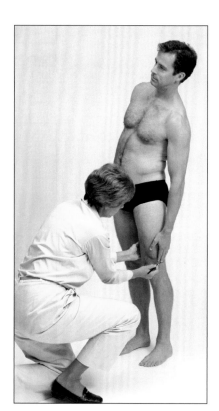

Figure 9-81 End position: trunk lateral flexion.

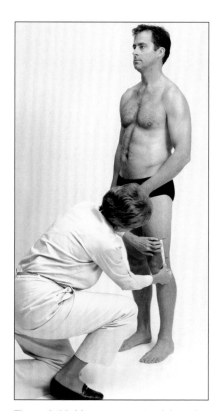

Figure 9-82 Measurement: trunk lateral flexion.

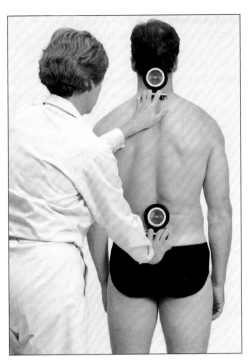

Figure 9-83 Inclinometer placement (spines of T1 and S2) for trunk lateral flexion.

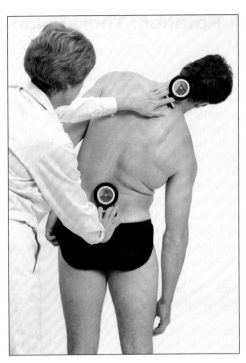

Figure 9-84 End position: trunk lateral flexion.

Universal Goniometer Measurement

Form 9-32

Start Position. Standing (Fig. 9-85).

Goniometer Axis. In the midline at the level of the PSIS (i.e., over the S2 spinous process).

Stationary Arm. Perpendicular to the floor.

Movable Arm. Points toward the spine of C7.

Lateral Flexion. The goniometer is realigned at the limit of trunk lateral flexion (Fig. 9-86). The number of degrees the movable arm lies away from the 0° position is recorded as the thoracolumbar lateral flexion ROM to the side measured.

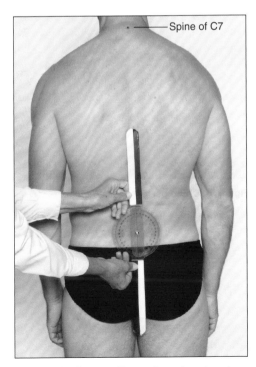

Figure 9-85 Start position: universal goniometer placement trunk lateral flexion.

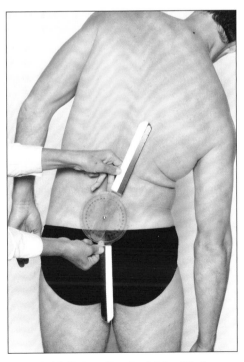

Figure 9-86 End position: trunk lateral flexion.

Trunk Rotation: Thoracolumbar Spine

Tape Measure Measurement

Start Position. The patient is sitting with the feet supported on a stool and the arms crossed in front of the chest. The patient holds the end of the tape measure on the lateral aspect of the acromion process. The therapist holds the other end of the tape measure on either the uppermost point of the iliac crest at the midaxillary line (not shown) or the upper border of the greater trochanter (Fig. 9-87). The distance between the lateral aspect of the acromion process and the uppermost point of the iliac crest at the midaxillary line or the upper border of the greater trochanter is measured.

Stabilization. The body weight on the pelvis; the therapist can also stabilize the pelvis.

Substitute Movement. Trunk flexion, trunk extension, and shoulder girdle protraction (on the side the tape measure is held).

End Position. The patient rotates the trunk to the limit of motion (Fig. 9-88). The distance between the lateral aspect of the acromion process and either the uppermost point of the iliac crest at the midaxillary line or the upper border of the greater trochanter is measured at the limit of rotation. The difference between the start position and end position measures is the thoracolumbar rotation ROM. The surface landmarks used in the assessment should be documented.

Frost and colleagues[37] described the use of the tape measure to measure trunk rotation (using the posterior clavicular prominence and the greater trochanter as landmarks) and noted that the accurate definition and palpation of the landmarks used in the assessment are critical for reliable assessment.

Clarkson recommends using the lateral aspect of the acromion process and the uppermost point of the iliac crest as the preferred surface landmarks, as these are easily palpated.

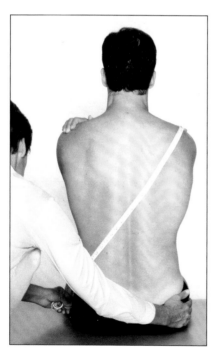

Figure 9-87 Start position: trunk rotation.

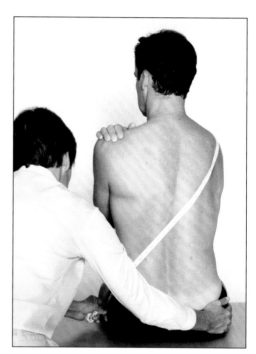

Figure 9-88 End position: trunk rotation.

Trunk Rotation: Thoracic Spine

Inclinometer Measurement

Form 9-34

Start Position. The patient is standing with the arms crossed in front of the chest. The patient leans forward with the head and trunk parallel to the floor or as close to this position as possible. The inclinometers are positioned and zeroed (Fig. 9-89).

Inclinometer Placement. *Superior*: On the spine of T1. *Inferior*: On the spine of T12.

End Positions. The patient rotates the trunk to the limit of motion (Fig. 9-90). At the end position, the therapist records the angle measurements from both inclinometers. The AROM for thoracic spine rotation is the difference between the inclinometer readings.

Substitute Movement. Trunk flexion and trunk extension. The range of trunk rotation when measured in the forward lean or stooped posture is less than when measured in sitting.[38] This may be caused by the contraction of the back muscles required to sustain the stooped posture that splint the spine and restrict trunk rotation.[38]

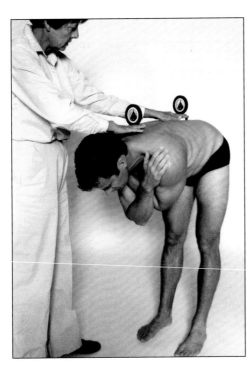

Figure 9-89 Start position: thoracic spine rotation with inclinometers placed over the spines of T1 and T12.

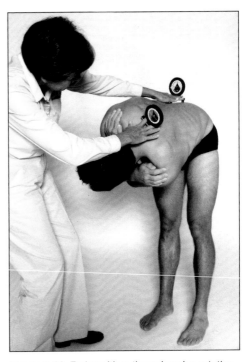

Figure 9-90 End position: thoracic spine rotation.

Chest Expansion

Tape Measure Measurement

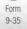

Form
9-35

Start Position. The patient is sitting. The patient makes a full expiration (Fig. 9-91).

End Position. The patient makes a full inspiration (Fig. 9-92).

Measurement. A tape measure is used to measure the circumference of the chest at the level of the xiphisternal joint. Measures are taken at full expiration and at full inspiration. The difference between the two measures is the chest expansion. The chest expansion may also be measured at the levels of the nipple line and anterior axillary fold. The chest expansion measured at the latter points is slightly less than that at the xiphisternal joint. It is recommended[39] that two measurement sites, specifically the xiphoid and axilla, and a consistent patient position be used to provide a thorough evaluation of pulmonary status. A wide range of normal values exists for normal chest expansion, and, beginning in the late 30s, chest expansion gradually decreases with increasing age.[40] Decreased chest expansion may indicate costovertebral joint involvement in certain pathological conditions[41] or may occur with chronic obstructive pulmonary disease (e.g., emphysema).

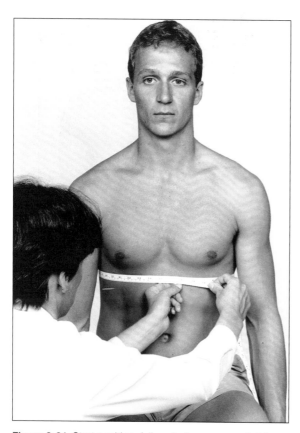

Figure 9-91 Start position: full expiration measured at the level of the xiphisternal joint.

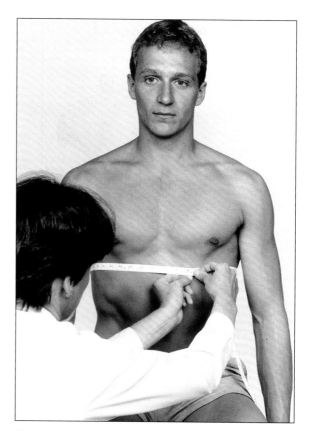

Figure 9-92 End position: full inspiration measured at the level of the xiphisternal joint.

Validity and Reliability: Measurement of the Thoracic and Lumbar Spine AROM

Littlewood and May[42] reviewed studies of the validity of low-tech clinical procedures, that is, clinically common, simple to use, and noninvasive methods, compared to x-ray (gold standard) measures of lumbar spine ROM in patients with nonspecific low-back pain. Only four studies were found that matched the criteria for inclusion for qualitative review. Littlewood and May[42] found limited evidence of validity of the modified-modified Schöber method for lumbar spine flexion ROM, and the double inclinometry method for measuring total lumbar flexion/extension, and lumbar extension ROM. There was also conflicting evidence of the validity of the double inclinometry method for lumbar flexion ROM. Therefore, Littlewood and May[42] were not able to make "convincing conclusions." These researchers indicate[42] that there is a need for high-quality meaningful research and reporting of the validity (using radiographic comparison) of low-tech clinical methods used to measure lumbar spine ROM in patient populations.

In a similar vein, Castro and colleagues[43] performed a systematic review of the literature to determine the criterion-concurrent validity of common clinical assessment procedures used to determine spinal ROM in patients with ankylosing spondylitis (e.g., the various Schöber tests, finger to floor distance, goniometry, and inclinometry) compared to radiographic measurements (the reference standard). Ten articles met the criteria for inclusion in this review, but only one article was considered of high quality, with some limitations. Castro and colleagues[43] found no high-quality studies to support the criterion-concurrent validity of common clinical assessment procedures used to evaluate spinal ROM in patients with ankylosing spondylitis and recommended the need for further research to identify clinical tests that accurately measure spinal ROM.

The *reliability* of tests of the low back assessment of ROM, strength, and endurance was reviewed by Essendrop, Maul, Läubli, et al.[44] This research team searched databases for studies published from 1980 until 1999 from the Danish, German, and English language literature. Only six studies that pertained to the reliability of tests of the low back assessment of ROM met the predetermined quality criteria and qualified for review. The most reliable methods of measuring mobility of the low back, when groups but not single individuals are compared, appeared to be the tape measure for trunk flexion, the tape measure and Cybex EDI 320 goniometric measurements for trunk lateral flexion, and no reliable measurement methods were found for trunk extension or rotation. Essendrop et al.[44] could not make a recommendation for consensus and indicate a need for more quality research and reporting of reliability studies of measures of low back function.

MUSCLE LENGTH ASSESSMENT AND MEASUREMENT: TRUNK

 Practice Makes Perfect

To aid you in practicing the skills covered in this section, or for a handy review, use the Summary & Evaluation Forms found at

http://thepoint.lww.com/ClarksonJM2e.

Trunk Extensors and Hamstrings (Toe-Touch Test)

Form 9-36

The trunk extensors are the erector spinae (iliocostalis thoracis and lumborum, longissimus thoracis, spinalis thoracis, semispinalis thoracis, and multifidus); the hip extensor and knee flexor muscles are the hamstrings (semitendinosus, semimembranosus, and biceps femoris). The toe-touch test provides a composite measure of hip, spine, and shoulder girdle ROM.

Start Position. The patient is standing (Fig. 9-93).

Substitute Movement. Knee flexion.

Stabilization. None.

End Position. The patient flexes the trunk and hips and reaches toward the toes to the limit of motion (Fig. 9-94).

Measurement. A tape measure is used to measure the distance between the floor and the most distant point reached by both hands. Normal ROM is present if the patient can touch the toes. If the patient can reach beyond floor level, the test can be carried out with the patient standing on a step or platform to measure reach distance beyond the supporting surface.

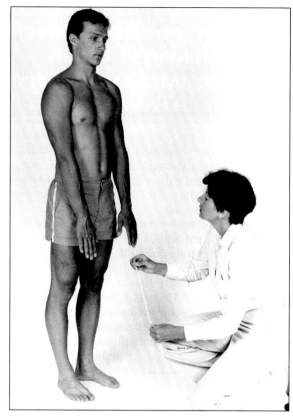

Figure 9-93 Start position: toe-touch test.

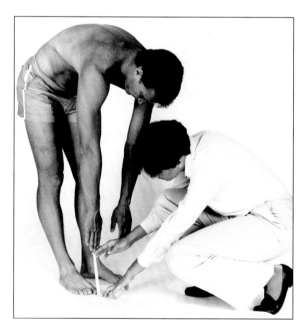

Figure 9-94 End position: trunk extensor and hamstring muscle length.

Functional Application: Neck and Trunk

Joint Function: Neck and Trunk

The trunk complex articulations include the vertebral column, sacrum and coccyx, ribs, costal cartilages, and sternum. The vertebral column and its system of linkages have particular significance in functional application of ROM and strength. The stability function of the spine includes resisting compressive forces; supporting the major portion of the body weight; supporting the head, arms, and trunk against the force of gravity; shock absorption; protection of the spinal cord; and providing a stable structure for movement of the extremities.[7,45]

The articulations at the intervertebral body and facet joints of the vertebral column permit movement in flexion, extension, lateral flexion, and rotation to allow neck and back mobility. The functional range of the lower region of the spine is increased by the tilt of the pelvis. The total motion of the spine is the result of the collective movements of the articulations of the various segments of the vertebral column[7,14,46] with functional ranges varying between individuals.[46] Restriction of motion at any level may result in increased motion at another level.[46] Mobility in all planes is the greatest at the cervical spine segment. The thoracic spine has limited mobility in all planes due to the limitations imposed by the thorax.[1,7,14] Through movements of the thoracic wall, intrathoracic volume is increased or decreased for inspiration and expiration. The lumbar spine is most mobile in the sagittal plane. Functional ROM is described for the cervical and the thoracic and lumbar spines.

Functional Range of Motion

Cervical Spine

The movement components of the cervical spine allow movement for functioning of the sense organs within the head[47] and expression of nonverbal communication, including affirmative (nodding) or negative responses. Maintenance of ROM in flexion, extension, lateral flexion, and rotation is of particular importance to the individual for interacting with the environment through the sense of vision. The significance of the interdependence between vision and neck movements is demonstrated in many self-care, leisure, and occupational tasks.

During ADL, neck flexion and extension are the most frequently performed neck movements, occurring twice as often as lateral flexion and rotation.[48] Full ROM in all planes is not required for most self-care activities (Table 9-4) (Figs. 9-95 and 9-96). The majority of neck ROM performed during normal daily activities is less than 15° (i.e., median ROM of 13° for flexion, extension, and rotation; and 10° for lateral flexion).[48]

Ranges approximating full values may be required for such activities as driving (in a left-hand drive car: neck rotation occasionally reaching 36° left and 43° right rotation[50]) (Fig. 9-97), painting a ceiling, placing an object on a high shelf (Fig. 9-98), gazing at the stars (extension), and many specific leisure and occupational tasks linking vision and neck movements. When eye mobility is restricted, greater cervical spine ROM may be required[52] or head posture may be affected[53] to accommodate for the restricted field of gaze.

Neck extension is required when drinking (Fig. 9-99). The shape of the body of the glass and the diameter of the rim are factors that determine the amount of neck extension required to drink from a glass.[54] "Pot-bellied" and narrow-rimmed glasses require more neck extension.[54] For example, nearly full neck extension (i.e., a mean of 40°) is required to

TABLE 9-4 **Cervical Spine ROM Required for Selected ADL**[49-51]				
Activity	Flexion ROM Max	Extension ROM Max	Rotation ROM Max	Lateral Flexion ROM Max
Cervical Spine ROM				
Shampooing hair[49]	46°	—	—	—
Washing face[49]	16°	—	—	—
Eating[49]	—	8°	—	—
Driving[50]* (left-hand drive car)	—	—	36° left 43° right	—
Lumbar Spine ROM				
Putting on a sock in sitting[51]*	48°	—	3°	4°

*Mean values from original source[50,51] rounded to the nearest degree.

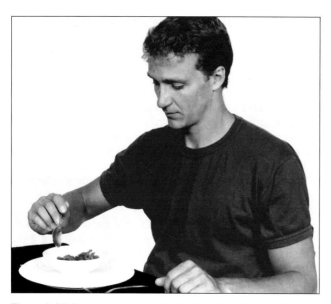

Figure 9-95 Eating: an activity requiring less than full neck flexion ROM.

drink from a narrow champagne flute compared to 0° for a saucer-shaped champagne glass.[54]

Thoracic and Lumbar Spines

Trunk rotation extends the reach of the hands beyond the contralateral side of the body, permits the individual to face different directions without foot movement (Fig. 9-100), and assists one to roll over while in the recumbent position. Rotation of the trunk is achieved through the movement components of the thoracic and lumbar spine and is coupled with slight lateral flexion.[45,46,55] Rotation is a movement that is most free in the upper spinal segments and progressively diminishes in the lower segments.[55]

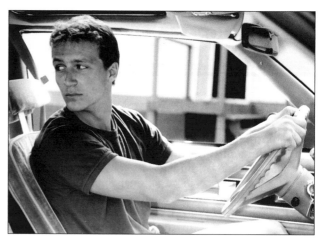

Figure 9-97 An activity requiring full neck rotation ROM.

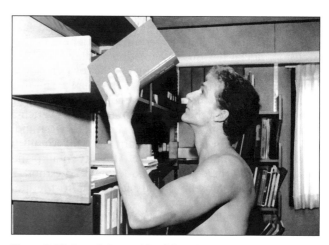

Figure 9-98 An activity requiring full neck extension ROM.

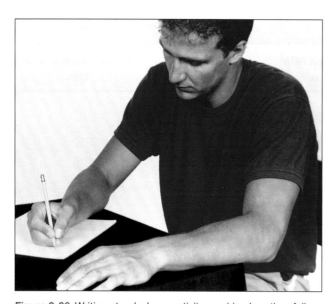

Figure 9-96 Writing at a desk: an activity requiring less than full neck flexion ROM.

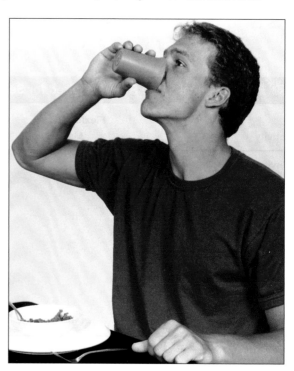

Figure 9-99 Drinking: an activity requiring neck extension.

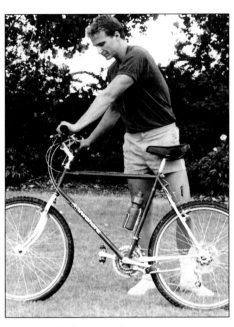

Figure 9-100 Trunk rotation.

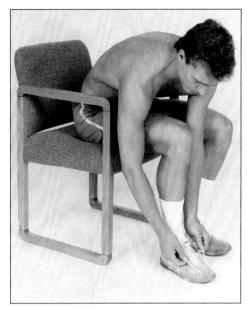

Figure 9-102 Tying a shoelace with the foot flat on the floor requires thoracic and lumbar flexion and neck extension.

The major contribution of the mobility in the lumbar spine to daily functioning is through flexion and extension movements. When combined with the thoracic and cervical segments, the individual can reach the more distal parts of the lower extremities and objects in the environment (Figs. 9-98, 9-101 to 9-103). The final degrees of functional range are achieved through the interaction of the pelvis and hip.[7,14]

When forward flexing to touch the toes (see Figs. 9-93 and 9-94), a coordinated pattern of movement occurs between the lumbar spine and pelvis, called "lumbar–pelvic rhythm,"[56] providing smooth movement and a large excursion of movement for the lower extremity and trunk. The lumbar spine and hip (i.e., as the pelvis moves on the femur) contribute an average of about 40° lumbar spine flexion and 70° hip flexion, respectively, to complete this

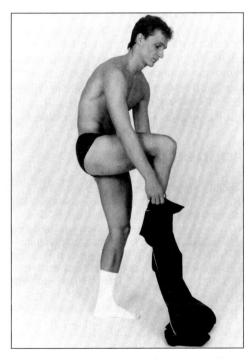

Figure 9-101 Donning a pair of trousers requires flexion of the thoracic and lumbar spines.

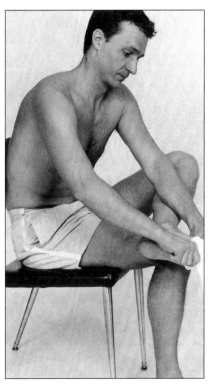

Figure 9-103 Lumbar flexion.

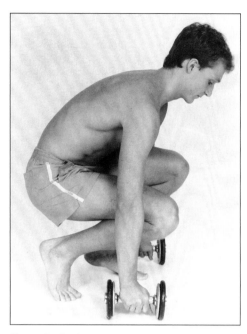

Figure 9-104 Squatting to pick up an object from the floor requires almost full lumbar flexion (i.e., about 95% of full flexion).[59]

forward bending motion.[57] Lumbar and pelvic motions are nearly simultaneous with varying degrees of contribution from the lumbar spine and pelvis throughout range.[57,58] Changing the speed of motion, lifting various size loads, and past history of low back pain may influence the lumbar–pelvic rhythm.[57,58]

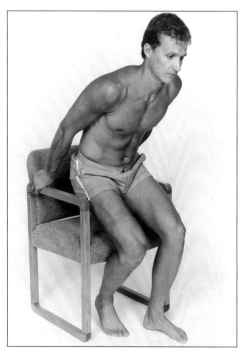

Figure 9-105 Moving from standing to sitting and returning to standing requires about 56% to 66% of full lumbar flexion ROM.[59]

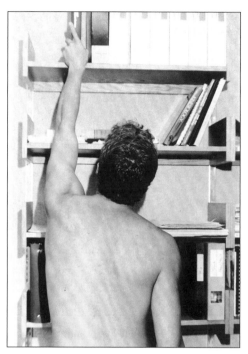

Figure 9-106 Reaching objects overhead requires trunk lateral flexion.

Normal ROM for lumbar spine flexion is about 60°.[59] Sitting to put on a sock (Fig. 9-103) and squatting to pick up an object from the floor (Fig. 9-104) are examples of activities that require almost full lumbar spine flexion (i.e., about 90% and 95% of full flexion, respectively).[59] Moving from standing to sitting and returning to standing position requires about 56% to 66% of full lumbar flexion ROM[59] (Fig. 9-105). The joints in the lumbar spine and L5/S1 approach full flexion in the slouched sitting position.[60]

Activities that require lateral flexion of the spine include reaching down to pick up an object from a low surface at one's side, moving from a side-lying position to sitting on the edge of a bed, and reaching objects overhead (Fig. 9-106). To mount a bicycle, one leg is lifted over the seat of the bicycle and the trunk is laterally flexed to the same side.

References

1. Kapandji IA. *The Physiology of the Joints. Vol 3. The Spinal Column, Pelvic Girdle and Head.* 6th ed. London, UK: Churchill Livingstone Elsevier; 2008.
2. Soames RW, ed. Skeletal system. Salmon S, ed. Muscle. In: *Gray's Anatomy.* 38th ed. New York, NY: Churchill Livingstone; 1995.
3. Berryman Reese N, Bandy WD. *Joint Range of Motion and Muscle Length Testing.* 2nd ed. St. Louis, MO: Saunders Elsevier; 2010.
4. Magee DJ. *Orthopedic Physical Assessment.* 4th ed. Philadelphia, PA: Saunders; 2002.
5. American Academy of Orthopaedic Surgeons. *Joint Motion: Method of Measuring and Recording.* Chicago, IL: AAOS; 1965.
6. Cyriax J. *Textbook of Orthopaedic Medicine. Vol 1. Diagnosis of Soft Tissue Lesions.* 8th ed. London, UK: Bailliere Tindall; 1982.
7. Levangie PK, Norkin CC. *Joint Structure & Function: A Comprehensive Analysis.* 3rd ed. Philadelphia, PA: FA Davis; 2001.

8. Daniels L, Worthingham C. *Muscle Testing: Techniques of Manual Examination.* 5th ed. Philadelphia, PA: WB Saunders; 1986.

9. Youdas JW, Garrett TR, Suman VJ, Bogard CL, Hallman HO, Carey JR. Normal range of motion of the cervical spine: an initial goniometric study. *Phys Ther.* 1992;72:770-780.

10. Balogun JA, Abereoje OK, Olaogun MO, Obajuluwa VA. Inter- and intratester reliability of measuring neck motions with tape measure and Myrin gravity-reference goniometer. *J Orthop Sports Phys Ther.* 1989;10:248-253.

11. Hsieh C-Y, Yeung BW. Active neck motion measurements with a tape measure. *J Orthop Sports Phys Ther.* 1986;8:88-92.

12. American Medical Association. *Guides to the Evaluation of Permanent Impairment.* 5th ed. Chicago, IL: AMA Press; 2001.

13. American Medical Association. *Guides to the Evaluation of Permanent Impairment.* 2nd ed. Chicago, IL: AMA Press; 1984.

14. Soderberg GL. *Kinesiology: Application to Pathological Motion.* 2nd ed. Baltimore, MD: Williams & Wilkins; 1997.

15. Iglarsh ZA, Snyder-Mackler L. Temporomandibular joint and the cervical spine. In: Richardson JK, Iglarsh ZA, eds. *Clinical Orthopaedic Physical Therapy.* Philadelphia, PA: WB Saunders; 1994.

16. Moskovich R. Biomechanics of the cervical spine. In: Nordin M, Frankel VH, eds. *Basic Biomechanics of the Musculoskeletal System.* 3rd ed. Philadelphia, PA: Lippincott Williams & Wilkins; 2001.

17. Performance Attainment Associates. *CROM Procedure Manual: Procedure for Measuring Neck Motion with the CROM.* St. Paul, MN: University of Minnesota; 1988 (copyright University of Minnesota).

18. Mayer TG, Kindraske G, Beals SB, Gatchel RJ. Spinal range of motion: accuracy and sources of error with inclinometric measurement. *Spine.* 1997;22:1976-1984.

19. Performance Attainment Associates, 958 Lydia Drive, Roseville, MN: 55113.

20. Calder I, Picard J, Chapman M, O'Sullivan C, Crockard HA. Mouth opening: a new angle. *Anesthesiology.* 2003;99:799-801.

21. Higbie EJ, Seidel-Cobb D, Taylor LF, Cummings GS. Effect of head position on vertical mandibular opening. *J Orthop Sports Phys Ther.* 1999;29:127-130.

22. Thurnwald PA. The effect of age and gender on normal temporomandibular joint movement. *Physiother Theory Pract.* 1991;7:209-221.

23. Venes D, ed. *Taber's Cyclopedic Medical Dictionary.* 19th ed. Philadelphia, PA: FA Davis; 2001.

24. American Medical Association. *Guides to the Evaluation of Permanent Impairment.* 3rd ed (Revised). Chicago, IL: AMA Press; 1990.

25. Walker N, Bohannon RW, Cameron D. Discriminant validity of temporomandibular joint range of motion measurements obtained with a ruler. *J Orthop Sports Phys Ther.* 2000;30:484-492.

26. Dijkstra PU, De Bont LGM, Stegenga B, Boering G. Temporomandibular joint mobility assessment: a comparison between four methods. *J Oral Rehabil.* 1995;22:439-444.

27. Dworkin SF, LeResche L, DeRouen T, VonKorff M. Assessing clinical signs of temporomandibular disorders: reliability of clinical examiners. *J Prosthet Dent.* 1990;63:574-579.

28. Al-Ani MZ, Gray RJ. Evaluation of three devices used for measuring mouth opening. *Dent Update.* 2004;31(6):346-348, 350.

29. Jordan K. Assessment of published reliability studies for cervical range-of-motion measurement tools. *J Manipulative Physiol Ther.* 2000;23:180-195.

30. de Koning CHP, van den Heuvel SP, Staal JB, Smits-Engelsman BCM, Hendriks EJM. Clinimetric evaluation of active range of motion measures in patients with non-specific neck pain: a systematic review. *Eur Spine J.* 2008;17:905-921.

31. Williams MA, McCarthy CJ, Chorti A, Cooke MW, Gates S. Literature Review. A systematic review of reliability and validity studies of methods for measuring active and passive cervical range of motion. *J Manipulative Physiol Ther.* 2010;33(2):138.

32. Rondoni A, Rossettini G, Ristori D, et al. Intrarater and inter-rater reliability of active cervical range of motion in patients with nonspecific neck pain measured with technological and common use devices: a systematic review with meta-regression. *J Manipulative Physiol Ther.* 2017;40(8):597-608.

33. White AA, Panjabi MM. *Clinical Biomechanics of the Spine.* Philadelphia, PA: JB Lippincott; 1978.

34. Neumann DA. *Kinesiology of the Musculoskeletal System: Foundations for Rehabilitation.* 2nd ed. St. Louis, MO: Mosby Elsevier; 2010.

35. van Adrichem JAM, van der Korst JK. Assessment of the flexibility of the lumbar spine. *Scand J Rheumatol.* 1973;2:87-91.

36. Mellin GP. Accuracy of measuring lateral flexion of the spine with a tape. *Clin Biomech (Bristol, Avon).* 1986;1:85-89.

37. Frost M, Stuckey S, Smalley LA, Dorman G. Reliability of measuring trunk motions in centimeters. *Phys Ther.* 1982;62:1431-1437.

38. Pearcy MJ. Twisting mobility of the human back in flexed postures. *Spine.* 1993;18:114-119.

39. Harris J, Johansen J, Pedersen S, LaPier TK. Site of measurement and subject position affect chest expansion measurements. *Cardiopulm Phys Ther J.* 1997;8:12-17.

40. Moll JMH, Wright V. An objective clinical study of chest expansion. *Ann Rheum Dis.* 1972;31:1-8.

41. Neustadt DH. Ankylosing spondylitis. *Postgrad Med.* 1977;61:124-135.

42. Littlewood C, May S. Measurement of range of movement in the lumbar spine—what methods are valid? A systematic review. *Physiotherapy.* 2007;93:201-211.

43. Castro MP, Stebbings SM, Milosavljevic S, Bussey MD. Criterion-concurrent validity of spinal mobility tests in ankylosing spondylitis: a systematic review of the literature. *J Rheumatol.* 2015;42(2):243-251.

44. Essendrop M, Maul I, Läubli T, Riihimäki H, Schibye B. Measures of low back function: a review of reproducibility studies. *Phys Ther Sport.* 2003;4:137-151. Reprinted from *Clinical Biomech.* 2002;17:235-249.

45. Smith LK, Weiss EL, Lemkuhl LD. *Brunnstrom's Clinical Kinesiology.* 5th ed. Philadelphia, PA: FA Davis; 1996.

46. Lindh M. Biomechanics of the lumbar spine. In: Nordin M, Frankel VH. *Basic Biomechanics of the Musculoskeletal System.* 2nd ed. Philadelphia, PA: Lea & Febiger; 1989.

47. Cailliet R. *Neck and Arm Pain.* 3rd ed. Philadelphia, PA: FA Davis; 1991.

48. Sterling AC, Cobian DG, Anderson PA, Heiderscheit C. Annual frequency and magnitude of neck motion in healthy individuals. *Spine.* 2008;33(17):1882-1888.

49. Henmi S, Yonenobu K, Masatomi T, Oda K. A biomechanical study of daily living using neck and upper limbs with an optical three-dimensional motion analysis system. *Mod Rheumatol.* 2006;16:289-293.

50. Shugg JAJ, Jackson CD, Dickey JP. Cervical spine rotation and range of motion: pilot measurements during driving. *Traffic Inj Prev.* 2011;12:82-87.

51. Shum GLK, Crosbie J, Lee RYW. Symptomatic and asymptomatic movement coordination of the lumbar spine and hip during an everyday activity. *Spine.* 2005;30(23):E697-E702.

52. Hutton JT, Shapiro I, Christians B. Functional significance of restricted gaze. *Arch Phys Med Rehabil.* 1982;63:617-619.

53. Muñoz M. Congenital absence of the inferior rectus muscle. *Am J Ophthalmol*. 1992;121:327-329.
54. Pemberton PL, Calder I, O'Sullivan C, Crockard HA. The champagne angle. *Anaesthesia*. 2002;57:402-403.
55. MacConaill MA, Basmajian JV. *Muscles and Movements: A Basis for Human Kinesiology*. Huntington, WV: RE Krieger; 1977.
56. Cailliet R. *Low Back Pain Syndrome*. 5th ed. Philadelphia, PA: FA Davis; 1995.
57. Esola M, McClure PW, Fitzgerald GK, Siegler S. Analysis of lumbar spine and hip motion during forward bending in subjects with and without a history of low back pain. *Spine*. 1996;21(1):71-78.
58. Granata KP, Sanford AH. Lumbar-pelvic coordination is influenced by lifting task parameters. *Spine*. 2000;25(11):1412-1418.
59. Hsieh CJ, Pringle RK. Range of motion of the lumbar spine required for four activities of daily living. *J Manipulative Physiol Ther*. 1994;17:353-358.
60. Dunk NM, Kedgley AE, Jenkyn TR, Callaghan JP. Evidence of a pelvis-driven flexion pattern: are the joints of the lower lumbar spine fully flexed in seated postures? *Clin Biomech (Bristol, Avon)*. 2009;24:164-168.

EXERCISES AND QUESTIONS

See the Answer Guide in Appendix E for suggested answers to the following exercises and questions.

1. PALPATION

A. For each of the spinal movements listed below:
   - Identify the anatomic landmarks used to measure the spinal ROM using a **tape measure**
   - Palpate these landmarks on a partner
   - Identify other spinal movements that also use all of the same anatomic landmarks to evaluate the spinal ROM.
     i.   Neck flexion
     ii. Neck lateral flexion
     iii. Thoracolumbar spine extension
     iv. Lumbar spine flexion
     v.   Trunk rotation

B. For each of the spinal movements listed below:
   - Identify the anatomic landmarks used to measure the spinal ROM using **inclinometers**
   - Palpate these landmarks on a partner
   - Identify other spinal movements that use all of the same anatomic landmarks to evaluate the spinal ROM.
     i.   Neck extension
     ii. Thoracolumbar spine extension
     iii. Lumbar spine flexion
     iv. Trunk lateral flexion
     v.   Thoracic spine rotation

C. Identify the surface anatomy locations the therapist would use when using the **CROM** to assess neck ROM.

2. ASSESSMENT AND MEASUREMENT OF AROM

For each of the movements listed below, demonstrate measurement of the AROM on a partner *using a tape measure* and answer the question(s) that follow. Have a third partner evaluate your performance using the appropriate Practice Makes Perfect Summary & Evaluation Forms at http://thepoint.lww.com/ClarksonJM2e.
   Record your findings on the recording form on page 312.

TMJ Movements
   i.   Identify the jaw movements that occur at the TMJs.
   ii. Describe the articular surfaces that make up the TMJs.
   iii. Identify the TMJ movements that can be measured using a ruler; demonstrate the measurement of these movements.
   iv. Describe how functional ROM can be determined for mouth opening.

Neck Extension
   If the mouth is open when measuring neck extension using a tape measure, what effect will this have on the ROM measurement?

Neck Left Lateral Flexion
   What substitute movements should be avoided when assessing neck lateral flexion?

Neck Right Rotation
   i.   If a therapist measures neck rotation using inclinometry, what is the start position for the measurement?
   ii. Where would the therapist position the inclinometer(s) to take the measurement for neck rotation?

Thoracolumbar Spine Flexion

Can thoracolumbar spine flexion be measured using inclinometers? If so, identify the inclinometer placements used to take the measurement.

Lumbar Spine Flexion

Lumbar spine flexion ROM can be measured using a tape measure. Identify other lumbar spine ROM that can be measured using a tape measure and the same anatomical landmarks.

Thoracolumbar Spine Extension (Prone Press-Up)

Identify factors that may result in inaccurate ROM measurements when measuring thoracolumbar spine extension ROM using the prone press-up position and a tape measure.

Thoracolumbar Spine Rotation

Identify the anatomic landmarks used to position the tape measure for the measurement of thoracolumbar spine rotation AROM.

Thoracolumbar Spine Lateral Flexion

i.   What substitute movements should be avoided when assessing thoracolumbar spine lateral flexion?

ii. Demonstrate the two different methods that may be used to assess thoracolumbar spine lateral flexion using a tape measure. Have a partner evaluate your performance using Practice Makes Perfect Summary & Evaluation Forms 9-29 and 9-30.

iii. Can thoracolumbar spine lateral flexion AROM be measured using inclinometers? If so, identify where the inclinometers would be placed to take the measurement.

AROM RECORDING FORM

Patient's Name _____   Age _____

Diagnosis _____   Date of Onset _____

Therapist Name _____   AROM Measurements

Therapist Signature _____   Measurement Instrument _____

				Left Side / Date of Measurement			Right Side		
	*		*	**Date of Measurement**	*		*		
				Head, Neck and Trunk					
				Mandible: Depression					
				Protrusion					
				Lateral deviation					
				Neck: Flexion (0–45°)					
				Extension (0–45°)					
				Lateral flexion (0–45°)					
				Rotation (0–60°)					
				Trunk: Flexion (0–80°, 10 cm)					
				Extension (0–20–30°)					
				Lateral flexion (0–35°)					
				Rotation (0–45°)					
				Hypermobility:					
				Comments:					

3. MUSCLE LENGTH ASSESSSMENT AND MEASUREMENT

Toe-Touch Test

   i.   The toe-touch test measures only hamstring muscle length. True or false?

   ii. The toe-touch test measures only spinal ROM. True or false?

  iii. The toe-touch test provides a composite measure of hip, spine, and shoulder girdle ROM. True or false?

4. FUNCTIONAL ROM AT THE HEAD, NECK, AND TRUNK

A. For each spinal motion listed below, identify three daily activities that require the specified movement:

   i.   thoracolumbar flexion

   ii. thoracolumbar extension

  iii. cervical spine rotation

  iv. cervical spine lateral flexion

B. Sit and keep your head in the anatomical position. Move your eyes to look up, down, and side to side. Note the range of your field of vision. If you could not move your neck, what strategies would you use to increase your field of vision?

C. Identify the TMJ, cervical, thoracic, and/or lumbar spine motion(s) required to perform the following activities:

   i.   sitting and tying a shoe with the foot flat on the floor

   ii. combing the hair on the back of the head

  iii. brushing one's teeth

  iv. reaching for a wallet in a back pocket

SECTION III

Appendices

Sample Numerical Recording Form: Range of Motion Assessment and Measurement

Patient's Name _____   Age _____

Diagnosis _____   Date of Onset _____

Therapist _____   AROM ☐   PROM ☐

Signature _____   Measurement Instrument _____

Recording:

1. The Neutral Zero Method defined by the American Academy of Orthopaedic Surgeons[1] is used for measurement and recording.

2. Average ranges defined by the American Academy of Orthopaedic Surgeons[1] are provided in parentheses.

3. The columns designated with asterisks (*) are used for indicating limitation of range of motion and referencing for summarization.

4. Space is left at the end of each section to record hypermobile ranges and comments regarding positioning of the patient or body part, measuring instrument, edema, pain, and/or end feel.

Patient's Name _____   Therapist _____

Left Side				Therapist Initials	Right Side			
	*		*	**Date of Measurement**		*		*
				Head, Neck, and Trunk				
				Mandible: Depression				
				Protrusion				
				Lateral deviation				
				Neck: Flexion (0–45°)				
				Extension (0–45°)				
				Lateral flexion (0–45°)				
				Rotation (0–60°)				
				Trunk: Flexion (0–80°, 10 cm)				
				Extension (0–20–30°)				
				Lateral flexion (0–35°)				
				Rotation (0–45°)				
				Hypermobility:				
				Comments:				

[1]American Academy of Orthopaedic Surgeons: Joint Motion: Method of Measuring and Recording. Chicago: AAOS; 1965.

Clarkson HM. *Joint Motion, Muscle Length, and Function Assessment: A Research-Based Practical Guide*. 2nd ed, Baltimore: Wolters Kluwer, 2020.

Patient's Name _____   Therapist _____

					Left Side				Right Side			
	*		*		**Therapist Initials**			*		*	
					Date of Measurement						
					Scapula						
					Elevation						
					Depression						
					Abduction						
					Adduction						
					Shoulder Complex						
					Elevation through Flexion (0–180°)						
					Elevation through Abduction (0–180°)						
					Shoulder (Glenohumeral) Joint						
					Flexion (0–120°)[2]						
					Abduction (0–90° to 120°)[2]						
					Extension (0–60°)						
					Horizontal abduction (0–45°)						
					Horizontal adduction (0–135°)						
					Internal rotation (0–70°)						
					External rotation (0–90°)						
					Hypermobility: Comments:						
					Elbow and Forearm						
					Flexion (0–150°)						
					Supination (0–80°)						
					Pronation (0–80°)						
					Hypermobility: Comments:						

Patient's Name _____   Therapist _____

Left Side					Right Side			
	*		*	**Therapist Initials**	*		*	
				Date of Measurement				
				Wrist				
				Flexion　　　　　(0–80°)				
				Extension　　　　(0–70°)				
				Ulnar deviation　(0–30°)				
				Radial deviation　(0–20°)				
				Hypermobility:				
				Comments:				
				Thumb				
				CM flexion　　　(0–15°)				
				CM extension　(0–20°)				
				CM abduction　(0–70°)				
				MCP flexion　　(0–50°)				
				IP flexion　　　(0–80°)				
				Opposition				
				Hypermobility:				
				Comments:				
				Fingers				
				MCP digit 2 flexion　　(0–90°)				
				extension　(0–45°)				
				abduction				
				adduction				
				MCP digit 3 flexion　　(0–90°)				
				extension　(0–45°)				
				abduction (radial)				
				adduction (ulnar)				
				MCP digit 4 flexion　　(0–90°)				
				extension　(0–45°)				
				abduction				
				adduction				

Clarkson HM. *Joint Motion, Muscle Length, and Function Assessment: A Research-Based Practical Guide*. 2nd ed, Baltimore: Wolters Kluwer, 2020.

Patient's Name _____   Therapist _____

				Therapist Initials				
	★		★	**Therapist Initials**	★		★	
				Date of Measurement				
				Fingers (continued)				
				MCP digit 5 flexion (0–90°)				
				extension (0–45°)				
				abduction				
				adduction				
				PIP digit 2 flexion (0–100°)				
				3 flexion (0–100°)				
				4 flexion (0–100°)				
				5 flexion (0–100°)				
				DIP digit 2 flexion (0–90°)				
				3 flexion (0–90°)				
				4 flexion (0–90°)				
				5 flexion (0–90°)				
				Composite finger abduction/thumb extension—Distance between:				
				Thumb–digit 2				
				Digit 2–digit 3				
				Digit 3–digit 4				
				Digit 4–digit 5				
				Composite flexion—Distance between:				
				Finger pulp-distal palmar crease				
				Finger pulp-proximal palmar crease				
				Hypermobility: Comments:				

Above the table: **Left Side** (left columns) / **Right Side** (right columns)

Patient's Name _____   Therapist _____

	Left Side					**Right Side**	
	*		*	**Therapist Initials**	*		*	
				Date of Measurement				
				Hip				
				Flexion (0–120°)				
				Extension (0–30°)				
				Abduction (0–45°)				
				Adduction (0–30°)				
				Internal rotation (0–45°)				
				External rotation (0–45°)				
				Hypermobility: Comments:				
				Knee				
				Flexion (0–135°)				
				Tibial rotation				
				Patellar mobility—Distal glide				
				Patellar mobility—Medial-lateral glide				
				Hypermobility: Comments:				
				Ankle				
				Dorsiflexion (0–20°)				
				Plantarflexion (0–50°)				
				Inversion (0–35°)				
				Eversion (0–15°)				
				Hypermobility: Comments:				

Clarkson HM. *Joint Motion, Muscle Length, and Function Assessment: A Research-Based Practical Guide*. 2nd ed, Baltimore: Wolters Kluwer, 2020.

Patient's Name _____   Therapist _____

				Left Side / Therapist Initials etc.		Right Side		
				Left Side		**Right Side**		
	*		*	**Therapist Initials**	*		*	
				Date of Measurement				
				Toes				
				MTP great toe flexion (0–45°)				
				extension (0–70°)				
				abduction				
				MTP digit 2 flexion (0–40°)				
				extension (0–40°)				
				MTP digit 3 flexion (0–40°)				
				extension (0–40°)				
				MTP digit 4 flexion (0–40°)				
				extension (0–40°)				
				MTP digit 5 flexion (0–40°)				
				extension (0–40°)				
				IP great toe flexion (0–90°)				
				PIP digit 2 flexion (0–35°)				
				PIP digit 3 flexion (0–35°)				
				PIP digit 4 flexion (0–35°)				
				PIP digit 5 flexion (0–35°)				
				Hypermobility: Comments:				

Summary of Limitation:

Additional Comments:

[1]American Academy of Orthopaedic Surgeons: *Joint Motion: Method of Measuring and Recording*. Chicago: AAOS; 1965.
[2]Levangie PK, Norkin CC. *Joint Structure and Function: A Comprehensive Analysis*. 3rd ed. Philadelphia: FA Davis; 2001.

Practice Makes Perfect–Summary & Evaluation Forms

Introduction

To become proficient in the clinical skills of assessment and measurement of joint ROM and muscle length requires knowledge, attention to detail, and practice.

This appendix contains Practice Makes Perfect–Summary & Evaluation Forms for the assessment and measurement of active range of motion (AROM) and passive range of motion (PROM) of the extremity joints, muscle length, and AROM of the temporomandibular joint (TMJ), neck, and trunk, as presented in Joint Motion, Muscle Length, and Function Assessment: A Research-Based Practical Guide, 2e.

The criteria used to perform these assessment and measurement techniques are listed in a chart/checklist format in each Practice Makes Perfect–Summary & Evaluation Form. These forms can be printed for use, or used on a computer or iPad by clicking on the boxes to insert an "X" in the box, when the criterion is met. The "Sample Numeric Recording Form: ROM Measurement" in Appendix A can be accessed at http://thepoint.lww.com/ClarksonJM2e and used to record the joint AROM, PROM, end feel, and/or muscle length findings.

The Summary & Evaluation Forms serve as:

i. excellent summaries and a quick clinical reference tool of the clinical skills presented in this textbook,

ii. a means to test your proficiency in the application of the clinical skills, and prepare for Practical Examinations and clinical practice,

iii. Practical Examination Forms for Faculty use in evaluating and grading student performance.

Preparing for practical examinations can be a stressful time, however, with the Practice Makes Perfect–Summary & Evaluations Forms you will have the main criteria Faculty use to evaluate your proficiency in the assessment and measurement of joint ROM and muscle length.

Practice Makes Perfect: Summary & Evaluation Forms can be used in the classroom, in study groups, or in Practical Examinations. In classroom or study group situations, a group of three persons is the ideal, one person to serve as an examiner another the patient, and the student whose proficiency is being evaluated.

Practice Makes Perfect: Summary & Evaluation Forms

PROM Assessment and Measurement: Shoulder Complex

Scapular Elevation 🔊 (Form 3-1)
Scapular Depression 🔊 (Form 3-2)
Scapular Abduction 🔊 (Form 3-3)
Scapular Adduction 🔊 (Form 3-4)
Shoulder Elevation Through Flexion 🔊 (Form 3-5)
Glenohumeral Joint Flexion 🔊 (Form 3-6)
Shoulder Extension 🔊 (Form 3-7)
Shoulder Elevation Through Abduction 🔊 (Form 3-8)
Glenohumeral Joint Abduction 🔊 (Form 3-9)
Shoulder Horizontal Abduction 🔊 (Form 3-10)
Shoulder Horizontal Adduction 🔊 (Form 3-11)
Shoulder Internal Rotation 🔊 (Form 3-12)
Shoulder External Rotation 🔊 (Form 3-13)

Muscle Length Assessment and Measurement: Shoulder Complex

Pectoralis Major 🔊 (Form 3-14)
Pectoralis Minor 🔊 (Form 3-15)

PROM Assessment and Measurement: Elbow and Forearm

Elbow Flexion 🔊 (Form 4-1)
Elbow Extension/Hyperextension 🔊 (Form 4-2)
Forearm Supination 🔊 (Form 4-3)
Forearm Pronation 🔊 (Form 4-4)

Muscle Length Assessment and Measurement: Elbow and Forearm

Biceps Brachii 🔊 (Form 4-5)
Triceps Brachii 🔊 (Form 4-6)

PROM Assessment and Measurement: Wrist and Hand

Wrist Flexion 🔊 (Form 5-1)
Wrist Extension 🔊 (Form 5-2)
Wrist Ulnar Deviation 🔊 (Form 5-3)
Wrist Radial Deviation 🔊 (Form 5-4)
Finger MCP Flexion 🔊 (Form 5-5)
Finger MCP Extension 🔊 (Form 5-6)
Finger MCP Abduction 🔊 (Form 5-7)
Finger MCP Adduction 🔊 (Form 5-8)
Finger IP Flexion 🔊 (Form 5-9)
Finger IP Extension 🔊 (Form 5-10)
Thumb CM Flexion 🔊 (Form 5-11)
Thumb CM Extension 🔊 (Form 5-12)
Thumb MCP Flexion 🔊 (Form 5-13)
Thumb MCP Extension 🔊 (Form 5-14)
Thumb IP Flexion 🔊 (Form 5-15)
Thumb IP Extension 🔊 (Form 5-16)
Thumb CM Abduction 🔊 (Form 5-17)
Thumb and Fifth Finger Opposition 🔊 (Form 5-18)

Muscle Length Assessment and Measurement: Wrist and Hand

Finger Flexors 🔊 (Form 5-19)

(i.e., Flexor Digitorum Superficialis, Flexor Digitorum Profundus, Flexor Digiti Minimi, and Palmaris Longus)

Finger Extensors 🔊 (Form 5-20)

(i.e., Extensor Digitorum Communis, Extensor Indicis Proprius, and Extensor Digiti Minimi)

Lumbricales 🔊 (Form 5-21)

PROM Assessment and Measurement: Hip

Hip Flexion 🔊 (Form 6-1)
Hip Extension 🔊 (Form 6-2)
Hip Abduction 🔊 (Form 6-3)
Hip Adduction 🔊 (Form 6-4)
Hip Internal Rotation 🔊 (Form 6-5)
Hip External Rotation 🔊 (Form 6-6)

Muscle Length Assessment and Measurement: Hip

Hamstrings Passive Straight Leg Raise (PSLR) 🔊 (Form 6-7)
Hip Flexors (Thomas Test) 🔊 (Form 6-8)
Hip Adductors 🔊 (Form 6-9)
Tensor Fascia Latae (Iliotibial Band) (Ober's Test) 🔊 (Form 6-10)
Tensor Fascia Latae (Iliotibial Band) (Ober's Test: Trunk Prone) 🔊 (Form 6-11)

PROM Assessment and Measurement: Knee

Knee Flexion 🔊 (Form 7-1)
Knee Extension/Hyperextension 🔊 (Form 7-2)
Patellar Distal Glide 🔊 (Form 7-3)
Patellar Medial-Lateral Glide 🔊 (Form 7-4)
Tibial Rotation 🔊 (Form 7-5)

Muscle Length Assessment and Measurement: Knee

Hamstrings Passive Knee Extension (PKE) Supine 🔊 (Form 7-6)
Hamstrings Alternate Position–Sitting 🔊 (Form 7-7)
Rectus Femoris (prone one foot on the floor) 🔊 (Form 7-8)
Rectus Femoris Alternate Position–Ely's Test 🔊 (Form 7-9)
Rectus Femoris Alternate Position–Thomas Test Position 🔊 (Form 7-10)

PROM Assessment and Measurement: Ankle and Foot

Ankle Dorsiflexion 🔊 (Form 8-1)
Ankle Plantarflexion 🔊 (Form 8-2)
AROM: Subtalar Inversion and Eversion 🔊 (Form 8-3)
Subtalar Inversion 🔊 (Form 8-4)
Subtalar Eversion 🔊 (Form 8-5)
Ankle and Foot Supination: Inversion Component 🔊 (Form 8-6)
Ankle and Foot Pronation: Eversion Component 🔊 (Form 8-7)
Great toe MTP Joint Flexion 🔊 (Form 8-8)
Great toe MTP Joint Extension 🔊 (Form 8-9)
Great toe MTP Joint Abduction 🔊 (Form 8-10)
Great toe MTP Joint Adduction 🔊 (Form 8-11)
Great toe IP Joint Flexion 🔊 (Form 8-12)
Great toe IP Joint Extension 🔊 (Form 8-13)

Muscle Length Assessment and Measurement: Ankle and Foot

Gastrocnemius 🔊 (Form 8-14)

AROM Assessment and Measurement: Head, Neck, and Trunk

TMJ: Occlusion and Depression of the Mandible 🔊 (Form 9-1)
TMJ: Protrusion of the Mandible 🔊 (Form 9-2)
TMJ: Lateral Deviation of the Mandible 🔊 (Form 9-3)
Neck Flexion:
Tape Measure (Form 🔊 9-4)
Inclinometer (Form 🔊 9-6)

CROM ◐ (Form 9-8)
Universal Goniometer ◐ (Form 9-10)
Neck Extension:
Tape Measure ◐ (Form 9-5)
Inclinometer ◐ (Form 9-7)
CROM ◐ (Form 9-9)
Universal Goniometer ◐ (Form 9-11)
Neck Lateral Flexion:
Tape Measure ◐ (Form 9-12)
Inclinometer ◐ (Form 9-13)
CROM ◐ (Form 9-14)
Universal Goniometer ◐ (Form 9-15)
Neck Rotation:
Tape Measure ◐ (Form 9-16)
Inclinometer ◐ (Form 9-17)
CROM ◐ (Form 9-18)
Universal Goniometer ◐ (Form 9-19)
Trunk Flexion—Thoracolumbar Spine:
Tape Measure ◐ (Form 9-20)
Inclinometer ◐ (Form 9-22)
Trunk Extension—Thoracolumbar Spine:
Tape Measure ◐ (Form 9-21)
Inclinometer ◐ (Form 9-23)
Trunk Extension—Thoracolumbar Spine (prone press-up):
Tape Measure ◐ (Form 9-24)

Trunk Flexion—Lumbar Spine:
Tape Measure (Modified Modified Schöber Method ◐ (Form 9-25)
Inclinometer ◐ (Form 9-27)
Trunk Extension—Lumbar Spine:
Tape Measure ◐ (Form 9-26)
Inclinometer ◐ (Form 9-28)
Trunk Lateral Flexion—Thoracolumbar Spine
Tape Measure—(Fingertip-to-Floor Method) ◐ (Form 9-29)
Tape Measure—(Thigh Method) ◐ (Form 9-30)
Inclinometer ◐ (Form 9-31)
Universal Goniometer ◐ (Form 9-32)
Trunk Rotation—Thoracolumbar Spine:
Tape Measure ◐ (Form 9-33)
Trunk Rotation—Thoracic Spine:
Inclinometer ◐ (Form 9-34)
Chest Expansion
Tape Measure ◐ (Form 9-35)

Muscle Length Assessment and Measurement: Trunk

Trunk Extensors and Hamstrings (Toe-Touch Test) ◐ (Form 9-36)

PROM Assessment and Measurement Testing: Shoulder Complex

Movement	Start Position	Stabilization	Therapist's Hand Placement	End Position	Recording	Instructions	Handling/ Comments
SCAPULAR ELEVATION Form 3-1	1. Side-ly, hips and knees flexed ☐ 2. Head supported on pillow ☐ 3. Arm at side ☐	1. Trunk stabilized ☐	1. One hand: on superior aspect of shoulder girdle ☐ 2. Other hand: cups inferior angle of scapula, while forearm supports patient's upper extremity ☐	1. Therapist elevates scapula to limit of motion ☐ 2. Full PROM achieved ☐ 3. Trunk stabilized ☐	1. Full PROM ☐ 2. End feel ☐	1. Verbal (clear/concise) ☐ 2. Demonstration (clear) ☐	1. Adequate support of limb/limb segment ☐ 2. Comfortable grip ☐ 3. Safe body mechanics of therapist ☐ Comments:
SCAPULAR DEPRESSION Form 3-2	1. Side-ly, hips and knees flexed ☐ 2. Head supported on pillow ☐ 3. Arm at side ☐	1. Trunk stabilized ☐	1. One hand: on superior aspect of shoulder girdle ☐ 2. Other hand: cups inferior angle of scapula, while forearm supports patient's upper extremity ☐	1. Therapist depresses scapula to limit of motion ☐ 2. Full PROM achieved ☐ 3. Trunk stabilized ☐	1. Full PROM ☐ 2. End feel ☐	1. Verbal (clear/concise) ☐ 2. Demonstration (clear) ☐	1. Adequate support of limb/limb segment ☐ 2. Comfortable grip ☐ 3. Safe body mechanics of therapist ☐ Comments:
SCAPULAR ABDUCTION Form 3-3	1. Side-ly, hips and knees flexed ☐ 2. Head supported on pillow ☐ 3. Arm at side ☐	1. Trunk stabilized ☐	1. One hand: on superior aspect of shoulder girdle ☐ 2. Other hand: grasps vertebral border and inferior angle of scapula, while forearm supports patient's upper extremity ☐	1. Therapist abducts scapula to limit of motion ☐ 2. Full PROM achieved ☐ 3. Trunk stabilized ☐	1. Full PROM ☐ 2. End feel ☐	1. Verbal (clear/concise) ☐ 2. Demonstration (clear) ☐	1. Adequate support of limb/limb segment ☐ 2. Comfortable grip ☐ 3. Safe body mechanics of therapist ☐ Comments:
SCAPULAR ADDUCTION Form 3-4	1. Side-ly, hips and knees flexed ☐ 2. Head supported on pillow ☐ 3. Arm at side ☐	1. Trunk stabilized ☐	1. One hand: on superior aspect of shoulder girdle ☐ 2. Other hand: grasps axillary border and inferior angle of scapula, while forearm supports patient's upper extremity ☐	1. Therapist adducts scapula to limit of motion ☐ 2. Full PROM achieved ☐ 3. Trunk stabilized ☐	1. Full PROM ☐ 2. End feel ☐	1. Verbal (clear/concise) ☐ 2. Demonstration (clear) ☐	1. Adequate support of limb/limb segment ☐ 2. Comfortable grip ☐ 3. Safe body mechanics of therapist ☐ Comments:

STEP 1 — **STEP 2**

PROM Measurement: Using a Universal Goniometer

Movement	PROM Assessment of End Feel	Start Position	Axis	Stationary Arm	End Position	Movable Arm	Recording	Instructions	Handling/Comments
SHOULDER ELEVATION THROUGH FLEXION Form 3-5	1. Start position ☐ 2. Stabilized ☐ 3. Therapist distal hand placement ☐ 4. End position (Full PROM achieved) ☐ 5. End Feel ☐	1. Crook ly ☐ 2. Arm at side, palm faces medially ☐ 3. Trunk stabilized ☐	1. Lateral aspect center humeral head ☐	1. Parallel lateral midline of trunk ☐ 2. Position maintained for start position ☐ 3. Position maintained for end position ☐	1. Humerus moved anteriorly and upward to limit of motion ☐ 2. Scapular and glenohumeral motion ☐ 3. Full PROM achieved ☐ 4. Trunk stabilized ☐	1. Parallel long axis of humerus ☐ 2. Position maintained for start position ☐ 3. Position maintained for end position ☐	1. Full PROM ☐ 2. End feel ☐	1. Verbal (clear/concise) ☐ 2. Demonstration (clear) ☐	1. Adequate support of limb/limb segment ☐ 2. Comfortable grip ☐ 3. Safe body mechanics of therapist ☐ Comments:
GLENO-HUMERAL JOINT FLEXION Form 3-6	1. Start position ☐ 2. Stabilized ☐ 3. Therapist distal hand placement ☐ 4. End position (Full PROM achieved) ☐ 5. End Feel ☐	1. Crook ly ☐ 2. Arm at side, palm faces medially ☐ 3. Trunk stabilized ☐ 4. Scapula stabilized ☐	1. Lateral aspect center humeral head ☐	1. Parallel lateral midline of trunk ☐ 2. Position maintained for start position ☐ 3. Position maintained for end position ☐	1. Humerus moved anteriorly and upward to limit of motion ☐ 2. Glenohumeral joint motion only ☐ 3. Full PROM achieved ☐ 4. Trunk stabilized ☐ 5. Scapula stabilized ☐	1. Parallel long axis of humerus ☐ 2. Position maintained for start position ☐ 3. Position maintained for end position ☐	1. Full PROM ☐ 2. End feel ☐	1. Verbal (clear/concise) ☐ 2. Demonstration (clear) ☐	1. Adequate support of limb/limb segment ☐ 2. Comfortable grip ☐ 3. Safe body mechanics of therapist ☐ Comments:
SHOULDER EXTENSION Form 3-7	1. Start position ☐ 2. Stabilized ☐ 3. Therapist distal hand placement ☐ 4. End position (Full PROM achieved) ☐ 5. End Feel ☐	1. Prone ☐ 2. Arm at side, palm faces medially ☐ 3. Scapula stabilized ☐	1. Lateral aspect center humeral head ☐	1. Parallel lateral midline of trunk ☐ 2. Position maintained for start position ☐ 3. Position maintained for end position ☐	1. Humerus moved posteriorly to limit of glenohumeral joint motion ☐ 2. Full PROM achieved ☐ 3. Scapula stabilized ☐	1. Parallel long axis of humerus, pointing to lateral epicondyle of humerus ☐ 2. Position maintained for start position ☐ 3. Position maintained for end position ☐	1. Full PROM ☐ 2. End feel ☐	1. Verbal (clear/concise) ☐ 2. Demonstration (clear) ☐	1. Adequate support of limb/limb segment ☐ 2. Comfortable grip ☐ 3. Safe body mechanics of therapist ☐ Comments:

(continues)

PROM Assessment and Measurement Testing: Shoulder Complex (*continued*)

STEP 1 — STEP 2

PROM Measurement: Using a Universal Goniometer

Movement	PROM Assessment of End Feel (STEP 1)	Start Position	Axis	Stationary Arm	End Position	Movable Arm	Recording	Instructions	Handling/Comments
SHOULDER ELEVATION THROUGH ABDUCTION Form 3-8	1. Start position ☐ 2. Stabilized ☐ 3. Therapist distal hand placement ☐ 4. End position (Full PROM achieved) ☐ 5. End Feel ☐	1. Supine ☐ 2. Arm at side, in adduction and external rotation ☐ 3. Trunk stabilized ☐	1. Midpoint anterior aspect glenohumeral joint, about 1.3 cm inferior and lateral to coracoid process ☐	1. Parallel sternum ☐ 2. Position maintained for start position ☐ 3. Position maintained for end position ☐	1. Humerus moved laterally and upward to limit of motion ☐ 2. Scapular and glenohumeral motion ☐ 3. Full PROM achieved ☐ 4. Trunk stabilized ☐	1. Parallel long axis of humerus ☐ 2. Position maintained for start position ☐ 3. Position maintained for end position ☐	1. Full PROM ☐ 2. End feel ☐	1. Verbal (clear/concise) ☐ 2. Demonstration (clear) ☐	1. Adequate support of limb/limb segment ☐ 2. Comfortable grip ☐ 3. Safe body mechanics of therapist ☐ Comments:
GLENOHUMERAL JOINT ABDUCTION Form 3-9	1. Start position ☐ 2. Stabilized ☐ 3. Therapist distal hand placement ☐ 4. End position (Full PROM achieved) ☐ 5. End feel ☐	1. Supine ☐ 2. Arm at side, elbow flexed to 90° ☐ 3. Scapula and clavicle stabilized ☐	1. Midpoint anterior aspect glenohumeral joint, about 1.3 cm inferior and lateral to coracoid process ☐	1. Parallel sternum ☐ 2. Position maintained for start position ☐ 3. Position maintained for end position ☐	1. Humerus moved laterally and upward to limit of motion ☐ 2. Glenohumeral joint motion only ☐ 3. Full PROM achieved ☐ 4. Scapula and clavicle stabilized ☐	1. Parallel long axis of humerus ☐ 2. Position maintained for start position ☐ 3. Position maintained for end position ☐	1. Full PROM ☐ 2. End feel ☐	1. Verbal (clear/concise) ☐ 2. Demonstration (clear) ☐	1. Adequate support of limb/limb segment ☐ 2. Comfortable grip ☐ 3. Safe body mechanics of therapist ☐ Comments:
SHOULDER HORIZONTAL ABDUCTION Form 3-10	1. Start position ☐ 2. Stabilized ☐ 3. Therapist distal hand placement ☐ 4. End position (full PROM achieved) ☐ 5. End feel ☐	1. Sitting ☐ 2. Shoulder abducted or flexed to 90° and neutral rotation ☐ 3. Elbow flexed, forearm midposition ☐ 4. Trunk stabilized ☐ 5. Scapula stabilized ☐	1. On top of acromion process ☐	1. Perpendicular to trunk ☐ 2. Position maintained for start position ☐ 3. Position maintained for end position ☐	1. Arm supported in abduction or flexion ☐ 2. Humerus moved posteriorly to limit of motion ☐ 3. Full PROM achieved ☐ 4. Trunk stabilized ☐ 5. Scapula stabilized ☐	1. Parallel long axis of humerus ☐ 2. Position maintained for start position ☐ 3. Position maintained for end position ☐	1. Full PROM ☐ 2. End feel ☐ 3. Start position recorded: shoulder 90° abduction or flexion ☐	1. Verbal (clear/concise) ☐ 2. Demonstration (clear) ☐	1. Adequate support of limb/limb segment ☐ 2. Comfortable grip ☐ 3. Safe body mechanics of therapist ☐ Comments:

STEP 1 — **STEP 2**

PROM Measurement: Using a Universal Goniometer

Movement	PROM Assessment of End Feel	Start Position	Axis	Stationary Arm	End Position	Movable Arm	Recording	Instructions	Handling/ Comments
SHOULDER HORIZONTAL ADDUCTION Form 3–11	1. Start position ☐ 2. Stabilized ☐ 3. Therapist distal hand placement ☐ 4. End position (Full PROM achieved) ☐ 5. End Feel ☐	1. Sitting ☐ 2. Shoulder abducted or flexed to 90° and neutral rotation ☐ 3. Elbow flexed, forearm midposition ☐ 4. Trunk stabilized ☐ 5. Scapula stabilized ☐	1. On top of acromion process ☐	1. Perpendicular to trunk ☐ 2. Position maintained for start position ☐ 3. Position maintained for end position ☐	1. Arm supported in abduction or flexion ☐ 2. Humerus moved anteriorly across chest to limit of motion ☐ 3. Full PROM achieved ☐ 4. Trunk stabilized ☐ 5. Scapula stabilized ☐	1. Parallel long axis of humerus ☐ 2. Position maintained for start position ☐ 3. Position maintained for end position ☐	1. Full PROM ☐ 2. End feel ☐ 3. Start position recorded: shoulder 90° abduction or flexion ☐	1. Verbal (clear/ concise) ☐ 2. Demonstration (clear) ☐	1. Adequate support of limb/limb segment ☐ 2. Comfortable grip ☐ 3. Safe body mechanics of therapist ☐ Comments:
SHOULDER INTERNAL ROTATION Form 3–12	1. Start position ☐ 2. Stabilized ☐ 3. Therapist distal hand placement ☐ 4. End position (Full PROM achieved) ☐ 5. End Feel ☐	1. Prone ☐ 2. Shoulder abducted 90°, elbow flexed 90°, forearm midposition ☐ 3. Pad under humerus ☐ 4. Scapula stabilized ☐	1. On olecranon process of ulna ☐	1. Perpendicular to floor ☐ 2. Position maintained for start position ☐ 3. Position maintained for end position ☐	1. Palm of hand moved toward ceiling to limit of motion ☐ 2. Full PROM achieved ☐ 3. Scapula stabilized ☐ 4. Position of humerus maintained ☐	1. Parallel long axis of ulna, pointing to ulnar styloid process ☐ 2. Position maintained for start position ☐ 3. Position maintained for end position ☐	1. Full PROM ☐ 2. End feel ☐	1. Verbal (clear/ concise) ☐ 2. Demonstration (clear) ☐	1. Adequate support of limb/limb segment ☐ 2. Comfortable grip ☐ 3. Safe body mechanics of therapist ☐ Comments:
SHOULDER EXTERNAL ROTATION Form 3–13	1. Start position ☐ 2. Stabilized ☐ 3. Therapist distal hand placement ☐ 4. End position (Full PROM achieved) ☐ 5. End Feel ☐	1. Supine ☐ 2. Shoulder abducted 90°, elbow flexed 90°, forearm midposition ☐ 3. Pad under humerus ☐ 4. Scapula stabilized ☐	1. On olecranon process of ulna ☐	1. Perpendicular to floor ☐ 2. Position maintained for start position ☐ 3. Position maintained for end position ☐	1. Dorsum of hand moved toward floor to limit of motion ☐ 2. Full PROM achieved ☐ 3. Scapula stabilized ☐ 4. Position of humerus maintained ☐	1. Parallel long axis of ulna, pointing to ulnar styloid process ☐ 2. Position maintained for start position ☐ 3. Position maintained for end position ☐	1. Full PROM ☐ 2. End feel ☐	1. Verbal (clear/ concise) ☐ 2. Demonstration (clear) ☐	1. Adequate support of limb/limb segment ☐ 2. Comfortable grip ☐ 3. Safe body mechanics of therapist ☐ Comments:

Muscle Length Assessment and Measurement Testing: Shoulder Complex

Muscle	Start Position	Stabilization	End Position	Measurement of Joint Position Using Universal Goniometer	Recording	Instructions	Handling/Comments
PECTORALIS MAJOR Form 3-14	1. Supine 2. Shoulder external rotation, 90° elevation through plane midway between flexion and abduction, elbow flexed 90° ☐	1. Therapist's hand on contralateral shoulder to stabilize trunk ☐	1. Shoulder moved to limit of horizontal abduction ☐ 2. Full PROM achieved ☐ 3. Trunk stabilized ☐	Shoulder horizontal abduction 1. Axis: on top of acromion process ☐ 2. Stationary arm: perpendicular to trunk ☐ 3. Movable arm: parallel long axis of humerus ☐	1. Full PROM ☐ 2. End feel ☐	1. Verbal (clear/concise) ☐ 2. Demonstration (clear) ☐	1. Adequate support of limb/limb segment ☐ 2. Comfortable grip ☐ 3. Safe body mechanics of therapist ☐ Comments:

Muscle	Start Position	Stabilization	End Position	Measurement of Muscle Length Using Tape Measure and Second Therapist	Recording	Instructions	Handling/Comments
PECTORALIS MINOR Form 3-15	1. Supine 2. Scapula over side of plinth ☐ 3. Shoulder external rotation and ~80° flexion, elbow flexed ☐	1. Trunk stabilized ☐	1. Therapist applies force through long axis of shaft of humerus to move shoulder girdle to limit of scapular retraction ☐ 2. Scapula moved to limit of retraction ☐ 3. Full PROM achieved ☐ 4. Trunk stabilized ☐	With muscle on stretch, therapist instructs a second therapist to: 1. Mark the: - inferomedial edge coracoid process ☐ - inferior edge 4th rib adjacent to sternum ☐ 2. Have patient exhale fully ☐ 3. Measure distance between marks ☐	1. Full PROM ☐ 2. End feel ☐	1. Verbal (clear/concise) ☐ 2. Demonstration (clear) ☐	1. Adequate support of limb/limb segment ☐ 2. Comfortable grip ☐ 3. Safe body mechanics of therapist ☐ Comments:

PROM Assessment and Measurement Testing: Elbow and Forearm

Movement	STEP 1	STEP 2 PROM Measurement: Using a Universal Goniometer							
	PROM Assessment of End Feel	Start Position	Axis	Stationary Arm	End Position	Movable Arm	Recording	Instructions	Handling/ Comments
ELBOW FLEXION Form 4-1	1. Start position ☐ 2. Stabilized ☐ 3. Therapist distal hand placement ☐ 4. End position (full PROM achieved) ☐ 5. End feel ☐	1. Supine ☐ 2. Shoulder and elbow in anatomical position ☐ 3. Towel under distal humerus ☐ 4. Humerus stabilized ☐	1. Over lateral epicondyle of humerus ☐	1. Parallel long axis humerus, pointing toward tip of acromion process ☐ 2. Position maintained for start position ☐ 3. Position maintained for end position ☐	1. Forearm moved anteriorly to limit of elbow flexion ☐ 2. Full PROM achieved ☐ 3. Humerus stabilized ☐	1. Parallel long axis of radius, pointing toward styloid process of radius ☐ 2. Position maintained for start position ☐ 3. Position maintained for end position ☐	1. Full PROM ☐ 2. End feel ☐	1. Verbal (clear/ concise) ☐ 2. Demon-stration (clear) ☐	1. Adequate support of limb/limb segment ☐ 2. Comfortable grip ☐ 3. Safe body mechanics of therapist ☐ Comments:
ELBOW EXTENSION/ HYPER-EXTENSION Form 4-2	1. Start position ☐ 2. Stabilized ☐ 3. Therapist distal hand placement ☐ 4. End position (full PROM achieved) ☐ 5. End feel ☐	1. Supine ☐ 2. Shoulder and elbow in anatomical position ☐ 3. Towel under distal humerus ☐ 4. Humerus stabilized ☐	1. Over lateral epicondyle of humerus ☐	1. Parallel long axis humerus, pointing toward tip of acromion process ☐ 2. Position maintained for start position ☐ 3. Position maintained for end position ☐	1. Forearm moved posteriorly to limit of elbow extension/ hyperextension ☐ 2. Full PROM achieved ☐ 3. Humerus stabilized ☐	1. Parallel long axis of radius, pointing toward styloid process of radius ☐ 2. Position maintained for start position ☐ 3. Position maintained for end position ☐	1. Full PROM ☐ 2. End feel ☐	1. Verbal (clear/ concise) ☐ 2. Demon-stration (clear) ☐	1. Adequate support of limb/limb segment ☐ 2. Comfortable grip ☐ 3. Safe body mechanics of therapist ☐ Comments:

(continues)

PROM Assessment and Measurement Testing: Elbow and Forearm (continued)

Movement	STEP 1		STEP 2 — PROM Measurement: Using a Universal Goniometer						
	PROM Assessment of End Feel	Start Position	Axis	Stationary Arm	End Position	Movable Arm	Recording	Instructions	Handling/Comments
FOREARM SUPINATION Form 4-3	1. Start position ☐ 2. Stabilized ☐ 3. Therapist distal hand placement ☐ 4. End position (full PROM achieved) ☐ 5. End feel ☐	1. Sitting ☐ 2. Arm at side, elbow flexed 90° ☐ 3. Forearm midposition ☐ 4. Pencil held tightly in hand, wrist in neutral position ☐ 5. Humerus stabilized ☐	1. Over head of third metacarpal ☐	1. Perpendicular to floor ☐ 2. Position maintained for start position ☐ 3. Position maintained for end position ☐	1. Forearm rotated so palm faces up toward ceiling ☐ 2. Full PROM achieved ☐ 3. Humerus stabilized ☐ 4. Position of pencil maintained ☐	1. Parallel to pencil ☐ 2. Position maintained for start position ☐ 3. Position maintained for end position ☐	1. Full PROM ☐ 2. End feel ☐	1. Verbal (clear/concise) ☐ 2. Demonstration (clear) ☐	1. Adequate support of limb/limb segment ☐ 2. Comfortable grip ☐ 3. Safe body mechanics of therapist ☐ Comments:
FOREARM PRONATION Form 4-4	1. Start position ☐ 2. Stabilized ☐ 3. Therapist distal hand placement ☐ 4. End position (full PROM achieved) ☐ 5. End feel ☐	1. Sitting ☐ 2. Arm at side, elbow flexed 90° ☐ 3. Forearm midposition ☐ 4. Pencil held tightly in hand, wrist in neutral position ☐ 5. Humerus stabilized ☐	1. Over head of third metacarpal ☐	1. Perpendicular to floor ☐ 2. Position maintained for start position ☐ 3. Position maintained for end position ☐	1. Forearm rotated so palm faces down toward floor ☐ 2. Full PROM achieved ☐ 3. Humerus stabilized ☐ 4. Position of pencil maintained ☐	1. Parallel to pencil ☐ 2. Position maintained for start position ☐ 3. Position maintained for end position ☐	1. Full PROM ☐ 2. End feel ☐	1. Verbal (clear/concise) ☐ 2. Demonstration (clear) ☐	1. Adequate support of limb/limb segment ☐ 2. Comfortable grip ☐ 3. Safe body mechanics of therapist ☐ Comments:

Muscle Length Assessment and Measurement Testing: Elbow and Forearm

Muscle	Start Position	Stabilization	End Position	Measurement of Joint Position Using Universal Goniometer	Recording	Instructions	Handling/Comments
BICEPS BRACHII Form 4-5	1. Supine ☐ 2. Shoulder in extension over edge of plinth ☐ 3. Elbow flexed, forearm pronated ☐	1. Humerus stabilized ☐	1. Elbow moved to limit of extension ☐ 2. Full PROM achieved ☐ 3. Humerus stabilized ☐	Elbow extension 1. Axis: over lateral epicondyle of humerus ☐ 2. Stationary arm: parallel long axis humerus pointing toward tip of acromion process ☐ 3. Movable arm: parallel long axis of radius, pointing toward styloid process of radius ☐	1. Full PROM ☐ 2. End feel ☐	1. Verbal (clear/concise) ☐ 2. Demonstration (clear) ☐	1. Adequate support of limb/limb segment ☐ 2. Comfortable grip ☐ 3. Safe body mechanics of therapist ☐ Comments:
TRICEPS Form 4-6	1. Sitting ☐ 2. Full shoulder elevation through flexion, and shoulder externally rotated ☐ 3. Elbow in anatomical position, forearm supinated ☐	1. Humerus stabilized ☐	1. Elbow moved to limit of flexion ☐ 2. Full PROM achieved ☐ 3. Humerus stabilized ☐	Elbow Flexion 1. Axis: over lateral epicondyle of humerus ☐ 2. Stationary arm: parallel long axis humerus pointing toward tip of acromion process ☐ 3. Movable arm: parallel long axis of radius, pointing toward styloid process of radius ☐	1. Full PROM ☐ 2. End feel ☐	1. Verbal (clear/concise) ☐ 2. Demonstration (clear) ☐	1. Adequate support of limb/limb segment ☐ 2. Comfortable grip ☐ 3. Safe body mechanics of therapist ☐ Comments:

PROM Assessment and Measurement Testing: Wrist and Hand

Movement	STEP 1 — PROM Assessment of End Feel	STEP 2 — PROM Measurement: Using a Universal Goniometer							
		Start Position	Axis	Stationary Arm	End Position	Movable Arm	Recording	Instructions	Handling/Comments
WRIST FLEXION Form 5-1	1. Start position ☐☐ 2. Stabilized ☐☐ 3. Therapist distal hand placement ☐ 4. End position (full PROM achieved) ☐☐ 5. End feel ☐☐	1. Sitting ☐ 2. Elbow flexed, forearm pronated, wrist in anatomical position, fingers relaxed ☐ 3. Forearm stabilized ☐	1. Medial aspect of wrist at level of ulnar styloid process ☐	1. Parallel long axis of ulna ☐ 2. Position maintained for start position ☐ 3. Position maintained for end position ☐	1. Wrist moved in anterior direction to limit of motion ☐ 2. Full PROM achieved ☐ 3. Forearm stabilized ☐	1. Parallel long axis of fifth metacarpal ☐ 2. Position maintained for start position ☐ 3. Position maintained for end position ☐	1. Full PROM ☐ 2. End feel ☐	1. Verbal (clear/concise) ☐ 2. Demonstration (clear) ☐	1. Adequate support of limb/limb segment ☐ 2. Comfortable grip ☐ 3. Safe body mechanics of therapist ☐ Comments:
WRIST EXTENSION Form 5-2	1. Start position ☐☐ 2. Stabilized ☐☐ 3. Therapist distal hand placement ☐ 4. End position (full PROM achieved) ☐☐ 5. End feel ☐☐	1. Sitting ☐ 2. Elbow flexed, forearm pronated, wrist in anatomical position, fingers relaxed ☐ 3. Forearm stabilized ☐	1. Medial aspect of wrist at level of ulnar styloid process ☐	1. Parallel long axis of ulna ☐ 2. Position maintained for start position ☐ 3. Position maintained for end position ☐	1. Wrist moved in posterior direction to limit of motion ☐ 2. Full PROM achieved ☐ 3. Forearm stabilized ☐	1. Parallel long axis of fifth metacarpal ☐ 2. Position maintained for start position ☐ 3. Position maintained for end position ☐	1. Full PROM ☐ 2. End feel ☐	1. Verbal (clear/concise) ☐ 2. Demonstration (clear) ☐	1. Adequate support of limb/limb segment ☐ 2. Comfortable grip ☐ 3. Safe body mechanics of therapist ☐ Comments:
WRIST ULNAR DEVIATION Form 5-3	1. Start position ☐☐ 2. Stabilized ☐☐ 3. Therapist distal hand placement ☐ 4. End position (full PROM achieved) ☐☐ 5. End feel ☐☐	1. Sitting ☐ 2. Elbow flexed, forearm pronated, palm of hand rests lightly on table ☐ 3. Wrist and fingers in anatomical position ☐ 4. Forearm stabilized ☐	1. Posterior aspect wrist over capitate ☐	1. Along midline of forearm ☐ 2. Position maintained for start position ☐ 3. Position maintained for end position ☐	1. Wrist ulnar deviated to limit of motion ☐ 2. Full PROM achieved ☐ 3. Forearm stabilized ☐	1. Parallel long axis shaft of third metacarpal ☐ 2. Position maintained for start position ☐ 3. Position maintained for end position ☐	1. Full PROM ☐ 2. End feel ☐	1. Verbal (clear/concise) ☐ 2. Demonstration (clear) ☐	1. Adequate support of limb/limb segment ☐ 2. Comfortable grip ☐ 3. Safe body mechanics of therapist ☐ Comments:

STEP 1 — STEP 2

PROM Measurement: Using a Universal Goniometer

Movement	PROM Assessment of End Feel	Start Position	Axis	Stationary Arm	End Position	Movable Arm	Recording	Instructions	Handling/Comments
WRIST RADIAL DEVIATION Form 5-4	1. Start position ☐ 2. Stabilized ☐ 3. Therapist distal hand placement ☐ 4. End position (full PROM achieved) ☐ 5. End feel ☐	1. Sitting ☐ 2. Elbow flexed, forearm pronated, palm of hand rests lightly on table ☐ 3. Wrist and fingers in anatomical position ☐ 4. Forearm stabilized ☐	1. Posterior aspect of wrist over capitate ☐	1. Along midline of forearm ☐ 2. Position maintained for start position ☐ 3. Position maintained for end position ☐	1. Wrist radially deviated to limit of motion ☐ 2. Full PROM achieved ☐ 3. Forearm stabilized ☐	1. Parallel long axis shaft of third metacarpal ☐ 2. Position maintained for start position ☐ 3. Position maintained for end position ☐	1. Full PROM ☐ 2. End feel ☐	1. Verbal (clear/concise) ☐ 2. Demonstration (clear) ☐	1. Adequate support of limb/limb segment ☐ 2. Comfortable grip ☐ 3. Safe body mechanics of therapist ☐ Comments:
FINGER MCP FLEXION Form 5-5	1. Start position ☐ 2. Stabilized ☐ 3. Therapist distal hand placement ☐ 4. End position (full PROM achieved) ☐ 5. End feel ☐	1. Sitting ☐ 2. Elbow flexed, forearm rests on table, wrist slightly extended, MCP joint of finger in anatomical position ☐ 3. Metacarpal stabilized ☐	1. On posterior aspect of MCP joint ☐	1. Parallel long axis shaft of metacarpal ☐ 2. Position maintained for start position ☐ 3. Position maintained for end position ☐	1. Proximal phalanx moved toward palm to limit of flexion ☐ 2. IP joints allowed to extend ☐ 3. Full PROM achieved ☐ 4. Metacarpal stabilized ☐	1. Parallel long axis of proximal phalanx ☐ 2. Position maintained for start position ☐ 3. Position maintained for end position ☐	1. Full PROM ☐ 2. End feel ☐	1. Verbal (clear/concise) ☐ 2. Demonstration (clear) ☐	1. Adequate support of limb/limb segment ☐ 2. Comfortable grip ☐ 3. Safe body mechanics of therapist ☐ Comments:
FINGER MCP EXTENSION Form 5-6	1. Start position ☐ 2. Stabilized ☐ 3. Therapist distal hand placement ☐ 4. End position (full PROM achieved) ☐ 5. End feel ☐	1. Sitting ☐ 2. Elbow flexed, forearm rests on table, wrist slightly flexed, MCP joint of finger in anatomical position ☐ 3. Metacarpal stabilized ☐	1. On anterior aspect of MCP joint ☐	1. Parallel long axis shaft of metacarpal ☐ 2. Position maintained for start position ☐ 3. Position maintained for end position ☐	1. Proximal phalanx moved in posterior direction to limit of extension ☐ 2. IP joints allowed to flex ☐ 3. Full PROM achieved ☐ 4. Metacarpal stabilized ☐	1. Parallel long axis of proximal phalanx ☐ 2. Position maintained for start position ☐ 3. Position maintained for end position ☐	1. Full PROM ☐ 2. End feel ☐	1. Verbal (clear/concise) ☐ 2. Demonstration (clear) ☐	1. Adequate support of limb/limb segment ☐ 2. Comfortable grip ☐ 3. Safe body mechanics of therapist ☐ Comments:

(continues)

PROM Assessment and Measurement Testing: Wrist and Hand (*continued*)

	STEP 1	STEP 2							
		PROM Measurement: Using a Universal Goniometer							
Movement	PROM Assessment of End Feel	Start Position	Axis	Stationary Arm	End Position	Movable Arm	Recording	Instructions	Handling/Comments
FINGER MCP ABDUCTION Form 5-7	1. Start position ☐ 2. Stabilized ☐ 3. Therapist distal hand placement ☐ 4. End position (Full PROM achieved) ☐ 5. End Feel ☐	1. Sitting ☐ 2. Elbow flexed, forearm pronated and palm of hand rests on table ☐ 3. Wrist and fingers in anatomical position ☐ 4. Metacarpals stabilized ☐	1. On posterior surface of MCP joint ☐	1. Parallel long axis of metacarpal ☐ 2. Position maintained for start position ☐ 3. Position maintained for end position ☐	1. Finger is moved away from midline of hand to limit of MCP abduction ☐ 2. Full PROM achieved ☐ 3. Metacarpals stabilized ☐	1. Parallel long axis of proximal phalanx ☐ 2. Position maintained for start position ☐ 3. Position maintained for end position ☐	1. Full PROM ☐ 2. End feel ☐	1. Verbal (clear/concise) ☐ 2. Demonstration (clear) ☐	1. Adequate support of limb/limb segment ☐ 2. Comfortable grip ☐ 3. Safe body mechanics of therapist ☐ Comments:
FINGER MCP ADDUCTION Form 5-8	1. Start position ☐ 2. Stabilized ☐ 3. Therapist distal hand placement ☐ 4. End position (Full PROM achieved) ☐ 5. End Feel ☐	1. Sitting ☐ 2. Elbow flexed, forearm pronated and palm of hand rests on table ☐ 3. Wrist and finger in anatomical position ☐ 4. Nontest fingers out of way ☐ 5. Metacarpals stabilized ☐	1. On posterior surface of MCP joint ☐	1. Parallel long axis of metacarpal ☐ 2. Position maintained for start position ☐ 3. Position maintained for end position ☐	1. Finger is moved toward midline of hand to limit of MCP adduction ☐ 2. Full PROM achieved ☐ 3. Metacarpals stabilized ☐	1. Parallel long axis of proximal phalanx ☐ 2. Position maintained for start position ☐ 3. Position maintained for end position ☐	1. Full PROM ☐ 2. End feel ☐	1. Verbal (clear/concise) ☐ 2. Demonstration (clear) ☐	1. Adequate support of limb/limb segment ☐ 2. Comfortable grip ☐ 3. Safe body mechanics of therapist ☐ Comments:
FINGER IP FLEXION Form 5-9	1. Start position ☐ 2. Stabilized ☐ 3. Therapist distal hand placement ☐ 4. End position (Full PROM achieved) ☐ 5. End Feel ☐	1. Sitting ☐ 2. Forearm rests on table, wrist and fingers in anatomical position ☐ 3. PIP joint: proximal phalanx stabilized DIP joint: middle phalanx stabilized ☐	1. Over posterior surface of IP joint ☐	1. Parallel long axis of: PIP joint: proximal phalanx DIP joint: middle phalanx ☐ 2. Position maintained for start position ☐ 3. Position maintained for end position ☐	1. PIP or DIP joint flexed to limit of motion ☐ 2. Full PROM achieved ☐ 3. PIP joint: proximal phalanx stabilized DIP joint: middle phalanx stabilized ☐	1. Parallel long axis of: PIP joint: middle phalanx DIP joint: distal phalanx ☐ 2. Position maintained for start position ☐ 3. Position maintained for end position ☐	1. Full PROM ☐ 2. End feel ☐	1. Verbal (clear/concise) ☐ 2. Demonstration (clear) ☐	1. Adequate support of limb/limb segment ☐ 2. Comfortable grip ☐ 3. Safe body mechanics of therapist ☐ Comments:

	STEP 1			STEP 2					
		PROM Measurement: Using a Universal Goniometer							
Movement	**PROM Assessment of End Feel**	**Start Position**	**Axis**	**Stationary Arm**	**End Position**	**Movable Arm**	**Recording**	**Instructions**	**Handling/Comments**
FINGER IP EXTENSION Form 5-10	1. Start position 2. Stabilized 3. Therapist distal hand placement 4. End position (full PROM achieved) 5. End feel	1. Sitting 2. Forearm rests on table, wrist and fingers in anatomical position 3. PIP joint: proximal phalanx stabilized DIP joint: middle phalanx stabilized	1. Over anterior surface of IP joint	1. Parallel long axis of: PIP joint: proximal phalanx DIP joint: middle phalanx 2. Position maintained for start position 3. Position maintained for end position	1. PIP or DIP joint extended to limit of motion 2. Full PROM achieved 3. PIP joint: proximal phalanx stabilized DIP joint: middle phalanx stabilized	1. Parallel long axis of: PIP joint: middle phalanx DIP joint: distal phalanx 2. Position maintained for start position 3. Position maintained for end position	1. Full PROM 2. End feel (clear)	1. Verbal (clear/concise) 2. Demonstration	1. Adequate support of limb/limb segment 2. Comfortable grip 3. Safe body mechanics of therapist Comments:
THUMB CM FLEXION Form 5-11	1. Start position 2. Stabilized 3. Therapist distal hand placement 4. End position (full PROM achieved) 5. End feel	1. Sitting 2. Elbow flexed, forearm in midposition, wrist neutral position 3. Thumb MCP and IP joints in anatomical position 4. Trapezium, wrist, and forearm stabilized	1. Over anterior aspect first CM joint	1. Parallel long axis of radius 2. Position maintained for start position 3. Position maintained for end position	1. Thumb CM joint flexed to limit of motion 2. Full PROM achieved 3. Trapezium, wrist, and forearm stabilized	1. Parallel long axis thumb metacarpal 2. Position maintained for start position 3. Position maintained for end position	1. Full PROM 2. End feel	1. Verbal (clear/concise) 2. Demonstration (clear)	1. Adequate support of limb/limb segment 2. Comfortable grip 3. Safe body mechanics of therapist Comments:
THUMB CM EXTENSION Form 5-12	1. Start position 2. Stabilized 3. Therapist distal hand placement 4. End position (full PROM achieved) 5. End feel	1. Sitting 2. Elbow flexed, forearm in midposition, wrist neutral position 3. Thumb MCP and IP joints in anatomical position 4. Trapezium, wrist, and forearm stabilized	1. Over anterior aspect first CM joint	1. Parallel long axis of radius 2. Position maintained for start position 3. Position maintained for end position	1. Thumb CM joint extended to limit of motion 2. Full PROM achieved 3. Trapezium, wrist, and forearm stabilized	1. Parallel long axis of thumb metacarpal 2. Position maintained for start position 3. Position maintained for end position	1. Full PROM 2. End feel	1. Verbal (clear/concise) 2. Demonstration (clear)	1. Adequate support of limb/limb segment 2. Comfortable grip 3. Safe body mechanics of therapist Comments:

(continues)

PROM Assessment and Measurement Testing: Wrist and Hand (continued)

	STEP 1	STEP 2							
		PROM Measurement: Using a Universal Goniometer							
Movement	**PROM Assessment of End Feel**	**Start Position**	**Axis**	**Stationary Arm**	**End Position**	**Movable Arm**	**Recording**	**Instructions**	**Handling/ Comments**
THUMB MCP FLEXION Form 5-13	1. Start position ☐ 2. Stabilized ☐ 3. Therapist distal hand placement ☐ 4. End position (full PROM achieved) ☐ 5. End feel ☐	1. Sitting ☐ 2. Elbow flexed, forearm rests on table in midposition, wrist, thumb and fingers in anatomical position ☐ 3. First metacarpal stabilized ☐	1. Over posterior or lateral aspect of MCP joint of thumb ☐	1. Parallel long axis of first metacarpal ☐ 2. Position maintained for start position ☐ 3. Position maintained for end position ☐	1. Proximal phalanx moved across palm to limit of MCP joint flexion ☐ 2. Full PROM achieved ☐ 3. First metacarpal stabilized ☐	1. Parallel long axis of proximal phalanx ☐ 2. Position maintained for start position ☐ 3. Position maintained for end position ☐	1. Full PROM ☐ 2. End feel ☐	1. Verbal (clear/ concise) ☐ 2. Demonstration (clear) ☐	1. Adequate support of limb/limb segment ☐ 2. Comfortable grip ☐ 3. Safe body mechanics of therapist ☐ Comments: ☐
THUMB MCP EXTENSION Form 5-14	1. Start position ☐ 2. Stabilized ☐ 3. Therapist distal hand placement ☐ 4. End position (full PROM achieved) ☐ 5. End feel ☐	1. Sitting ☐ 2. Elbow flexed, forearm rests on table in midposition, wrist, thumb and fingers in anatomical position ☐ 3. First metacarpal stabilized ☐	1. Over anterior or lateral aspect of MCP joint of thumb ☐	1. Parallel long axis of first metacarpal ☐ 2. Position maintained for start position ☐ 3. Position maintained for end position ☐	1. Proximal phalanx moved to limit of MCP joint extension ☐ 2. Full PROM achieved ☐ 3. First metacarpal stabilized ☐	1. Parallel long axis of proximal phalanx ☐ 2. Position maintained for start position ☐ 3. Position maintained for end position ☐	1. Full PROM ☐ 2. End feel ☐	1. Verbal (clear/ concise) ☐ 2. Demonstration (clear) ☐	1. Adequate support of limb/limb segment ☐ 2. Comfortable grip ☐ 3. Safe body mechanics of therapist ☐ Comments: ☐
THUMB IP FLEXION Form 5-15	1. Start position ☐ 2. Stabilized ☐ 3. Therapist distal hand placement ☐ 4. End position (full PROM achieved) ☐ 5. End feel ☐	1. Sitting ☐ 2. Elbow flexed, forearm rests on table in midposition, wrist, thumb and fingers in anatomical position ☐ 3. Proximal phalanx stabilized ☐	1. Over posterior or lateral aspect of IP joint of thumb ☐	1. Parallel long axis proximal phalanx of thumb ☐ 2. Position maintained for start position ☐ 3. Position maintained for end position ☐	1. IP joint flexed to limit of motion ☐ 2. Full PROM achieved ☐ 3. Proximal phalanx stabilized ☐	1. Parallel long axis of distal phalanx ☐ 2. Position maintained for start position ☐ 3. Position maintained for end position ☐	1. Full PROM ☐ 2. End feel ☐	1. Verbal (clear/ concise) ☐ 2. Demonstration (clear) ☐	1. Adequate support of limb/limb segment ☐ 2. Comfortable grip ☐ 3. Safe body mechanics of therapist ☐ Comments: ☐

STEP 1 — STEP 2

PROM Measurement: Using a Universal Goniometer

Movement	PROM Assessment of End Feel	Start Position	Axis	Stationary Arm	End Position	Movable Arm	Recording	Instructions	Handling/Comments
THUMB IP EXTENSION Form 5-16	1. Start position ☐ 2. Stabilized ☐ 3. Therapist distal hand placement ☐ 4. End position (full PROM achieved) ☐ 5. End feel ☐	1. Sitting ☐ 2. Elbow flexed, forearm rests on table in midposition, wrist, thumb and fingers in anatomical position ☐ 3. Proximal phalanx stabilized ☐	1. Over anterior or lateral aspect of IP joint of thumb ☐	1. Parallel long axis of proximal phalanx of thumb ☐ 2. Position maintained for start position ☐ 3. Position maintained for end position ☐	1. IP joint extended to limit of motion ☐ 2. Full PROM achieved ☐ 3. Proximal phalanx stabilized ☐	1. Parallel long axis of distal phalanx ☐ 2. Position maintained for start position ☐ 3. Position maintained for end position ☐	1. Full PROM ☐ 2. End feel ☐	1. Verbal (clear/concise) ☐ 2. Demonstration (clear) ☐	1. Adequate support of limb/limb segment ☐ 2. Comfortable grip ☐ 3. Safe body mechanics of therapist ☐ Comments:
THUMB CM ABDUCTION Form 5-17	1. Start position ☐ 2. Stabilized ☐ 3. Therapist distal hand placement ☐ 4. End position (full PROM achieved) ☐ 5. End feel ☐	1. Sitting ☐ 2. Elbow flexed, forearm in midposition, wrist and fingers in anatomical position ☐ 3. Thumb in contact along side of index finger ☐ 4. Second metacarpal stabilized ☐	1. Posterior aspect, junction at bases of first and second metacarpals ☐	1. Parallel long axis second metacarpal ☐ 2. Position maintained for start position ☐ 3. Position maintained for end position ☐	1. First metacarpal moved in plane perpendicular to palm to limit of CM joint abduction ☐ 2. Full PROM achieved ☐ 3. Second metacarpal stabilized ☐	1. Parallel long axis first metacarpal ☐ 2. Position maintained for start position ☐ 3. Position maintained for end position ☐	1. Full PROM ☐ 2. End feel ☐	1. Verbal (clear/concise) ☐ 2. Demonstration (clear) ☐	1. Adequate support of limb/limb segment ☐ 2. Comfortable grip ☐ 3. Safe body mechanics of therapist ☐ Comments:
THUMB AND FIFTH FINGER OPPOSITION Form 5-18		1. Sitting ☐ 2. Elbow flexed, forearm supinated, wrist in anatomical position ☐ 3. Fingers and thumb relaxed ☐ 4. Forearm stabilized ☐			1. Active thumb and fifth finger opposition to limit of motion (so pads of thumb and finger in same plane) ☐ 2. Forearm stabilized ☐	1. Linear measurement between center tip of thumb pad and center tip of fifth finger pad ☐	1. Full AROM ☐	1. Verbal (clear/concise) ☐ 2. Demonstration (clear) ☐	1. Adequate support of limb/limb segment ☐ 2. Comfortable grip ☐ 3. Safe body mechanics of therapist ☐ Comments:

Muscle Length Assessment and Measurement Testing: Wrist and Hand

Muscle	Start Position	Stabilization	End Position	Measurement of Joint Position Using Universal Goniometer	Recording	Instructions	Handling/Comments
FINGER FLEXORS Form 5-19	1. Supine 2. Elbow extended, forearm supinated, wrist in anatomical position, fingers extended ☐	1. Humerus stabilized ☐ 2. Radius and ulna stabilized ☐	1. With fingers held in extension, wrist moved to limit of extension ☐ 2. Full PROM achieved ☐ 3. Humerus stabilized ☐ 4. Radius and ulna stabilized ☐	Wrist extension 1. Axis: medial aspect wrist at level of ulnar styloid process ☐ 2. Stationary arm: parallel long axis of ulna ☐ 3. Movable arm: parallel long axis of fifth metacarpal ☐	1. Full PROM ☐ 2. End feel ☐	1. Verbal (clear/concise) ☐ 2. Demonstration (clear ☐	1. Adequate support of limb/limb segment ☐ 2. Comfortable grip ☐ 3. Safe body mechanics of therapist ☐ Comments:
FINGER EXTENSORS Form 5-20	1. Sitting 2. Elbow extended, forearm pronated, wrist in anatomical position, fingers flexed ☐	1. Radius and ulna stabilized ☐	1. With fingers held in flexion, wrist moved to limit of flexion ☐ 2. Full PROM achieved ☐ 3. Radius and ulna stabilized ☐	Wrist flexion 1. Axis: medial aspect of wrist at level of ulnar styloid process ☐ 2. Stationary arm: parallel long axis of ulna ☐ 3. Movable arm: parallel long axis of fifth metacarpal ☐	1. Full PROM ☐ 2. End feel ☐	1. Verbal (clear/concise) ☐ 2. Demonstration (clear) ☐	1. Adequate support of limb/limb segment ☐ 2. Comfortable grip ☐ 3. Safe body mechanics of therapist ☐ Comments:
LUMBRICALES Form 5-21	1. Sitting 2. Elbow flexed, forearm in midposition or supinated, wrist extended, IP joints of fingers flexed ☐	1. Metacarpals stabilized ☐	1. With IP joints held in flexion, MCP joints moved to limit of extension ☐ 2. Full PROM achieved ☐ 3. Metacarpals stabilized ☐	MCP joint extension 1. Axis: lateral to MCP joint of index finger or medial to MCP joint of little finger ☐ 2. Stationary arm: parallel long axis of metacarpal ☐ 3. Movable arm: parallel long axis of proximal phalanx ☐	1. Full PROM ☐ 2. End feel ☐	1. Verbal (clear/concise) ☐ 2. Demonstration (clear) ☐	1. Adequate support of limb/limb segment ☐ 2. Comfortable grip ☐ 3. Safe body mechanics of therapist ☐ Comments:

PROM Assessment and Measurement Testing: Hip

	STEP 1	STEP 2 — PROM Measurement: Using A Universal Goniometer							
Movement	PROM Assessment of End Feel	Start Position	Axis	Stationary Arm	End Position	Movable Arm	Recording	Instructions	Handling/ Comments
HIP FLEXION Form 6-1	1. Start position ☐ 2. Stabilized ☐ 3. Therapist distal hand placement ☐ 4. End position (full PROM achieved) ☐ 5. End feel ☐	1. Supine ☐ 2. Test side hip and knee in anatomical position ☐ 3. Pelvis in neutral position ☐ 4. Trunk and pelvis stabilized ☐	1. Over greater trochanter ☐	1. Parallel midaxillary line of trunk ☐ 2. Position maintained for start position ☐ 3. Position maintained for end position ☐	1. With knee flexed, hip is flexed to limit of motion ☐ 2. Full PROM achieved ☐ 3. Trunk and pelvis stabilized ☐	1. Parallel long axis of femur, pointing toward lateral epicondyle ☐ 2. Position maintained for start position ☐ 3. Position maintained for end position ☐	1. Full PROM ☐ 2. End feel ☐	1. Verbal (clear/ concise) ☐ 2. Demonstration (clear) ☐	1. Adequate support of limb/limb segment ☐ 2. Comfortable grip ☐ 3. Safe body mechanics of therapist ☐ Comments:
HIP EXTENSION Form 6-2	1. Start position ☐ 2. Stabilized ☐ 3. Therapist distal hand placement ☐ 4. End position (full PROM achieved) ☐ 5. End feel ☐	1. Prone ☐ 2. Hips and knees in anatomical position ☐ 3. Feet over end of plinth ☐ 4. Pelvis stabilized with strap or by second therapist ☐	1. Over greater trochanter ☐	1. Parallel midaxillary line of trunk ☐ 2. Position maintained for start position ☐ 3. Position maintained for end position ☐	1. With knee in extension, hip is extended to limit of motion ☐ 2. Full PROM achieved ☐ 3. Pelvis stabilized ☐	1. Parallel long axis of femur, pointing toward lateral epicondyle ☐ 2. Position maintained for start position ☐ 3. Position maintained for end position ☐	1. Full PROM ☐ 2. End feel ☐	1. Verbal (clear/ concise) ☐ 2. Demonstration (clear) ☐	1. Adequate support of limb/limb segment ☐ 2. Comfortable grip ☐ 3. Safe body mechanics of therapist ☐ Comments:
HIP ABDUCTION Form 6-3	1. Start position ☐ 2. Stabilized ☐ 3. Therapist distal hand placement ☐ 4. End position (full PROM achieved) ☐ 5. End feel ☐	1. Supine ☐ 2. Hip and knee in anatomical position ☐ 3. Pelvis is level ☐ 4. Pelvis stabilized ☐	1. Over ipsilateral ASIS ☐	1. Along line joining the two ASISs ☐ 2. Position maintained for start position ☐ 3. Position maintained for end position ☐	1. Hip is abducted to limit of motion ☐ 2. Full PROM achieved ☐ 3. Pelvis stabilized ☐	1. Parallel long axis of femur pointing to midline of patella ☐ 2. Position maintained for start position ☐ 3. Position maintained for end position ☐	1. Full PROM ☐ 2. End feel ☐	1. Verbal (clear/ concise) ☐ 2. Demonstration (clear) ☐	1. Adequate support of limb/limb segment ☐ 2. Comfortable grip ☐ 3. Safe body mechanics of therapist ☐ Comments:

(continues)

PROM Assessment and Measurement Testing: Hip (*continued*)

Movement	STEP 1 — PROM Assessment of End Feel	STEP 2 — PROM Measurement: Using A Universal Goniometer							
		Start Position	Axis	Stationary Arm	End Position	Movable Arm	Recording	Instructions	Handling/Comments
HIP ADDUCTION Form 6-4	1. Start position ☐ 2. Stabilized ☐ 3. Therapist distal hand placement ☐ 4. End position (full PROM achieved) ☐ 5. End feel ☐	1. Supine 2. Hip and knee in anatomical position ☐ 3. Pelvis is level ☐ 4. Contralateral hip abducted ☐ 5. Pelvis stabilized ☐	1. Over ipsilateral ASIS ☐	1. Along line joining the two ASISs ☐ 2. Position maintained for start position ☐ 3. Position maintained for end position ☐	1. Hip adducted to limit of motion ☐ 2. Full PROM achieved ☐ 3. Pelvis stabilized ☐	1. Parallel long axis of femur pointing to midline of patella ☐ 2. Position maintained for start position ☐ 3. Position maintained for end position ☐	1. Full PROM ☐ 2. End feel ☐	1. Verbal (clear/ concise) ☐ 2. Demonstration (clear) ☐	1. Adequate support of limb/limb segment ☐ 2. Comfortable grip ☐ 3. Safe body mechanics of therapist ☐ Comments:
HIP INTERNAL ROTATION Form 6-5	1. Start position ☐ 2. Stabilized ☐ 3. Therapist distal hand placement ☐ 4. End position (full PROM achieved) ☐ 5. End feel ☐	1. Sitting grasping edge of plinth ☐ 2. Pad is placed under thigh to keep thigh horizontal ☐ 3. Contralateral hip abducted and foot supported ☐ 4. Pelvis and femur stabilized ☐	1. Over midpoint of patella ☐	1. Perpendicular to floor ☐ 2. Position maintained for start position ☐ 3. Position maintained for end position ☐	1. Hip internally rotated to limit of motion ☐ 2. Full PROM achieved ☐ 3. Pelvis and femur stabilized ☐	1. Parallel anterior midline of tibia ☐ 2. Position maintained for start position ☐ 3. Position maintained for end position ☐	1. Full PROM ☐ 2. End feel ☐	1. Verbal (clear/ concise) ☐ 2. Demonstration (clear) ☐	1. Adequate support of limb/limb segment ☐ 2. Comfortable grip ☐ 3. Safe body mechanics of therapist ☐ Comments:
HIP EXTERNAL ROTATION Form 6-6	1. Start position ☐ 2. Stabilized ☐ 3. Therapist distal hand placement ☐ 4. End position (full PROM achieved) ☐ 5. End feel ☐	1. Sitting grasping edge of plinth ☐ 2. Pad is placed under thigh to keep thigh horizontal ☐ 3. Contralateral hip abducted and foot supported ☐ 4. Pelvis and femur stabilized ☐	1. Over midpoint of patella ☐	1. Perpendicular to floor ☐ 2. Position maintained for start position ☐ 3. Position maintained for end position ☐	1. Hip externally rotated to limit of motion ☐ 2. Full PROM achieved ☐ 3. Pelvis and femur stabilized ☐	1. Parallel anterior midline of tibia ☐ 2. Position maintained for start position ☐ 3. Position maintained for end position ☐	1. Full PROM ☐ 2. End feel ☐	1. Verbal (clear/ concise) ☐ 2. Demonstration (clear) ☐	1. Adequate support of limb/limb segment ☐ 2. Comfortable grip ☐ 3. Safe body mechanics of therapist ☐ Comments:

Muscle Length Assessment and Measurement Testing: Hip

Muscle	Start Position	Stabilization	End Position	Measurement of Joint Position Using Universal Goniometer	Recording	Instructions	Handling/Comments
HAMSTRINGS (PSLR) Form 6-7	1. Supine ☐ 2. Low back and sacrum flat on plinth ☐ 3. Ankle relaxed in plantarflexion ☐	1. Nontest thigh stabilized on plinth ☐ 2. Excessive anterior or posterior pelvic tilt avoided ☐	1. Hip flexed to limit of motion ☐ 2. Knee maintained in extension ☐ 3. Ankle relaxed in plantarflexion ☐ 4. Full PROM achieved ☐ 5. Nontest thigh stabilized on plinth ☐ 6. Excessive pelvic tilt avoided ☐	Hip flexion 1. Axis: over greater trochanter ☐ 2. Stationary arm: parallel midaxillary line of trunk ☐ 3. Movable arm: parallel long axis of femur, pointing toward lateral epicondyle ☐	1. Full PROM ☐ 2. End feel ☐	1. Verbal (clear/concise) ☐ 2. Demonstration (clear) ☐	1. Adequate support of limb/limb segment ☐ 2. Comfortable grip ☐ 3. Safe body mechanics of therapist ☐ Comments:
HIP FLEXORS (THOMAS TEST) Form 6-8	1. Sitting, with edge of plinth at midthigh level ☐ 2. Patient assisted into supine ☐ 3. Nontest hip held in flexion ☐ 4. Sacrum and lumbar spine flat on plinth ☐	1. Pelvis and lumbar spine stabilized ☐ 2. Anterior pelvic tilt avoided ☐	1. Leg falls toward plinth in neutral rotation ☐ 2. Hip is extended to limit of motion ☐ 3. Knee free to extend ☐ 4. Full PROM achieved ☐ 5. Pelvis and lumbar spine stabilized ☐ 6. Anterior pelvic tilt avoided ☐	Hip extension 1. Axis: over greater trochanter ☐ 2. Stationary arm: parallel midaxillary line of trunk ☐ 3. Movable arm: parallel long axis of femur, pointing toward lateral epicondyle ☐	1. Full PROM ☐ 2. End feel ☐	1. Verbal (clear/concise) ☐ 2. Demonstration (clear) ☐	1. Adequate support of limb/limb segment ☐ 2. Comfortable grip ☐ 3. Safe body mechanics of therapist ☐ Comments:
HIP ADDUCTORS Form 6-9	1. Supine ☐ 2. Hip and knee in anatomical position ☐ 3. Nontest hip abducted, knee flexed, and foot rests on stool beside plinth ☐ 4. Pelvis is level ☐	1. Pelvis stabilized ☐	1. Hip is abducted to limit of motion ☐ 2. Full PROM achieved ☐ 3. Pelvis stabilized ☐	Hip abduction 1. Axis: over ipsilateral ASIS ☐ 2. Stationary arm: along line joining the two ASISs ☐ 3. Movable arm: parallel along axis of femur, pointing to midline of patella ☐	1. Full PROM ☐ 2. End feel ☐	1. Verbal (clear/concise) ☐ 2. Demonstration (clear) ☐	1. Adequate support of limb/limb segment ☐ 2. Comfortable grip ☐ 3. Safe body mechanics of therapist ☐ Comments:

(continues)

Muscle Length Assessment and Measurement Testing: Hip (continued)

Muscle	Start Position	Stabilization	End Position	Measurement of Joint Position Using Universal Goniometer	Recording	Instructions	Handling/Comments
TENSOR FASCIA LATAE (ILIOTIBIAL BAND) (OBER'S TEST) Form 6-10	1. Sidelly on nontest side ☐ 2. Patient holds nontest hip and knee in flexion ☐ 3. Hip abducted and extended, in neutral rotation ☐ 4. Knee flexed 90° ☐	1. Therapist stands against buttocks ☐ 2. Pelvis stabilized downward at iliac crest ☐	1. Pelvis stabilized ☐ 2. Hip maintained in extension and neutral rotation ☐ 3. Leg allowed to fall toward plinth ☐ 4. Hip is adducted to limit of motion ☐ 5. Full PROM achieved ☐	Hip adduction Second therapist instructed to measure joint position: 1. Axis: over ipsilateral ASIS ☐ 2. Stationary arm: Along line joining the two ASISs ☐ 3. Movable arm: parallel long axis of femur, pointing to midline of patella ☐	1. Full PROM ☐ 2. End feel ☐	1. Verbal (clear/ concise) ☐ 2. Demonstration (clear) ☐	1. Adequate support of limb/limb segment ☐ 2. Comfortable grip ☐ 3. Safe body mechanics of therapist ☐ Comments:
TENSOR FASCIA LATAE (ILIOTIBIAL BAND) (OBER'S TEST: TRUNK PRONE) Form 6-11	1. Prone over end of plinth with nontest hip and knee flexed, foot on floor under plinth ☐ 2. Arms overhead grasp plinth ☐ 3. Hip abducted and extended, in neutral rotation ☐ 4. Knee flexed 90° ☐	1. Therapist stabilizes pelvis ☐	1. Pelvis stabilized ☐ 2. Hip maintained in extension and neutral rotation ☐ 3. Hip is adducted to limit of motion ☐ 4. Full PROM achieved ☐	Hip adduction Second therapist instructed to measure joint position: 1. Axis: posterior aspect of pelvis over projected location of ipsilateral ASIS ☐ 2. Stationary arm: Along line joining the two ASISs projected to posterior aspect of pelvis ☐ 3. Movable arm: parallel long axis of femur ☐	1. Full PROM ☐ 2. End feel ☐	1. Verbal (clear/ concise) ☐ 2. Demonstration (clear) ☐	1. Adequate support of limb/limb segment ☐ 2. Comfortable grip ☐ 3. Safe body mechanics of therapist ☐ Comments:

PROM Assessment and Measurement Testing: Knee

STEP 1 ── ── STEP 2

Movement	PROM Assessment of End Feel	Start Position	Axis	Stationary Arm	End Position	Movable Arm	Recording	Instructions	Handling/ Comments
				PROM Measurement: Using A Universal Goniometer					
KNEE FLEXION Form 7-1	1. Start position ☐ 2. Stabilized ☐ 3. Therapist distal hand placement ☐ 4. End position (full PROM achieved) ☐ 5. End feel ☐	1. Supine ☐ 2. Hip and knee in anatomical position ☐ 3. Towel under distal thigh ☐ 4. Pelvis and femur stabilized ☐	1. Over lateral epicondyle of femur ☐	1. Parallel longitudinal axis of femur, pointing toward greater trochanter ☐ 2. Position maintained for start position ☐ 3. Position maintained for end position ☐	1. Hip and knee flexed ☐ 2. Heel moved toward buttock to limit of knee flexion ☐ 3. Full PROM achieved ☐ 4. Pelvis and femur stabilized ☐	1. Parallel long axis of fibula, pointing toward the lateral malleolus ☐ 2. Position maintained for start position ☐ 3. Position maintained for end position ☐	1. Full PROM ☐ 2. End feel ☐	1. Verbal (clear/ concise) ☐ 2. Demonstration (clear) ☐	1. Adequate support of limb/limb segment ☐ 2. Comfortable grip ☐ 3. Safe body mechanics of therapist ☐ Comments:
KNEE EXTENSION/ HYPER- EXTENSION Form 7-2	1. Start position ☐ 2. Stabilized ☐ 3. Therapist distal hand placement ☐ 4. End position (full PROM achieved) ☐ 5. End feel ☐	1. Supine ☐ 2. Hip and knee in anatomical position ☐ 3. Towel under distal thigh ☐ 4. Femur stabilized ☐	1. Over lateral epicondyle of femur ☐	1. Parallel longitudinal axis of femur, pointing toward greater trochanter ☐ 2. Position maintained for start position ☐ 3. Position maintained for end position ☐	1. Knee extended/ hyper- extended to limit of motion ☐ 2. Full PROM achieved ☐ 3. Femur stabilized ☐	1. Parallel long axis of fibula, pointing toward the lateral malleolus ☐ 2. Position maintained for start position ☐ 3. Position maintained for end position ☐	1. Full PROM ☐ 2. End feel ☐	1. Verbal (clear/ concise) ☐ 2. Demonstration (clear) ☐	1. Adequate support of limb/limb segment ☐ 2. Comfortable grip ☐ 3. Safe body mechanics of therapist ☐ Comments:

(continues)

PROM Assessment and Measurement Testing: Knee (continued)

Movement	Start Position	Stabilization	Therapist's Hand Placement	End Position	Recording	Instructions	Handling/Comments
PATELLAR DISTAL GLIDE Form 7-3	1. Supine 2. Roll supports knee in slight flexion	1. Femur stabilized ☐	1. Heel of hand against base of patella, forearm lies along thigh ☐ 2. Palm of other hand placed on top of first hand ☐	1. Patella moved distally ☐ 2. Patellar compression against femur avoided ☐ 3. Full PROM achieved ☐ 4. Femur stabilized ☐	1. Full PROM ☐ 2. End feel ☐	1. Verbal (clear/concise) ☐ 2. Demonstration (clear) ☐	1. Adequate support of limb/limb segment ☐ 2. Comfortable grip ☐ 3. Safe body mechanics of therapist ☐ Comments:
PATELLAR MEDIAL-LATERAL GLIDE Form 7-4	1. Supine 2. Roll supports knee in slight flexion	1. Femur and tibia stabilized ☐	1. Palmar aspect of thumbs positioned along lateral border of patella ☐ 2. Pads of index fingers on medial border of patella ☐	1. Patella moved medially ☐ 2. Patella moved laterally ☐ 3. Patellar compression against femur avoided ☐ 4. Full PROM achieved ☐ 5. Femur and tibia stabilized ☐	1. Full PROM ☐ 2. End feel ☐	1. Verbal (clear/concise) ☐ 2. Demonstration (clear) ☐	1. Adequate support of limb/limb segment ☐ 2. Comfortable grip ☐ 3. Safe body mechanics of therapist ☐ Comments:
TIBIAL ROTATION Form 7-5	1. Sitting 2. Pad placed under distal thigh to maintain thigh in horizontal position ☐ 3. Knee flexed 90° ☐ 4. Tibia in full internal rotation ☐	1. Femur stabilized ☐	1. Distal tibia and fibula ☐	1. Tibia externally rotated to the limit of motion ☐ 2. Full PROM achieved ☐ 3. Femur stabilized ☐	1. Full PROM ☐ 2. End feel ☐	1. Verbal (clear/concise) ☐ 2. Demonstration (clear) ☐	1. Adequate support of limb/limb segment ☐ 2. Comfortable grip ☐ 3. Safe body mechanics of therapist ☐ Comments:

Muscle Length Assessment and Measurement Testing: Knee

Muscle	Start Position	Stabilization	End Position	Measurement of Joint Position Using Universal Goniometer	Recording	Instructions	Handling/Comments
HAMSTRINGS PASSIVE KNEE EXTENSION (PKE) SUPINE *Form 7-6*	1. Supine ☐ 2. Hip flexed 90°, patient holds distal thigh to maintain position ☐ 3. Knee flexed ☐ 4. Ankle relaxed in plantarflexion ☐	1. Thigh stabilized in 90° hip flexion ☐ 2. Posterior pelvic tilt avoided ☐ 3. If necessary nontest thigh stabilized on plinth ☐	1. Knee extended to limit of motion ☐ 2. Ankle relaxed in plantarflexion ☐ 3. Full PROM achieved ☐ 4. Thigh stabilized ☐ 5. Posterior pelvic tilt avoided ☐	Knee flexion 1. Axis: over the lateral epicondyle of the femur ☐ 2. Stationary arm: parallel longitudinal axis of femur, pointing toward greater trochanter ☐ 3. Movable arm: parallel long axis of fibula, pointing toward lateral malleolus ☐	1. Full PROM ☐ 2. End feel ☐	1. Verbal (clear/concise) ☐ 2. Demonstration (clear) ☐	1. Adequate support of limb/limb segment ☐ 2. Comfortable grip ☐ 3. Safe body mechanics of therapist ☐ Comments:
HAMSTRINGS (SITTING) *Form 7-7*	1. Sitting grasping edge of plinth ☐ 2. Towel placed under distal thigh ☐ 3. Ankle relaxed in plantarflexion ☐ 4. Nontest leg: foot supported on stool ☐	1. Pelvis and femur stabilized ☐	1. Knee extended to limit of motion ☐ 2. Full PROM achieved ☐ 3. Pelvis and femur stabilized ☐	Knee extension 1. Axis: over the lateral epicondyle of the femur ☐ 2. Stationary arm: parallel longitudinal axis of femur, pointing toward greater trochanter ☐ 3. Movable arm: parallel longitudinal axis of fibula, pointing toward lateral malleolus ☐	1. Full PROM ☐ 2. End feel ☐	1. Verbal (clear/concise) ☐ 2. Demonstration (clear) ☐	1. Adequate support of limb/limb segment ☐ 2. Comfortable grip ☐ 3. Safe body mechanics of therapist ☐ Comments:

(continues)

Muscle Length Assessment and Measurement Testing: Knee (*continued*)

Muscle	Start Position	Stabilization	End Position	Measurement of Joint Position Using Universal Goniometer	Recording	Instructions	Handling/Comments
RECTUS FEMORIS (PRONE ONE FOOT ON FLOOR) Form 7-8	1. Prone ☐ 2. Hip and knee in anatomical position ☐ 3. Towel placed under distal thigh ☐ 4. Nontest leg over side of plinth, with hip flexed and foot on floor ☐	1. Pelvis and femur stabilized ☐	1. Knee flexed to limit of motion ☐ 2. Full PROM achieved ☐ 3. Pelvis and femur stabilized ☐	Knee flexion 1. Axis: over the lateral epicondyle of the femur ☐ 2. Stationary arm: parallel longitudinal axis of femur, pointing toward greater trochanter ☐ 3. Movable arm: parallel longitudinal axis of fibula, pointing toward lateral malleolus ☐	1. Full PROM ☐ 2. End feel ☐	1. Verbal (clear/concise) ☐ 2. Demonstration (clear) ☐	1. Adequate support of limb/limb segment ☐ 2. Comfortable grip ☐ 3. Safe body mechanics of therapist ☐ Comments:
RECTUS FEMORIS (ELY'S TEST) Form 7-9	1. Prone ☐ 2. Towel placed under distal thigh ☐	1. Pelvis and femur stabilized ☐	1. Knee flexed to limit of motion ☐ 2. Full PROM achieved ☐ 3. Pelvis and femur stabilized ☐	Knee flexion 1. Axis: over the lateral epicondyle of the femur ☐ 2. Stationary arm: parallel longitudinal axis of femur, pointing toward greater trochanter ☐ 3. Movable arm: parallel longitudinal axis of fibula, pointing toward lateral malleolus ☐	1. Full PROM ☐ 2. End feel ☐	1. Verbal (clear/concise) ☐ 2. Demonstration (clear) ☐	1. Adequate support of limb/limb segment ☐ 2. Comfortable grip ☐ 3. Safe body mechanics of therapist ☐ Comments:
RECTUS FEMORIS (THOMAS TEST POSITION) Form 7-10	1. Sitting, with edge of plinth at midthigh level ☐ 2. Patient assisted into supine ☐ 3. Nontest hip held in flexion ☐ 4. Sacrum and lumbar spine flat on plinth ☐ 5. With hip abducted on test side, hip is extended to limit of motion ☐	1. Pelvis and lumbar spine stabilized ☐ 2. Anterior pelvic tilt avoided ☐ 3. Femur stabilized ☐	1. Knee is flexed to limit of motion ☐ 2. Full PROM achieved ☐ 3. Pelvis and lumbar spine stabilized ☐ 4. Anterior pelvic tilt avoided ☐ 5. Femur stabilized ☐	Knee flexion 1. Axis: over the lateral epicondyle of the femur ☐ 2. Stationary arm: parallel longitudinal axis of femur, pointing toward greater trochanter ☐ 3. Movable arm parallel longitudinal axis of fibula, pointing toward lateral malleolus ☐	1. Full PROM ☐ 2. End feel ☐	1. Verbal (clear/concise) ☐ 2. Demonstration (clear) ☐	1. Adequate support of limb/limb segment ☐ 2. Comfortable grip ☐ 3. Safe body mechanics of therapist ☐ Comments:

PROM Assessment and Measurement Testing: Ankle and Foot

STEP 1 | STEP 2

Movement	PROM Assessment of End Feel	Start Position	PROM Measurement: Using A Universal Goniometer						Handling/Comments
			Axis	Stationary Arm	End Position	Movable Arm	Recording	Instructions	
ANKLE DORSIFLEXION Form 8-1	1. Start position ☐ 2. Stabilized ☐ 3. Therapist distal hand placement ☐ 4. End position (full PROM achieved) ☐ 5. End feel ☐	1. Supine ☐ 2. Roll under knee (about 20–30° knee flexion) ☐ 3. Ankle in anatomical position ☐ 4. Tibia and fibula stabilized ☐	1. Inferior to the lateral malleolus ☐	1. Parallel longitudinal axis of fibula pointing to fibular head ☐ 2. Position maintained for start position ☐ 3. Position maintained for end position ☐	1. Ankle dorsiflexed to limit of motion ☐ 2. Full PROM achieved ☐ 3. Tibia and fibula stabilized ☐	1. Parallel to sole of heel ☐ 2. Position maintained for start position ☐ 3. Position maintained for end position ☐	1. Full PROM ☐ 2. End feel ☐	1. Verbal (clear/concise) ☐ 2. Demonstration (clear) ☐	1. Adequate support of limb/limb segment ☐ 2. Comfortable grip ☐ 3. Safe body mechanics of therapist ☐ Comments:
ANKLE PLANTARFLEXION Form 8-2	1. Start position ☐ 2. Stabilized ☐ 3. Therapist distal hand placement ☐ 4. End position (full PROM achieved) ☐ 5. End feel ☐	1. Supine ☐ 2. Roll under knee (about 20–30° knee flexion) ☐ 3. Ankle in anatomical position ☐ 4. Tibia and fibula stabilized ☐	1. Inferior to the lateral malleolus ☐	1. Parallel longitudinal axis of fibula pointing to fibular head ☐ 2. Position maintained for start position ☐ 3. Position maintained for end position ☐	1. Ankle plantarflexed to limit of motion ☐ 2. Full PROM achieved ☐ 3. Tibia and fibula stabilized ☐	1. Parallel to sole of heel ☐ 2. Position maintained for start position ☐ 3. Position maintained for end position ☐	1. Full PROM ☐ 2. End feel ☐	1. Verbal (clear/concise) ☐ 2. Demonstration (clear) ☐	1. Adequate support of limb/limb segment ☐ 2. Comfortable grip ☐ 3. Safe body mechanics of therapist ☐ Comments:

(continues)

PROM Assessment and Measurement Testing: Ankle and Foot (continued)

Movement	Start Position	Inversion End Position	Eversion End Position	Measurement and Recording	Instructions	Handling/ Comments

AROM: SUBTALAR IN-VERSION AND EVER-SION
 	
Form 8-3
	1. Supine ☐
	2. Paper adhered to flat surface placed under heel ☐
	3. Ankle and foot in anatomical position ☐
	4. Flat-surfaced object placed against sole of foot and line drawn along surface ☐
	5. Tibia and fibula stabilized ☐
		1. Tibia and fibula stabilized ☐
		2. Foot inverted to limit of motion ☐
		3. Full AROM achieved, patient holds position ☐
		4. Flat-surfaced object placed against sole of foot in inversion and line drawn along surface and labeled "Inv" ☐
			1. Tibia and fibula stabilized ☐
			2. Foot everted to limit of motion ☐
			3. Full AROM achieved, patient holds position ☐
			4. Flat-surfaced object placed against sole of foot in eversion and line drawn along surface and labeled "Ev" ☐
				Goniometer placed on line graphics:
				1. Inversion AROM angle correctly:
				  a. Measured ☐
				  b. Recorded ☐
				2. Eversion AROM angle correctly:
				  a. Measured ☐
				  b. Recorded ☐
					1. Verbal (clear/ concise) ☐
					2. Demonstration (clear) ☐
						1. Adequate support of limb/limb segment ☐
						2. Comfortable grip ☐
						3. Safe body mechanics of therapist ☐
						Comments:

STEP 1

STEP 2

PROM Measurement: Using A Universal Goniometer						
Movement	PROM Assessment of End Feel	Start Position	Axis	Stationary Arm	End Position	Movable Arm	Recording	Instructions	Handling/ Comments
SUBTALAR INVER-SION Form 8-4	1. Start position ☐ 2. Stabilized ☐ 3. Therapist distal hand placement ☐ 4. End position (full PROM achieved) ☐ 5. End feel ☐	1. Prone with feet off end of plinth ☐ 2. Ankle in anatomical position ☐ 3. Tibia and fibula stabilized ☐	1. Over mark placed at midline of superior aspect of calcaneus ☐	1. Parallel longitudinal axis of lower leg ☐ 2. Position maintained for start position ☐ 3. Position maintained for end position ☐	1. Calcaneus inverted to limit of motion ☐ 2. Full PROM achieved ☐ 3. Tibia and fibula stabilized ☐	1. Aligned with mark over midline, posterior aspect of calcaneus ☐ 2. Position maintained for start position ☐ 3. Position maintained for end position ☐	1. Full PROM ☐ 2. End feel ☐	1. Verbal (clear/ concise) ☐ 2. Demonstration (clear) ☐	1. Adequate support of limb/limb segment ☐ 2. Comfortable grip ☐ 3. Safe body mechanics of therapist ☐ Comments:

— STEP 1 —   STEP 2 —

PROM Measurement: Using A Universal Goniometer

Movement	PROM Assessment of End Feel	Start Position	Axis	Stationary Arm	End Position	Movable Arm	Recording	Instructions	Handling/Comments
SUBTALAR EVERSION Form 8-5	1. Start position ☐ 2. Stabilized ☐ 3. Therapist distal hand placement ☐ 4. End position (full PROM achieved) ☐ 5. End feel ☐	1. Prone with feet off end of plinth ☐ 2. Ankle in anatomical position ☐ 3. Tibia and fibula stabilized ☐	1. Over mark placed at midline of superior aspect of calcaneus ☐	1. Parallel longitudinal axis of lower leg ☐ 2. Position maintained for start position ☐ 3. Position maintained for end position ☐	1. Calcaneus everted to limit of motion ☐ 2. Full PROM achieved ☐ 3. Tibia and fibula stabilized ☐	1. Aligned with mark over midline, posterior aspect of calcaneus ☐ 2. Position maintained for start position ☐ 3. Position maintained for end position ☐	1. Full PROM ☐ 2. End feel ☐	1. Verbal (clear/concise) ☐ 2. Demonstration (clear) ☐	1. Adequate support of limb/limb segment ☐ 2. Comfortable grip ☐ 3. Safe body mechanics of therapist ☐ Comments:
ANKLE & FOOT SUPINATION: INVERSION COMPONENT Form 8-6	1. Start position ☐ 2. Stabilized ☐ 3. Therapist distal hand placement ☐ 4. End position (full PROM achieved) ☐ 5. End feel ☐	1. Sitting ☐ 2. Ankle and foot in anatomical position ☐ 3. Tibia and fibula stabilized ☐	1. Anterior ankle joint midway between medial and lateral malleoli ☐	1. Parallel midline of tibia ☐ 2. Position maintained for start position ☐ 3. Position maintained for end position ☐	1. Ankle and foot inversion to limit of motion ☐ 2. Full PROM achieved ☐ 3. Tibia and fibula stabilized ☐	1. Parallel to midline of second metatarsal ☐ 2. Position maintained for start position ☐ 3. Position maintained for end position ☐	1. Full PROM ☐ 2. End Feel ☐	1. Verbal (clear/concise) ☐ 2. Demonstration (clear) ☐	1. Adequate support of limb/limb segment ☐ 2. Comfortable grip ☐ 3. Safe body mechanics of therapist ☐ Comments:
ANKLE & FOOT PRONATION: EVERSION COMPONENT Form 8-7	1. Start position ☐ 2. Stabilized ☐ 3. Therapist distal hand placement ☐ 4. End position (full PROM achieved) ☐ 5. End feel ☐	1. Sitting ☐ 2. Ankle and foot in anatomical position ☐ 3. Tibia and fibula stabilized ☐	1. Anterior ankle joint midway between medial and lateral malleoli ☐	1. Parallel midline of tibia ☐ 2. Position maintained for start position ☐ 3. Position maintained for end position ☐	1. Ankle and foot eversion to limit of motion ☐ 2. Full PROM achieved ☐ 3. Tibia and fibula stabilized ☐	1. Parallel to midline of second metatarsal ☐ 2. Position maintained for start position ☐ 3. Position maintained for end position ☐	1. Full PROM ☐ 2. End Feel ☐	1. Verbal (clear/concise) ☐ 2. Demonstration (clear) ☐	1. Adequate support of limb/limb segment ☐ 2. Comfortable grip ☐ 3. Safe body mechanics of therapist ☐ Comments:

(continues)

PROM Assessment and Measurement Testing: Ankle and Foot (continued)

	STEP 1	STEP 2						
		PROM Measurement: Using A Universal Goniometer						
Movement	PROM Assessment of End Feel	Start Position	Axis	Stationary Arm	End Position	Movable Arm	Recording	Instructions	Handling/Comments

Movement	PROM Assessment of End Feel	Start Position	Axis	Stationary Arm	End Position	Movable Arm	Recording	Instructions	Handling/Comments
GREAT TOE MTP JOINT FLEXION Form 8-8	1. Start position ☐☐ 2. Stabilized ☐☐ 3. Therapist distal hand placement ☐ 4. End position (full PROM achieved) ☐☐ 5. End feel ☐☐	1. Supine 2. Ankle and toes in anatomical position ☐ 3. First metatarsal stabilized ☐	1. Over dorsum or over medial aspect of first MTP joint ☐	1. Parallel longitudinal axis of first metatarsal ☐ 2. Position maintained for start position ☐ 3. Position maintained for end position ☐	1. MTP joint flexed to limit of motion 2. Full PROM achieved ☐ 3. First metatarsal stabilized ☐	1. Parallel longitudinal axis of proximal phalanx of great toe ☐ 2. Position maintained for start position ☐ 3. Position maintained for end position ☐	1. Full PROM ☐ 2. End feel ☐	1. Verbal (clear/concise) ☐ 2. Demonstration (clear) ☐	1. Adequate support of limb/limb segment ☐ 2. Comfortable grip ☐ 3. Safe body mechanics of therapist ☐ Comments:
GREAT TOE MTP JOINT EXTENSION Form 8-9	1. Start position ☐☐ 2. Stabilized ☐☐ 3. Therapist distal hand placement ☐ 4. End position (full PROM achieved) ☐☐ 5. End feel ☐☐	1. Supine 2. Ankle and toes in anatomical position ☐ 3. First metatarsal stabilized ☐	1. Over plantar aspect or over medial aspect of first MTP joint ☐	1. Parallel longitudinal axis of first metatarsal ☐ 2. Position maintained for start position ☐ 3. Position maintained for end position ☐	1. MTP joint extended to limit of motion 2. Full PROM achieved ☐ 3. First metatarsal stabilized ☐	1. Parallel longitudinal axis of proximal phalanx of great toe ☐ 2. Position maintained for start position ☐ 3. Position maintained for end position ☐	1. Full PROM ☐ 2. End feel ☐	1. Verbal (clear/concise) ☐ 2. Demonstration (clear) ☐	1. Adequate support of limb/limb segment ☐ 2. Comfortable grip ☐ 3. Safe body mechanics of therapist ☐ Comments:
GREAT TOE MTP JOINT ABDUCTION Form 8-10	1. Start position ☐☐ 2. Stabilized ☐☐ 3. Therapist distal hand placement ☐ 4. End position (full PROM achieved) ☐☐ 5. End feel ☐☐	1. Supine 2. Ankle and great toe in anatomical position ☐ 3. First metatarsal stabilized ☐	1. Over dorsum of first MTP joint ☐	1. Parallel longitudinal axis of first metatarsal ☐ 2. Position maintained for start position ☐ 3. Position maintained for end position ☐	1. MTP joint abducted to limit of motion 2. Full PROM achieved ☐ 3. First metatarsal stabilized ☐	1. Parallel longitudinal axis of proximal phalanx of great toe ☐ 2. Position maintained for start position ☐ 3. Position maintained for end position ☐	1. Full PROM ☐ 2. End feel ☐	1. Verbal (clear/concise) ☐ 2. Demonstration (clear) ☐	1. Adequate support of limb/limb segment ☐ 2. Comfortable grip ☐ 3. Safe body mechanics of therapist ☐ Comments:

STEP 1 — **STEP 2**

PROM Measurement: Using A Universal Goniometer

Movement	STEP 1: PROM Assessment of End Feel	STEP 2: Start Position	Axis	Stationary Arm	End Position	Movable Arm	Recording	Instructions	Handling/Comments
GREAT TOE MTP JOINT ADDUCTION Form 8-11	1. Start position ☐ 2. Stabilized ☐ 3. Therapist distal hand placement ☐ 4. End position (full PROM achieved) ☐ 5. End feel ☐	1. Supine 2. Ankle and great toe in anatomical position ☐ 3. First metatarsal stabilized ☐	1. Over dorsum of first MTP joint ☐	1. Parallel longitudinal axis of first metatarsal ☐ 2. Position maintained for start position ☐ 3. Position maintained for end position ☐	1. MTP joint adducted to limit of motion ☐ 2. Full PROM achieved ☐ 3. First metatarsal stabilized ☐	1. Parallel longitudinal axis of proximal phalanx of great toe ☐ 2. Position maintained for start position ☐ 3. Position maintained for end position ☐	1. Full PROM ☐ 2. End feel ☐	1. Verbal (clear/concise) ☐ 2. Demonstration (clear) ☐	1. Adequate support of limb/limb segment ☐ 2. Comfortable grip ☐ 3. Safe body mechanics of therapist ☐ Comments:
GREAT TOE IP JOINT FLEXION Form 8-12	1. Start position ☐ 2. Stabilized ☐ 3. Therapist distal hand placement ☐ 4. End position (full PROM achieved) ☐ 5. End feel ☐	1. Supine 2. Ankle and great toe in anatomical position ☐ 3. Proximal phalanx of great toe stabilized ☐	1. Over dorsal or medial aspect of IP joint of great toe ☐	1. Parallel longitudinal axis of proximal phalanx of great toe ☐ 2. Position maintained for start position ☐ 3. Position maintained for end position ☐	1. IP joint flexed to limit of motion ☐ 2. Full PROM achieved ☐ 3. Proximal phalanx of great toe stabilized ☐	1. Parallel longitudinal axis of distal phalanx of great toe ☐ 2. Position maintained for start position ☐ 3. Position maintained for end position ☐	1. Full PROM ☐ 2. End feel ☐	1. Verbal (clear/concise) ☐ 2. Demonstration (clear) ☐	1. Adequate support of limb/limb segment ☐ 2. Comfortable grip ☐ 3. Safe body mechanics of therapist ☐ Comments:
GREAT TOE IP JOINT EXTENSION Form 8-13	1. Start position ☐ 2. Stabilized ☐ 3. Therapist distal hand placement ☐ 4. End position (full PROM achieved) ☐ 5. End feel ☐	1. Supine 2. Ankle and great toe in anatomical position ☐ 3. Proximal phalanx of great toe stabilized ☐	1. Over plantar or medial aspect of IP joint of great toe ☐	1. Parallel longitudinal axis of proximal phalanx of great toe ☐ 2. Position maintained for start position ☐ 3. Position maintained for end position ☐	1. IP joint extended to limit of motion ☐ 2. Full PROM achieved ☐ 3. Proximal phalanx of great toe stabilized ☐	1. Parallel longitudinal axis of distal phalanx of great toe ☐ 2. Position maintained for start position ☐ 3. Position maintained for end position ☐	1. Full PROM ☐ 2. End feel ☐	1. Verbal (clear/concise) ☐ 2. Demonstration (clear) ☐	1. Adequate support of limb/limb segment ☐ 2. Comfortable grip ☐ 3. Safe body mechanics of therapist ☐ Comments:

Muscle Length Assessment and Measurement Testing: Ankle and Foot

Muscle	Start Position	Stabilization	End Position	Measurement of Joint Position Using Universal Goniometer	Recording	Instructions	Handling/ Comments
GASTROCNEMIUS Form 8-14	1. Standing ☐ 2. Lower extremity in anatomical position ☐ 3. Facing a stable plinth or wall ☐	1. Foot and toes point forward and remain flat on floor ☐	1. Patient steps ahead with nontest leg ☐ 2. Patient leans forward to place hands on stable plinth or wall ☐ 3. Knee remains extended as patient leans forward ☐ 4. Ankle dorsiflexed to limit of motion ☐ 5. Foot and toes point forward and remain flat on floor ☐	Ankle dorsiflexion 1. Axis: inferior to the lateral malleolus ☐ 2. Stationary arm: parallel longitudinal axis of fibula pointing to head of fibula ☐ 3. Movable arm: parallel to sole of heel ☐	1. Full PROM ☐ 2. End feel ☐	1. Verbal (clear/concise) ☐ 2. Demonstration (clear) ☐	1. Adequate support of limb/limb segment ☐ 2. Comfortable grip ☐ 3. Safe body mechanics of therapist ☐ Comments:

AROM Assessment and Measurement Testing: Head, Neck

Movement	Start Position	Stabilization	End Position	Measurement	Recording	Instructions	Comments
TMJ: OCCLUSION AND DEPRESSION OF THE MANDIBLE Form 9-1	1. Sitting ☐ 2. Head and neck in anatomical position, TMJ in resting position ☐	1. Patient instructed to keep head, neck and trunk in anatomical position ☐	1. Lower jaw elevated, teeth in contact ☐ 2. Mouth opened to limit of motion ☐ 3. Full AROM achieved ☐	1. Occlusion: relative position of mandibular and maxillary teeth observed ☐ 2. Depression: distance measured between edges of upper and lower central incisors ☐	1. Full AROM recorded ☐	1. Verbal (clear/concise) ☐ 2. Demonstration (clear) ☐ 3. Substitute movement avoided ☐	
TMJ: PROTRUSION OF THE MANDIBLE Form 9-2	1. Sitting ☐ 2. Head and neck in anatomical position, TMJ in resting position ☐	1. Patient instructed to keep head, neck and trunk in anatomical position ☐	1. Lower jaw protruded, lower teeth beyond upper teeth ☐ 2. Full AROM achieved ☐	1. Distance measured between upper and lower central incisor teeth ☐	1. Full AROM recorded ☐	1. Verbal (clear/concise) ☐ 2. Demonstration (clear) ☐ 3. Substitute movement avoided ☐	
TMJ: LATERAL DEVIATION OF THE MANDIBLE Form 9-3	1. Sitting ☐ 2. Head and neck in anatomical position, TMJ in resting position ☐	1. Patient instructed to keep head, neck and trunk in anatomical position ☐	1. Lower jaw deviated to right ☐ 2. Lower jaw deviated to left ☐ 3. Full AROM achieved ☐	1. Distance measured between two selected points that are level (e.g. space between central incisors) ☐	1. Full AROM recorded ☐	1. Verbal (clear/concise) ☐ 2. Demonstration (clear) ☐ 3. Substitute movement avoided ☐	
NECK FLEXION (TAPE MEASURE) Form 9-4	1. Sitting ☐ 2. Head and neck in anatomical position ☐	1. Patient instructed on how to stabilize shoulder girdle and avoid thoracic and lumbar spine movements ☐	1. Neck flexed to limit of motion ☐ 2. Full AROM achieved ☐	1. Distance measured between tip of chin and suprasternal notch ☐	1. Full AROM recorded ☐	1. Verbal (clear/concise) ☐ 2. Demonstration (clear) ☐ 3. Substitute movement avoided ☐	

(continues)

AROM Assessment and Measurement Testing: Head, Neck (*continued*)

Movement	Start Position	Stabilization	End Position	Measurement	Recording	Instructions	Comments
NECK EXTENSION (TAPE MEASURE) Form 9-5	1. Sitting ☐ 2. Head and neck in anatomical position ☐	1. Patient instructed on how to stabilize shoulder girdle and avoid thoracic and lumbar spine movements ☐	1. Neck extended to limit of motion ☐ 2. Full AROM achieved ☐	1. Distance measured between tip of chin and suprasternal notch ☐	1. Full AROM recorded ☐	1. Verbal (clear/concise) ☐ 2. Demonstration (clear) ☐ 3. Substitute movement eliminated ☐	

Movement	Start Position	Inclinometer Placement	End Position	Recording	Instructions	Comments
NECK FLEXION (INCLINOMETER) Form 9-6	1. Sitting ☐ 2. Head and neck in anatomical position ☐ 3. Trunk and shoulder girdles stabilized ☐ 4. Inclinometers zeroed in start position ☐	1. Superior inclinometer: on vertex of head ☐ 2. Inferior inclinometer: a. on spine of T1 ☐ OR b. over spine of scapula ☐	1. Full neck flexion AROM achieved ☐ 2. Measurement recorded from superior inclinometer ☐ 3. Measurement recorded from inferior inclinometer ☐	1. Difference between two inclinometer readings recorded for neck flexion AROM ☐	1. Verbal (clear/concise) ☐ 2. Demonstration (clear) ☐ 3. Substitute movement eliminated ☐	
NECK EXTENSION (INCLINOMETER) Form 9-7	1. Sitting ☐ 2. Head and neck in anatomical position ☐ 3. Trunk and shoulder girdles stabilized ☐ 4. Inclinometers zeroed in start position ☐	1. Superior inclinometer: on vertex of head ☐ 2. Inferior inclinometer: a. on spine of T1 ☐ OR b. over spine of scapula ☐	1. Full neck extension AROM achieved ☐ 2. Measurement recorded from superior inclinometer ☐ 3. Measurement recorded from inferior inclinometer ☐	1. Difference between two inclinometer readings recorded for neck extension AROM ☐	1. Verbal (clear/concise) ☐ 2. Demonstration (clear) ☐ 3. Substitute movement eliminated ☐	

Movement	Start Position	CROM Placement	End Position	Recording	Instructions	Comments
NECK FLEXION (CROM) Form 9-8	1. Sitting ☐ 2. Head and neck in anatomical position ☐ 3. Trunk and shoulder girdles stabilized ☐	1. CROM positioned on head ☐ 2. Inclinometer on lateral aspect of head zeroed in start position ☐	1. Full neck flexion AROM achieved ☐	1. Inclinometer reading recorded for neck flexion AROM ☐	1. Verbal (clear/concise) ☐ 2. Demonstration (clear) ☐ 3. Substitute movement eliminated ☐	
NECK EXTENSION (CROM) Form 9-9	1. Sitting ☐ 2. Head and neck in anatomical position ☐ 3. Trunk and shoulder girdles stabilized ☐	1. CROM positioned on head ☐ 2. Inclinometer on lateral aspect of head zeroed in start position ☐	1. Full neck extension AROM achieved ☐	1. Inclinometer reading recorded for neck extension AROM ☐	1. Verbal (clear/concise) ☐ 2. Demonstration (clear) ☐ 3. Substitute movement eliminated ☐	

Movement	Start Position	Axis	Stationary Arm	End Position	Movable Arm	Recording	Instructions/Comments
NECK FLEXION (UNIVERSAL GONIOMETER) Form 9-10	1. Sitting ☐ 2. Head and neck in anatomical position ☐ 3. Trunk and shoulder girdles stabilized ☐	1. Over lobule of ear ☐	1. Perpendicular to floor ☐ 2. Position maintained for start position ☐ 3. Position maintained for end position ☐	1. Full neck flexion AROM ☐ 2. Trunk and shoulder girdles stabilized ☐	1. Parallel base of nares ☐ 2. Position maintained for start position ☐ 3. Position maintained for end position ☐	1. Full neck flexion AROM recorded ☐	1. Verbal (clear/concise) ☐ 2. Demonstration (clear) ☐ 3. Substitute movement eliminated ☐ Comments:
NECK EXTENSION (UNIVERSAL GONIOMETER) Form 9-11	1. Sitting ☐ 2. Head and neck in anatomical position ☐ 3. Trunk and shoulder girdles stabilized ☐	1. Over lobule of ear ☐	1. Perpendicular to floor ☐ 2. Position maintained for start position ☐ 3. Position maintained for end position ☐	1. Full neck extension AROM ☐ 2. Trunk and shoulder girdles stabilized ☐	1. Parallel base of nares ☐ 2. Position maintained for start position ☐ 3. Position maintained for end position ☐	1. Full neck extension AROM recorded ☐	1. Verbal (clear/concise) ☐ 2. Demonstration (clear) ☐ 3. Substitute movement eliminated ☐ Comments:

(continues)

AROM Assessment and Measurement Testing: Head, Neck (continued)

Movement	Start Position	Stabilization	End Position	Measurement	Recording	Instructions	Comments
NECK LATERAL FLEXION (TAPE MEASURE) Form 9-12	1. Sitting ☐ 2. Head and neck in anatomical position ☐	1. Patient instructed on how to stabilize shoulder girdle and avoid thoracic and lumbar spine movements ☐	1. Neck laterally flexed to limit of motion ☐ 2. Full AROM achieved ☐	1. Distance measured between mastoid process and acromion process ☐	1. Full AROM recorded ☐	1. Verbal (clear/concise) ☐ 2. Demonstration (clear) ☐ 3. Substitute movement avoided ☐	

Movement	Start Position	Inclinometer Placement	End Position	Recording	Instructions	Comments
NECK LATERAL FLEXION (INCLINOMETER) Form 9-13	1. Sitting ☐ 2. Head and neck in anatomical position ☐ 3. Trunk and shoulder girdles stabilized ☐ 4. Inclinometers zeroed in start position ☐	1. Superior inclinometer: on vertex of head ☐ 2. Inferior inclinometer: on spine of T1 ☐	1. Full neck lateral flexion AROM achieved ☐ 2. Measurement recorded from superior inclinometer ☐ 3. Measurement recorded from inferior inclinometer ☐	1. Difference between two inclinometer readings recorded for neck lateral flexion AROM ☐	1. Verbal (clear/concise) ☐ 2. Demonstration (clear) ☐ 3. Substitute movement eliminated ☐	

Movement	Start Position	CROM Placement	End Position	Recording	Instructions	Comments
NECK LATERAL FLEXION (CROM) Form 9-14	1. Sitting ☐ 2. Head and neck in anatomical position ☐ 3. Trunk and shoulder girdles stabilized ☐	1. CROM positioned on head ☐ 2. Inclinometer on anterior aspect of head zeroed in start position ☐	1. Full neck lateral flexion AROM achieved ☐	1. Inclinometer reading recorded for neck lateral flexion AROM ☐	1. Verbal (clear/concise) ☐ 2. Demonstration (clear) ☐ 3. Substitute movement eliminated ☐	

NECK LATERAL FLEXION (UNIVERSAL GONIOMETER) — Form 9-15

Movement	Start Position	Axis	Stationary Arm	End Position	Movable Arm	Recording	Instructions/Comments
NECK LATERAL FLEXION (UNIVERSAL GONIOMETER) Form 9-15	1. Sitting ☐ 2. Head and neck in anatomical position ☐ 3. Trunk and shoulder girdles stabilized ☐	1. Over C7 spinous process ☐	1. Along the spine perpendicular to floor ☐ 2. Position maintained for start position ☐ 3. Position maintained for end position ☐	1. Full neck lateral flexion AROM ☐ 2. Trunk and shoulder girdles stabilized ☐	1. Points toward midpoint of head ☐ 2. Position maintained for start position ☐ 3. Position maintained for end position ☐	1. Full neck lateral flexion AROM recorded ☐	1. Verbal (clear/concise) ☐ 2. Demonstration (clear) ☐ 3. Substitute movement eliminated ☐ Comments:

NECK ROTATION (TAPE MEASURE) — Form 9-16

Movement	Start Position	Stabilization	End Position	Measurement	Recording	Instructions	Comments
NECK ROTATION (TAPE MEASURE) Form 9-16	1. Sitting ☐ 2. Head and neck in anatomical position ☐	1. Patient instructed on how to stabilize shoulder girdle and avoid thoracic and lumbar spine movements ☐	1. Neck rotated to limit of motion ☐ 2. Full AROM achieved ☐	1. Distance measured between tip of chin and lateral edge of acromion process ☐	1. Full AROM recorded ☐	1. Verbal (clear/concise) ☐ 2. Demonstration (clear) ☐ 3. Substitute movement avoided ☐	

NECK ROTATION (INCLINOMETER) — Form 9-17

Movement	Start Position	Inclinometer Placement	End Position	Recording	Instructions
NECK ROTATION (INCLINOMETER) Form 9-17	1. Sitting ☐ 2. Head and neck in anatomical position ☐ 3. Trunk and shoulder girdles stabilized ☐ 4. Inclinometer zeroed in start position ☐	1. Inclinometer: in midline at base of forehead ☐	1. Neck rotated to limit of motion ☐ 2. Full AROM achieved ☐	1. Inclinometer reading recorded for neck rotation AROM ☐	1. Verbal (clear/concise) ☐ 2. Demonstration (clear) ☐ 3. Substitute movement eliminated ☐

(continues)

AROM Assessment and Measurement Testing: Head, Neck (continued)

Movement	Start Position	CROM Placement	End Position	Recording	Instructions	Comments
NECK ROTATION (CROM) Form 9-18	1. Sitting ☐ 2. Head and neck in anatomical position ☐ 3. Trunk and shoulder girdles stabilized ☐	1. CROM positioned on head ☐ 2. Magnetic yoke positioned over shoulders ☐ 3. Head positioned with anterior and lateral inclinometers zeroed ☐ 4. Compass on superior aspect of head zeroed in start position ☐	1. Neck rotated to limit of motion ☐ 2. Full AROM achieved ☐	1. Compass reading recorded for neck rotation AROM ☐	1. Verbal (clear/concise) ☐ 2. Demonstration (clear) ☐ 3. Substitute movement eliminated ☐	

Movement	Start Position	Axis	Stationary Arm	End Position	Movable Arm	Recording	Instructions/Comments
NECK ROTATION (UNIVERSAL GONIOMETER) Form 9-19	1. Sitting ☐ 2. Head and neck in anatomical position ☐ 3. Trunk and shoulder girdles stabilized ☐	1. Over midpoint of top of head ☐	1. Parallel to line joining two acromion processes ☐ 2. Position maintained for start position ☐ 3. Position maintained for end position ☐	1. Neck rotated to limit of motion ☐ 2. Full AROM achieved ☐ 3. Trunk and shoulder girdles stabilized ☐	1. Aligned with nose ☐ 2. Position maintained for start position ☐ 3. Position maintained for end position ☐	1. Full neck rotation AROM recorded ☐	1. Verbal (clear/concise) ☐ 2. Demonstration (clear) ☐ 3. Substitute movement eliminated ☐ **Comments:**

AROM Assessment and Measurement Testing: Trunk

Movement	Start Position	End Position	Measurement	Recording	Instructions	Comments
TRUNK FLEXION-THORACOLUMBAR SPINE (TAPE MEASURE) Form 9-20	1. Standing, feet shoulder width apart, knees straight ☐	1. Trunk flexed to limit of motion for thoracolumbar flexion ☐ 2. Full AROM achieved ☐	1. Distance measured between C7 and S2 at start position ☐ 2. Distance measured between C7 and S2 at end position ☐	1. Difference between start and end measures recorded for AROM ☐	1. Verbal (clear/concise) ☐ 2. Demonstration (clear) ☐ 3. Substitute movement avoided ☐	
TRUNK EXTENSION-THORACOLUMBAR SPINE (TAPE MEASURE) Form 9-21	1. Standing, feet shoulder width apart, knees straight ☐ 2. Hands on iliac crests and small of back ☐	1. Trunk extended to limit of motion for thoracolumbar extension ☐ 2. Full AROM achieved ☐	1. Distance measured between C7 and S2 at start position ☐ 2. Distance measured between C7 and S2 at end position ☐	1. Difference between start and end measures recorded for AROM ☐	1. Verbal (clear/concise) ☐ 2. Demonstration (clear) ☐ 3. Substitute movement avoided ☐	

Movement	Start Position	Inclinometer Placement	End Position	Recording	Instructions	Comments
TRUNK FLEXION – THORACOLUMBAR SPINE (INCLINOMETER) Form 9-22	1. Standing, feet shoulder width apart, knees straight ☐ 2. Inclinometers zeroed in start position ☐	1. Superior inclinometer: on spine of C7 ☐ 2. Inferior inclinometer: on spine of S2 ☐	1. Full thoracolumbar spine flexion AROM to limit of motion ☐ 2. Measurement recorded from superior inclinometer ☐ 3. Measurement recorded from inferior inclinometer ☐	1. Difference between two inclinometer readings recorded for thoracolumbar flexion AROM ☐	1. Verbal (clear/concise) ☐ 2. Demonstration (clear) ☐ 3. Substitute movement eliminated ☐	

(continues)

AROM Assessment and Measurement Testing: Trunk (*continued*)

Movement	Start Position	Inclinometer Placement	End Position	Recording	Instructions	Comments
TRUNK EXTENSION – THORACOLUMBAR SPINE (INCLINOMETER) Form 9-23	1. Standing, feet shoulder width apart, knees straight ☐ 2. Hands on iliac crests and small of back ☐ 3. Inclinometers zeroed in start position ☐	1. Superior inclinometer: on spine of C7 ☐ 2. Inferior inclinometer: on spine of S2 ☐	1. Full thoracolumbar spine extension AROM to limit of motion ☐ 2. Measurement recorded from superior inclinometer ☐ 3. Measurement recorded from inferior inclinometer ☐	1. Difference between two inclinometer readings recorded for thoracolumbar extension AROM ☐	1. Verbal (clear/concise) ☐ 2. Demonstration (clear) ☐ 3. Substitute movement eliminated ☐	

Movement	Start Position	Stabilization	End Position	Measurement	Recording	Instructions	Comments
TRUNK EXTENSION-THORACOLUMBAR SPINE (PRONE PRESS-UP) Form 9-24	1. Prone ☐ 2. Hands positioned on plinth at shoulder level ☐	1. Strap used to stabilize pelvis ☐	1. Patient extends elbows to raise trunk and extend thoracolumbar spine to limit of motion ☐ 2. Full AROM achieved ☐	1. Perpendicular distance measured between suprasternal notch and plinth ☐	1. Distance measured recorded for ROM ☐	1. Verbal (clear/concise) ☐ 2. Demonstration (clear) ☐ 3. Substitute movement eliminated ☐	
TRUNK FLEXION-LUMBAR SPINE (MODIFIED MODIFIED SCHÖBER METHOD) (TAPE MEASURE) Form 9-25	1. Standing, feet shoulder width apart ☐ 2. Mark placed over spine 15 cm above spinous process of S2 at start position ☐		1. Trunk flexed to limit of motion for lumbar flexion ☐ 2. Full AROM achieved ☐	1. Distance measured between 15 cm mark and S2 at end position ☐	1. Difference between start and end measures recorded for AROM ☐	1. Verbal (clear/concise) ☐ 2. Demonstration (clear) ☐ 3. Substitute movement eliminated ☐	

Movement	Start Position	Stabilization	End Position	Measurement	Recording	Instructions	Comments
TRUNK EXTENSION– LUMBAR SPINE (TAPE MEASUER) Form 9-26	1. Standing, feet shoulder width apart ☐ 2. Hands on iliac crests and small of back ☐ 3. Mark placed over spine 15 cm above spinous process of S2 at start position ☐		1. Trunk extended to limit of motion for lumbar extension ☐ 2. Full AROM achieved ☐	1. Distance measured between 15 cm mark and S2 at end position ☐	1. Difference between start and end measures recorded for AROM ☐	1. Verbal (clear/concise) ☐ 2. Demonstration (clear) ☐ 3. Substitute movement eliminated ☐	

Movement	Start Position	Inclinometer Placement	End Position	Recording	Instructions	Comments
TRUNK FLEXION – LUMBAR SPINE (INCLINOMETER) Form 9-27	1. Standing, feet shoulder width apart, knees straight ☐ 2. Inclinometers zeroed in start position ☐	1. Superior inclinometer: on a mark 15 cm above the spinous process of S2 ☐ 2. Inferior inclinometer: on spine of S2 ☐	1. Full lumbar spine flexion AROM to limit of motion ☐ 2. Measurement recorded from superior inclinometer ☐ 3. Measurement recorded from inferior inclinometer ☐	1. Difference between two inclinometer readings recorded for lumbar flexion AROM ☐	1. Verbal (clear/concise) ☐ 2. Demonstration (clear) ☐ 3. Substitute movement eliminated ☐	
TRUNK EXTENSION – LUMBAR SPINE (INCLINOMETER) Form 9-28	1. Standing, feet shoulder width apart, knees straight ☐ 2. Hands on iliac crests and small of back ☐ 3. Inclinometers zeroed in start position ☐	1. Superior inclinometer: on a mark 15 cm above the spinous process of S2 ☐ 2. Inferior inclinometer: on spine of S2 ☐	1. Full lumbar spine extension AROM to limit of motion ☐ 2. Measurement recorded from superior inclinometer ☐ 3. Measurement recorded from inferior inclinometer ☐	1. Difference between two inclinometer readings recorded for lumbar extension AROM ☐	1. Verbal (clear/concise) ☐ 2. Demonstration (clear) ☐ 3. Substitute movement eliminated ☐	

(continues)

AROM Assessment and Measurement Testing: Trunk (*continued*)

Movement	Start Position	End Position	Measurement	Recording	Instructions	Comments
TRUNK LATERAL FLEXION-THORACOLUMBAR SPINE (FINGERTIP-TO-FLOOR METHOD) (TAPE MEASURE) Form 9-29	1. Standing, feet shoulder width apart, knees straight, feet flat on floor ☐	1. Trunk laterally flexed to limit of motion ☐ 2. Full AROM achieved ☐	1. Distance measured between tip of third digit and floor ☐	1. Distance measured recorded	1. Verbal (clear/concise) ☐ 2. Demonstration (clear) ☐ 3. Substitute movement eliminated ☐	
TRUNK LATERAL FLEXION-THORACOLUMBAR SPINE (THIGH MEASUREMENT METHOD) (TAPE MEASURE) Form 9-30	1. Standing, feet shoulder width apart, knees straight, feet flat on floor ☐ 2. Arms at sides, mark on thigh at level of tip of middle finger ☐	1. Trunk laterally flexed to limit of motion ☐ 2. Full AROM achieved ☐ 3. Mark on thigh at level of tip of middle finger ☐	1. Distance measured between marks placed on thigh at start and end positions ☐	1. Distance measured recorded	1. Verbal (clear/concise) ☐ 2. Demonstration (clear) ☐ 3. Substitute movement eliminated ☐	

Movement	Start Position	Inclinometer Placement	End Position	Recording	Instructions	Comments
TRUNK LATERAL FLEXION (INCLINOMETER) Form 9-31	1. Standing, feet shoulder width apart, knees straight, feet flat on floor ☐ 2. Inclinometers zeroed in start position ☐	1. Superior inclinometer: on spine of T1 ☐ 2. Inferior inclinometer: on spine of S2 ☐	1. Full thoracolumbar spine lateral flexion AROM to limit of motion ☐ 2. Measurement recorded from superior inclinometer ☐ 3. Measurement recorded from inferior inclinometer ☐	1. Difference between two inclinometer readings recorded	1. Verbal (clear/concise) ☐ 2. Demonstration (clear) ☐ 3. Substitute movement eliminated ☐	

Movement	Start Position	Axis	Stationary Arm	End Position	Movable Arm	Recording	Instructions
TRUNK LATERAL FLEXION (UNIVERSAL GONIOMETER) Form 9-32	1. Standing, feet shoulder width apart, knees straight, feet flat on floor ☐	1. In midline at level of the PSIS (i.e. over S2 spinous process) ☐	1. Perpendicular to floor ☐ 2. Position maintained for start position ☐ 3. Position maintained for end position ☐	1. Full trunk lateral flexion AROM ☐	1. Points toward spine of C7 ☐ 2. Position maintained for start position ☐ 3. Position maintained for end position ☐	1. Full trunk lateral flexion AROM recorded ☐	1. Verbal (clear/ concise) ☐ 2. Demon-stration (clear) ☐ 3. Substitute movement eliminated ☐ **Comments:**

Movement	Start Position	Stabilization	End Position	Measurement	Recording	Instructions	Comments
TRUNK ROTATION - THORACOLUMBAR SPINE (TAPE MEASURE) Form 9-33	1. Sitting feet supported ☐ 2. Arms crossed in front of chest ☐ 3. Patient holds end of tape measure on lateral aspect of acromion process ☐ 4. Therapist holds other end of tape measure on contralateral iliac crest at midaxillary line or on upper border of greater trochanter ☐	1. Pelvis stabilized ☐	1. Trunk rotated to limit of motion ☐ 2. Full AROM achieved ☐ 3. Pelvis stabilized ☐	1. Distance measured between acromion process and iliac crest or greater trochanter at start position ☐ 2. Distance measured between acromion process and iliac crest or greater trochanter at end position ☐	1. Difference between start and end measures recorded ☐ 2. Surface landmarks used to measure AROM recorded ☐	1. Verbal (clear/concise) ☐ 2. Demonstration (clear) ☐ 3. Substitute movement eliminated ☐	

(continues)

AROM Assessment and Measurement Testing: Trunk (*continued*)

Movement	Start Position	Inclinometer Placement	End Position	Recording	Instructions	Comments
TRUNK ROTATION – THORACIC SPINE (INCLINOMETER) Form 9-34	1. Standing, forward flexed with head and trunk parallel to floor, with arms crossed in front of chest ☐ 2. Inclinometers zeroed in start position ☐	1. Superior inclinometer: on spine of T1 ☐ 2. Inferior inclinometer: on spine of T12 ☐	1. Full thoracic spine rotation AROM to limit of motion ☐ 2. Measurement recorded from superior inclinometer ☐ 3. Measurement recorded from inferior inclinometer ☐	1. Difference between two inclinometer readings recorded for thoracic rotation AROM ☐	1. Verbal (clear/concise) ☐ 2. Demonstration (clear) ☐ 3. Substitute movement eliminated ☐	

Movement	Start Position	End Position	Measurement	Recording	Instructions	Comments
CHEST EXPANSION Form 9-35	1. Sitting ☐ 2. Tape measure position around chest at level of xiphisternum ☐ 3. Full expiration made ☐	1. Full inspiration made ☐	1. Chest circumference at full expiration ☐ 2. Chest circumference at full inspiration ☐	1. Difference between two measures of circumference recorded ☐	1. Verbal (clear/concise) ☐ 2. Demonstration (clear) ☐ 3. Substitute movement eliminated ☐	

Muscle Length Assessment and Measurement Testing: Trunk and Hamstrings

| Muscle | Start Position | End Position | Measurement of Joint Position Using Tape | | Recording | Instructions | Comments |
			Measure				
TRUNK EXTENSORS-AND HAMSTRINGS (TOE-TOUCH TEST) Form 9-36	1. Standing, knees straight ☐	1. Trunk and hips flexed as patient reaches toward toes to limit of motion ☐ 2. Full AROM achieved ☐ 3. Knees maintained in extension ☐	1. Distance measured between most distant point reached by both hands and floor ☐		1. Distance measured recorded	1. Verbal (clear/concise) ☐ 2. Demonstration (clear) ☐ 3. Substitute movement eliminated ☐	

Summary of Patient Positioning for the Assessment and Measurement of Joint Range of Motion and Muscle Length

This summary chart is a resource the therapist may use to facilitate an organized and efficient assessment of joint range of motion (ROM) and muscle length, to avoid unnecessary patient position changes and fatigue.

The assessment and measurement of joint motion, that is, joint ROM and muscle length, presented in this book, first shows the *preferred start position* for these assessment techniques based on the position that offers the best stabilization. In some instances, *alternate start positions* are documented if commonly used in clinical practice. If these start positions are impractical or contraindicated for a patient, the therapist must determine the best approach based on the given patient parameters.

The following chart summarizes the *preferred (P)* and *alternate (A)* start positions that can be used by the therapist when assessing and measuring joint motion or muscle length.

Joint Motion/Muscle Length	Sitting	Supine	Prone	Sidely	Standing
Shoulder Complex					
Scapular movements	P			P	
Elevation through flexion	A	P			
Glenohumeral joint flexion		P			
Extension	A		P		
Elevation through abduction	A	P			
Glenohumeral joint abduction	A	P			
Adduction	A	P			
Horizontal adduction/ abduction	P				
Internal rotation	A		P		
External rotation	A	P			
Pectoralis major length		P			
Pectoralis minor length		P			
Elbow and Forearm					
Flexion/extension	A	P			
Supination/pronation	P				

Joint Motion/Muscle Length	Sitting	Supine	Prone	Sidely	Standing
Biceps brachii length		P			
Triceps length	P	A			
Wrist and Hand					
All wrist movements	P				
All finger and thumb movements	P				
Long finger flexors length	A	P			
Long finger extensors length	P				
Lumbricales length	P				
Hip					
Flexion		P			
Extension			P		
Abduction/adduction		P			
Internal/external rotation	P	A	A		
Hamstrings length (PSLR)		P			
Hip flexors length (Thomas Test)		P			
Hip adductors length		P			
Tensor fascia latae length (Ober's Test)				P	
Tensor fascia latae length (Ober's Test: Trunk Prone)			P		
Knee					
Flexion/extension		P			
Patellar glides		P			
Tibial rotation	P				
Hamstrings length (Passive Knee Extension (PKE) Supine)		P			
Hamstrings (Alternate Position – Sitting)	P				

Joint Motion/Muscle Length	Sitting	Supine	Prone	Sidely	Standing
Rectus femoris length (Prone one foot on floor)			P		
Rectus femoris length (Ely's Test)			P		
Rectus femoris length (Alternate Position – Thomas Test Position)		P			
Ankle and Foot					
Dorsiflexion	A	P			A
Plantarflexion	A	P			
Subtalar joint inversion/eversion		P	P		
Supination/pronation: Inversion/eversion components	P				
All toe movements		P			
Gastrocnemius length		A			P
Soleus length					P
Spine					
Flexion					P
Extension			P		A
Rotation	P				A
Lateral flexion					P
Trunk extensors & Hamstrings (Toe-touch test)					P
Neck					
Flexion/extension	P				
Lateral flexion	P				
Rotation	P	A			
TMJ					
All TMJ movements	P				

Gait

Introduction

The gait cycle consists of a series of motions that occur be-tween consecutive initial contacts of one leg.[1] The gait cycle is divided into two phases: the stance phase, when the foot is in contact with the ground and the body advances over the weight-bearing limb, and the swing phase, when the limb is unweighted and advanced forward in preparation for the next stance phase. Each phase is further subdivided into a total of eight instants[1] or freeze frames. Five instants occur in the stance phase and three occur in the swing phase of the gait cycle. The description of the normal gait pattern is provided so that the implications of the findings on assess-ment of joint range of motion and manual muscle strength can be understood in relation to gait. The average positions and the motions of the joints during the gait cycle that are reported in this appendix were adapted from the Rancho Los Amigos gait analysis forms as cited in Levangie and Norkin.[2] The right leg is used to illustrate the joint positions and mo-tions of the lower limb throughout the gait cycle.

Stance Phase

The lower limb is advanced in front of the body during the swing phase, and the stance phase begins at initial contact (Fig. D-1) when the heel makes the first contact between the foot and the ground. At initial contact, the pelvis is rotated forward and the trunk is rotated backward on the stance side. The rotation of the pelvis counteracts the trunk rotation to prevent excessive trunk motion. On the opposite side the upper extremity is flexed at the shoulder. As the body advances over the supporting limb through the stance phase, the pelvis rotates backward and the trunk rotates forward on the swing side. As the weight-bearing leg extends at the hip, the upper limb on the opposite side extends. The average joint positions and the motions of the right lower limb in the sagittal plane are described and illustrated.

Motion from *A* to *B* (Figs. D-1 and D-2)—*hip:* extension (from 30° to 25° flexion); *knee:* flexion (from 0° to 15° flexion); *ankle:* plantarflexion (from 0° to 15° plantarflexion); *MTP joints of toes:* 0°.

Motion from *B* to *C* (Figs. D-2 and D-3)—*hip:* extension (from 25° to 0° flexion); *knee:* extension (from 15° to 5° flexion); *ankle:* dorsiflexion (from 15° plantarflexion to 5° to 10° dorsiflexion); *MTP joints of toes:* remain at 0°.

Motion from *C* to *D* (Figs. D-3 and D-4)—*hip:* extension (from 0° flexion to 10° to 20° extension); *knee:* extension (from 5° flexion to 0°); *ankle:* dorsiflexion (from 5° to 10° dorsiflexion to 0° dorsiflexion); *MTP joints of toes:* extension (from 0° to 20° extension).

Motion from *D* to *E* (Figs. D-4 and D-5)—*hip:* flexion (from 10° to 20° extension to 0°); *knee:* flexion (from 0° to 30° flexion); *ankle:* plantarflexion (from 0° to 20° plantarflexion *MTP joints of toes:* extension (from 30° extension to 50° to 60° extension).

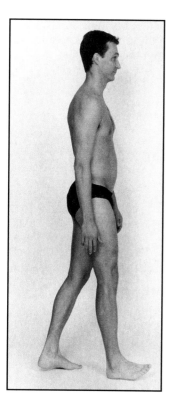

Figure D-1 Initial contact (*A*).

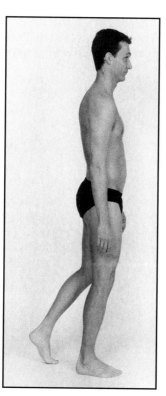

Figure D-2 Loading response (*B*).

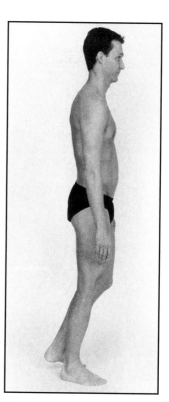

Figure D-3 Midstance (*C*).

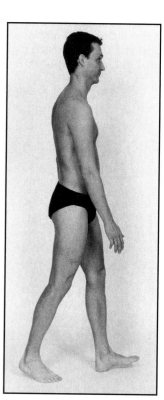

Figure D-4 Terminal stance (*D*).

Swing Phase

The swing phase begins after preswing when the foot leaves the ground and is advanced forward in the line of progression in preparation for initial contact. The positions and motions of the right lower limb are described and illustrated.

Motion from *E* to *F* (Figs. D-5 and D-6)—*hip:* flexion (from 0° to 20° flexion); *knee:* flexion (from 30° flexion to 60° flexion); *ankle:* dorsiflexion (from 20° plantarflexion to 10° plantarflexion).

Motion from *F* to *G* (Figs. D-6 and D-7)—*hip:* flexion (from 20° flexion to 30° flexion); *knee:* extension (from 60° flexion to 30° flexion); *ankle:* dorsiflexion (from 10° plantarflexion to 0°).

Motion from *G* to *H* (Figs. D-7 and D-8)—*hip:* remains flexed at 30°; *knee:* extension (from 30° flexion to 0°); *ankle:* remains at 0°.

Motion from *H* to *A* (Figs. D-8 and D-1)—*hip:* remains flexed at 30°; *knee:* remains extended at 0°; *ankle:* remains at 0°.

References

1. Koerner I. *Observation of Human Gait*. Edmonton, Alberta: Health Sciences Media Services and Development, University of Alberta; 1986.
2. Levangie PK, Norkin CC. *Joint Structure & Function: A Comprehensive Analysis*. 3rd ed. Philadelphia, PA: FA Davis; 2001.

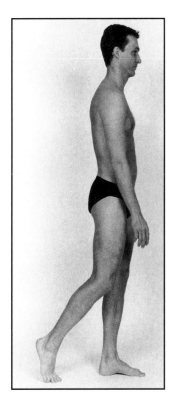

Figure D-5 Preswing (*E*).

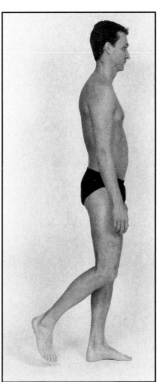

Figure D-6 Initial swing (*F*).

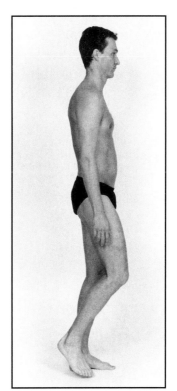

Figure D-7 Midswing (*G*).

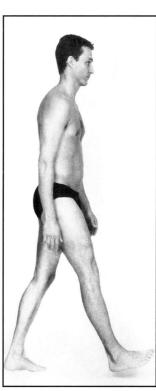

Figure D-8 Terminal swing (*H*).

Answer Guides for Chapter Exercises and Questions

Introduction

This appendix contains answers to the exercises and questions at the end of each chapter. In some cases, it is possible to provide concrete answers to the exercises and questions, but for some exercises and questions, there may be suitable alternate answers not identified here.

Chapter 1: Principles and Methods

1. Joint Movements

i. Flexion: Bending of a part so that the anterior surfaces come closer together; extension; sagittal plane, frontal axis.

ii. Abduction: movement away from the midline of the body or body part; adduction; frontal plane, sagittal axis.

iii. Internal rotation: turning of the anterior surface of a part toward the midline of the body; external rotation; horizontal plane, vertical/longitudinal axis.

iv. Lateral flexion: trunk or neck bending movements that occur in a lateral direction either to the right or left; lateral flexion to the opposite side; frontal plane, sagittal axis.

v. Horizontal adduction: starting with the shoulder or hip at 90° flexion or 90° abduction, movement of the arm or thigh, respectively, in either an anterior direction or toward the midline of the body; horizontal abduction; horizontal plane, vertical axis.

2. Osteokinematics and Arthrokinematics

A. *Osteokinematics* is the study of the movement of the bone in space.[1] *Arthrokinematics* is the study of the movement occurring between the articular surfaces of the bones, within the joint.[1]

B. *Osteokinematics:* To assess knee joint flexion PROM, the therapist stabilizes the femur and moves the tibia in a posterior direction to the limit of motion; observes, measures, and records the limited posterior movement of the tibia (i.e., limited knee flexion PROM); and considers the impact of the decreased knee flexion PROM on the patient's ADL.

C. *Arthrokinematics:* with the above knowledge, the therapist, knowing that the tibial articular surface is concave, applies the concave–convex rule: with the femur stabilized as the knee is flexed, the tibia moves in a posterior direction, and the concave tibial articular surface will glide in the same direction as the tibia moves (i.e., posterior). The therapist may conclude that the decreased posterior motion of the tibia (i.e., limited knee flexion PROM) is caused by a decreased posterior glide of the tibial articular surface. The therapist may decide that treatment is needed to restore posterior glide of the tibial articular surface to increase knee flexion PROM.

3. Contraindications and Precautions for ROM Assessment

A. AROM and PROM assessment techniques are contraindicated when muscle contraction (AROM) or motion (AROM and PROM) of the part could disrupt the healing process or result in injury or deterioration of the patient's condition.

B. The therapist would likely not perform an assessment of AROM and PROM in this case because the patient is under the influence of alcohol and may not be able to respond appropriately during the assessment.

If alcohol were not a factor, the therapist would consider the following precautions: status of fracture healing unknown, osteoporosis (general and upper extremity bone density), degree of pain experienced, and psychological state. The therapist may proceed with caution, carefully monitoring the patient's response to assessment.

4. The Rationale for the Assessment of AROM and PROM

A. i. The defined zero position is the anatomical position for the knee and ankle (see Figs. 1-14 through 1-16).

ii. The hamstrings could restrict knee extension AROM because the muscles are already lengthened over the flexed hip joint in high sitting.

Alternate start position: from the sitting position, the patient could backward lean (see Fig. 7-21) or lie supine with the knee remaining flexed over the edge of the plinth to place the hamstrings on slack at the nontest (i.e., hip) joint.

iii. Assessing Mr. Fitzgerald's AROM would provide the therapist with information about his ability to follow directions, attention span, and willingness to move; coordination; movements that cause or increase pain; ability to move the part through a full ROM; and ability to perform ADL.

iv. The therapist could not determine the reason for the decreased movement from the AROM assessment alone. The therapist must perform additional assessment techniques, such as assessment of the PROM, muscle strength, and special tests as required. Assessment of PROM will indicate if there is lack of movement at the joint; muscle strength testing will indicate if the muscle is too weak to move the limb through the PROM available at the joint. Special tests may also be necessary to determine the reason for the limited movement.

v. Mr. Fitzgerald's PROM would be assessed to determine the amount of movement possible at the joint, the quality of movement throughout the ROM, what structure(s) limit the movement by assessing the end feel, the presence or absence of pain, and whether a capsular or noncapsular pattern of movement exists.

B. Knee flexion AROM = PROM and the empty end feel with the complaint of knee pain indicates the joint cannot be moved through more than 60° flexion due to pain. Further assessment of the knee is required to determine the cause of the knee pain.

Knee extension AROM < PROM and the end feel is firm. Full extension PROM is possible at the knee joint and the end feel is normal, but the patient cannot actively move the knee into full knee extension. This is probably due to the knee extensor muscles being too weak to move the knee through the available full knee extension PROM.

Ankle dorsiflexion: the limited AROM is only slightly less than the limited PROM. The firm end feel and pulling sensation over the calf indicate that the resistance of the stretched calf muscles limits the ankle ROM.

5. Assessment and Measurement of AROM and PROM Using the Universal Goniometer

A. ii. a) You may have used some or all of the following substitute movements: trunk extension, scapular depression, shoulder flexion, wrist flexion.

b) Substitute motion can be avoided if the therapist provides appropriate instruction to the patient, manually stabilizes the proximal joint segment

(i.e., humerus in this case), and/or positions the patient to prevent unwanted movement.

c) The change in position from sitting to supine lying should have reduced the possible substitute movement, as the trunk and scapula are better stabilized.

6. Validity and Reliability: Universal Goniometer

A. *Validity* is "the degree to which an instrument measures what it is supposed to measure"[2 (p. 171)]. *Reliability* is "the extent to which the instrument yields the same measurement on repeated uses either by the same operator (intraobserver reliability) or by different operators (interobserver reliability)"[3 (p. 49)].

B. Reliable joint ROM measurements are best obtained by having the same therapist take the repeated measures, using a rigid standardized measurement protocol.

This involves using the same goniometer in the same clinical setting; assessing the patient at the same time of day and in a consistent manner relative to the application of treatment techniques; and using the same patient position, instructions, and accurate method of applying and reading the goniometer.

8. Using the OB "Myrin" Goniometer to Measure Joint ROM

i. The OB goniometer consists of a fluid-filled rotatable container consisting of a compass needle to measure movements in a horizontal plane, and an inclination needle to measure movements in a vertical plane. The floor of the container has a scale marked in 2° increments. The OB goniometer is attached via Velcro straps and plastic extension plates to the limb segment at a predetermined position in relation to bony landmarks, either proximal or distal to the joint being assessed.

With the patient in the start position, the fluid-filled container is rotated until the 0° arrow lines up directly underneath the needle used for the measurement. The patient moves through the ROM, and the number of degrees the needle moves away from the 0° arrow on the scale is recorded as the joint ROM.

ii. The *advantages* of using the OB goniometer to measure joint ROM compared to the universal goniometer are as follows:

It is not necessary to align the inclinometer with the joint axis.

Rotational movements using a compass inclinometer are measured with ease.

Assessment of trunk and neck ROM is done easily.

There is little change in the alignment of the goniometer throughout the ROM.

PROM is more easily assessed using the OB goniometer, as the therapist does not have to hold the goniometer and can stabilize the proximal joint segment with one hand while passively moving the distal segment with the other hand.

The *disadvantages* of using the OB goniometer compared to the universal goniometer are as follows:

It is expensive and bulky compared to the universal goniometer.

It cannot be used to measure the small joints of the hand and foot.

Magnetic fields, other than those of Earth, will cause the compass needle to deviate and must be avoided.

References

1. MacConaill MA, Basmajian JV. *Muscles and Movements: A Basis for Human Kinesiology*. 2nd ed. New York, NY: Robert E. Krieger; 1977.
2. Currier DP. *Elements of Research in Physical Therapy*. 3rd ed. Baltimore, MD: Williams & Wilkins; 1990.
3. Sim J, Arnell P. Measurement validity in physical therapy research. *Phys Ther*. 1993;73:48-56.

Chapter 2: Relating Treatment to Assessment

1. *Purpose*: The therapist selects assessment or treatment based on the outcome required.

   General Procedure: The therapist employs the general procedure as follows:

   Explanation and instruction: to explain and demonstrate the assessment or treatment to the patient and obtain the patient's informed consent.

   Expose the region to be assessed or treated and drape the patient as required.

   Start position: appropriate for the assessment or treatment; ensures the patient is safe, comfortable, and adequately supported.

   Stabilization: to allow only the desired movement.

   Movement: the appropriate movement is performed.

   Assistance: provided for passive movement.

   End position is achieved.

   Substitute movement: ensure no substitute movement.

   Purpose-Specific Procedure: Purpose-specific procedure is carried out to meet the purpose of the assessment or treatment.

   Charting: For assessment, record deviations from standardized testing procedure and assessment findings. For treatment, record purpose-specific procedures used in treatment and any change in the patient's condition.

2. The purpose for which assessment and treatment are used is different. Assessment is used to assess deficiencies. Treatment is used to alleviate deficiencies. Therefore, after employing the general procedure used for similar assessment and treatment, purpose-specific procedures are used to meet the purpose of either the assessment or the treatment used.

3. When applying similar assessments and treatments the key steps that are the same are those included under the general procedure (i.e., explanation and instruction, expose region, start position, stabilization, movement, assistance, end position, and substitute movement).

   When applying similar assessments and treatments the key steps that are different include the: purpose, purpose-specific procedure, and charting.

4. A. Active exercise
   B. Relaxed passive movement
   C. Prolonged passive stretch

5. A. Muscle length assessment
   B. Prolonged passive stretch
   C. The general procedure for the treatment is identical to the general procedure used to assess muscle length for the hip adductors. Therefore, either the:
      i. description for assessment of muscle length for the hip adductors (Chapter 6, page 193), or
      ii. the Practice Makes Perfect 🔍 Form 6-9 for the assessment of muscle length of the hip adductors can be used to check the correctness of the general procedure used to treat and increase the length of the hip adductors.

      To meet the specific purpose of the treatment (i.e., to increase muscle length), the muscle would be held on stretch for a prescribed length of time.

6. A. PROM assessment
   B. Relaxed passive movement
   C. The general procedure for the treatment is identical to the general procedure used to assess PROM for hip flexion. Therefore, either the:
      i. description for hip flexion PROM Assessment (Chapter 6, page 179), or
      ii. Practice Makes Perfect 🔍 Form 6-1 for assessment of hip flexion PROM could be used to check the correctness of the general procedure used to treat and maintain the hip flexion ROM.

      The passive movement would then be performed according to the treatment prescription (i.e., a prescribed number of repetitions, a prescribed number of times a day).

7. A. AROM assessment
   B. Active exercise
   C. The general procedure for the treatment is identical to the general procedure used to assess AROM for elbow flexion. The general treatment procedure specific to maintaining or increasing elbow flexion AROM would be performed according to the exercise prescription (i.e., a prescribed number of repetitions, a prescribed number of times a day).

Chapter 3: Shoulder Complex

1. Palpation

A. i. Horizontal abduction and adduction; axis.

    Shoulder elevation through flexion/glenohumeral joint flexion and extension; axis (i.e., 2.5 cm inferior to the lateral aspect of the acromion process).

ii. Shoulder elevation through flexion/glenohumeral joint flexion and extension; stationary arm.

iii. Shoulder internal and external rotation; axis.

iv. Shoulder elevation through flexion/glenohumeral joint flexion and extension; moveable arm.

Shoulder elevation through abduction/glenohumeral joint abduction/adduction; moveable arm. Horizontal abduction and adduction; moveable arm.

2. Assessment of AROM at the Shoulder Complex

A. i. The <u>shoulder complex</u> is made up of the sternoclavicular, acromioclavicular, scapulothoracic, and glenohumeral articulations.

ii. The <u>shoulder girdle</u> is made up of the sternoclavicular, acromioclavicular, and scapulothoracic articulations.

iii. The <u>shoulder joint</u> is made up of the glenohumeral joint (the shoulder joint can also be referred to as the glenohumeral joint).

B. True

C. Refer to the section in Chapter 3 titled "General Scan: Upper Extremity Active Range of Motion."

D. i. Elevation, depression, protraction, retraction, medial (downward) rotation, and lateral (upward) rotation.

Elevation—movement of the scapula in an upward or cranial direction.

Depression—movement of the scapula in a downward or caudal direction.

Protraction—movement of the scapula in a lateral direction over the thorax.

Retraction—movement of the scapula in a medial direction over the thorax.

Medial (downward) rotation—movement of the inferior angle of the scapula toward the midline and movement of the glenoid cavity in a downward (caudal) direction.

Lateral (upward) rotation—movement of the inferior angle of the scapula away from the midline and movement of the glenoid cavity in an upward (cranial) direction.

ii. Scapular medial (downward) rotation—shoulder extension and adduction to place the hand across the small of the back.

Scapular lateral (upward) rotation—shoulder elevation through flexion or abduction.

E. i. Extension: Scapular anterior tilting, scapular elevation, and shoulder abduction. In sitting, trunk flexion and ipsilateral trunk rotation may also occur.

ii. Abduction: Contralateral trunk lateral flexion, scapular elevation, and shoulder flexion.

iii. External rotation: In supine with the shoulder in 90° abduction: elbow extension, scapular depression, and shoulder adduction. In sitting with the arm at the side: scapular depression, shoulder adduction, and trunk rotation.

iv. Horizontal abduction: Scapular retraction, ipsilateral trunk rotation.

3. Assessment and Measurement of PROM at the Shoulder Complex

Scapular Elevation

i. Motion could be decreased at any of the following articulations: the scapulothoracic, acromioclavicular, and/or sternoclavicular articulations.

ii. Elevation of the clavicle is associated with scapular elevation.

iii. <u>Inferior</u> glide would be decreased—because the medial end of the clavicle is a convex surface vertically, and the manubrial surface of the sternoclavicular joint is reciprocally concave. Based on the concave/convex theory of movement, a convex surface will glide in the opposite direction to the movement of the bony segment it is a part of. If the manubrium is fixed and the lateral end of the clavicle moves upward (superiorly), the articular surface of the clavicle will glide downward (inferiorly) at the sternoclavicular joint.

Shoulder Elevation Through Flexion and Through Abduction

i. The glenohumeral, scapulothoracic, acromioclavicular, and sternoclavicular articulations all participate in shoulder elevation through either flexion or abduction.

ii. Glenohumeral joint:

proximal component—glenoid cavity of the scapula, concave;

distal component—head of the humerus, convex.

Sternoclavicular joint:

medial component—lateral aspect of the manubrium sternum and the adjacent superior surface of the first costal cartilage; convex horizontally, concave vertically;

lateral component—medial end of the clavicle; concave horizontally, convex vertically.

Glenohumeral (GH) Joint Abduction

i. The therapist places one hand on the superior aspect of the ipsilateral shoulder girdle (i.e., over the scapula and clavicle) to stabilize the shoulder girdle and isolate motion at the GH joint.

ii. Inferior glide of the humeral head would be decreased. The head of the humerus is convex and articulates with the concave glenoid cavity. Based on the concave/convex theory of movement, a convex surface will glide in the opposite direction to the movement of the bony segment it is a part of. If the humerus moves superiorly with glenohumeral joint abduction, the convex head of the humerus will glide inferiorly at the joint during this movement.

Shoulder Extension

The elbow should be in flexion to prevent restriction of shoulder extension due to passive insufficiency of the two-joint biceps brachii muscle.[1]

Shoulder Horizontal Adduction

i. Start positions: The patient is sitting. The shoulder is in neutral rotation and in either 90° abduction or 90° flexion. The elbow is flexed, and the forearm is in midposition. The start position of the shoulder should be recorded.

Shoulder horizontal abduction would also be assessed using the above start positions.

ii. Posterior glide of the humeral head would be restricted because the head of the humerus is convex and articulates with the concave glenoid cavity. Based on the concave/convex theory of movement, a convex surface will glide in the opposite direction to the movement of the bony segment it is a part of. If the humerus moves anteriorly with glenohumeral joint horizontal adduction, the convex head of the humerus will glide posteriorly at the joint during this movement.

Shoulder Internal Rotation

i. Motion would be decreased at the glenohumeral joint.

ii. PROM would be assessed to determine end feel for shoulder internal rotation.

iii. If your partner presented with a full PROM for shoulder internal rotation and the end feel was firm, this end feel would be considered a normal end feel. However, if your partner presented with a decreased PROM and the end feel was firm, this end feel would be considered abnormal.

iv. Normal limiting factors that would create a normal firm end feel for shoulder internal rotation are tension in the posterior glenohumeral joint capsule, infraspinatus, and teres minor.

Other Questions

A. Glenohumeral joint movements of abduction, flexion, extension, horizontal abduction and adduction, internal and external rotation

B. i. The AROM may be less than the PROM because the patient may not understand the movement to be performed; may be unwilling to move through the full available ROM; may experience pain that stops the movement when performed actively; or may have muscle weakness that prevents moving the part through the full available PROM.

ii. If AROM = PROM as described, this may indicate a restriction in mobility at the glenohumeral joint. The cause of this restriction is determined by identifying the end feel at 30° flexion PROM. Possible causes of the restricted ROM could include pain, soft tissue (capsule, ligament, muscle) stretch, bone contacting bone, soft tissue swelling, joint effusion, spasm, or an internal derangement of the joint.

4. Muscle Length Assessment and Measurement

Pectoralis Major

i. Origin[2]—Clavicular head: anterior border of the sternal half of the clavicle; Sternal head: ipsilateral half of the anterior surface of the sternum; cartilage of the first 6 or 7 ribs; sternal end of 6th rib; aponeurosis of the external abdominal oblique.

Insertion[2]—Lateral lip of the intertubercular groove of the humerus.

ii. Shoulder horizontal abduction and external rotation are the movements that would position the origin and insertion farther apart and place the muscle on stretch.

iii. The therapist would note a firm end feel if the pectoralis major is shortened.

iv. If the pectoralis major is shortened, shoulder horizontal abduction ROM will be restricted proportional to the decrease in muscle length. To assess this restriction, the goniometer axis is placed *on top of the acromion process,* the stationary arm is aligned *perpendicular to the trunk,* and the movable arm is aligned parallel to the *longitudinal axis of the humerus.*

Pectoralis Minor

i. Origin[2]—Outer surfaces of ribs 2 to 4 or 3 to 5 near the costal cartilages; fascia over corresponding external intercostals.

Insertion[2]—Medial border and upper surface of the coracoid process of the scapula.

ii. Scapular elevation and retraction would place the muscle on stretch.

iii. If the pectoralis minor is shortened, with the patient in supine, the therapist, standing at the head of the plinth, will observe the shoulder girdle on the affected side to be resting in a protracted position away from the surface of the plinth.

5. Functional ROM at the Shoulder Complex

A. The function of the shoulder complex is to position or move the arm in space for the purpose of hand function.

B. i. It would not be possible to complete any of the activities with the glenohumeral joint fixed in anatomical position without employing compensatory movement of other body parts.

ii. Reach to the midline of your chest to do up buttons – (shoulder internal rotation), elbow flexion and extension; forearm supination and pronation; wrist flexion, extension, radial and ulnar deviation.

Combing hair—(shoulder internal and external rotation), neck flexion, side flexion and rotation; shoulder girdle elevation; elbow flexion; wrist flexion, extension, radial and ulnar deviation.

Brushing teeth—(shoulder internal rotation), neck flexion, side flexion and rotation; shoulder girdle elevation; elbow flexion; wrist flexion, extension, radial and ulnar deviation.

Eat soup with a spoon – (shoulder internal rotation), neck flexion; elbow flexion and extension; forearm supination and pronation; wrist flexion and extension, radial and ulnar deviation.

C. i. Extension: Pulling a window down to close it; pushing oneself up on the sides of the tub to get out of the bathtub.

ii. Elevation through flexion: Reaching to place an object on a high shelf; changing a light bulb on the ceiling.

iii. Flexion below shoulder level: Eating with a spoon or fork; drinking from a cup.

iv. External rotation: Combing the hair; manipulating the clasp of a necklace behind the neck.

v. Horizontal adduction: Washing the axilla and the skin over the scapula on the contralateral side of the body; writing on a blackboard at shoulder level.

D. i. Scapulohumeral rhythm is the coordinated movement pattern achieved through scapulothoracic and glenohumeral movement.[3–6]

ii. The ratio of glenohumeral motion to scapular motion is 2:1—that is, 2° of glenohumeral motion to every degree of scapular motion.[3,5,7,8]

iii. Factors affecting the rhythm are the plane of elevation, arc of elevation, amount of load on the arm, and individual differences.[9]

iv. Movement occurs at the glenohumeral, sternoclavicular, acromioclavicular, scapulothoracic, and spinal joints.

v. Setting phase: 0°–60° shoulder flexion; 0°–30° shoulder abduction. The scapula remains relatively stationary, or slightly medially (downward) or laterally (upward) rotates. Most movement occurs at the glenohumeral joint.

vi. From the end of the setting phase to 170° of motion, there is a predictable scapulohumeral rhythm of 2° glenohumeral joint motion for every 1° of scapular motion. Scapular motion includes lateral (upward) rotation, accompanied by secondary rotations of posterior tilting (sagittal plane) and posterior rotation (transverse plane).[10] Full shoulder elevation through abduction depends on full external rotation of the humerus. Full shoulder elevation through flexion depends on the ability to rotate the humerus internally through range.[11] The final degrees of elevation beyond 170° are achieved through contralateral trunk lateral flexion and/or trunk extension.

References

1. Gajdosik RL, Hallett JP, Slaughter LL. Passive insufficiency of two-joint shoulder muscles. *Clin Biomech*. 1994;9:377-378.

2. Standring S, ed. *Gray's Anatomy: The Anatomical Basis of Clinical Practice*. 39th ed. London, UK: Elsevier Churchill Livingstone; 2005.

3. Levangie PK, Norkin CC. *Joint Structure & Function: A Comprehensive Analysis*. 3rd ed. Philadelphia, PA: FA Davis; 2001.

4. Smith LK, Lawrence Weiss E, Lehmkuhl LD. *Brunnstrom's Clinical Kinesiology*. 5th ed. Philadelphia, PA: FA Davis; 1996.

5. Cailliet R. *Shoulder Pain*. 3rd ed. Philadelphia, PA: FA Davis; 1991.

6. Soderberg GL. *Kinesiology: Application to Pathological Motion*. 2nd ed. Baltimore, MD: Williams & Wilkins; 1997.

7. Rosse C. The shoulder region and the brachial plexus. In: Rosse C, Clawson DK, eds. *The Musculoskeletal System in Health and Disease*. New York, NY: Harper & Row; 1980.

8. Inman VT, Saunders M, Abbot LC. Observations on the function of the shoulder joint. *J Bone Joint Surg*. 1944;26:1-30.

9. Matsen FA, Lippitt SB, Sidles JA, Harryman DT. *Practical Evaluation and Management of the Shoulder*. Philadelphia, PA: WB Saunders; 1994.

10. Peat M. The shoulder complex: a review of some aspects of functional anatomy. *Physiother Canada*. 1977;29:241-246.

11. Mallon WJ, Herring CL, Sallay PI, et al. Use of vertebral levels to measure presumed internal rotation at the shoulder: a radiologic analysis. *J Shoulder Elbow Surg*. 1996;5:299-306.

Chapter 4: Elbow and Forearm

1. Palpation

A. i. Elbow flexion/extension: Goniometer axis—lateral epicondyle of the humerus; stationary arm—tip of the acromion process; moveable arm—styloid process of the radius.

ii. Forearm supination/pronation: Goniometer axis – a. head of the third metacarpal, b. tip of the middle digit, c. ulnar styloid process;

Stationary arm – a. none (perpendicular to the floor), b. none (perpendicular to the floor), c. none (perpendicular to the floor);

Moveable arm – a. none (parallel to the pencil), b. parallel to the tips of the four extended fingers, c. against the anterior (supination) or posterior (pronation) aspects of the distal forearm in line with the ulnar styloid process.

2. Assessment Process

Records patient's history

Explains rationale and component parts of assessment

Observation

Assessment of AROM

Measurement of AROM, as required

Assessment of PROM

Measurement of PROM, as required

Assessment and measurement of muscle length, as required

Assessment of muscle strength

Application of other assessment techniques, as required

3. Assessment of AROM at the Elbow and Forearm Articulations

A. Proximal components of the elbow joint: trochlea of the humerus (convex anteroposteriorly); capitulum of the humerus (convex)

Distal components of the elbow joint: trochlea notch of the ulna (concave); proximal aspect of the head of the radius (concave)

Superior radioulnar joint (located within the capsule of the elbow joint): radial head (convex); radial notch of the ulna (concave)

Inferior radioulnar joint: ulnar head (convex); ulnar notch of the radius (concave)

B. i. Elbow flexion: Bending of the elbow so that the anterior surface of the forearm moves toward the anterior surface of the arm. Elbow extension: Straightening of the elbow. These movements occur around a frontal axis in the sagittal plane.

ii. Forearm supination: Rotation of the forearm so that the palm faces upward toward the ceiling. Forearm pronation: rotation of the forearm so that the palm faces downward toward the floor.
a) With the elbow flexed 90°, these movements occur around the axis for supination and pronation (see Fig. 4-2) (i.e., the longitudinal axis, in the frontal plane).
b) With the elbow in anatomical position, these movements occur in the transverse plane around a longitudinal axis. Shoulder internal rotation augments forearm pronation, and shoulder external rotation augments supination, with the elbow joint at 0°.

C. i. Forearm supination: ipsilateral trunk lateral flexion, shoulder adduction, and shoulder external rotation.

ii. Elbow extension: trunk flexion, shoulder extension, scapular elevation, and wrist extension.

iii. Elbow flexion: trunk extension, shoulder flexion, scapular depression, and wrist flexion.

iv. Forearm pronation: contralateral trunk lateral flexion, shoulder abduction, and shoulder internal rotation.

D. AROM may be less than PROM because the patient may not understand the movement to be performed, be unwilling to move through the full available PROM, experience pain that stops the movement when performed actively, or have muscle weakness that prevents moving the part through the full available PROM.

4. Assessment and Measurement of PROM at the Elbow and Forearm

Elbow Flexion

i. A soft or firm or hard end feel are the normal end feels expected when assessing elbow flexion.

ii. True

iii. Refer to Table 4-1.

Elbow Extension/Hyperextension

i. Biceps brachii. The muscle is placed on stretch if the shoulder is in *extension*, and the forearm is *pronated*. Therefore, the therapist ensures the forearm is *supinated* and the shoulder is in *anatomical* (i.e., 0°) to avoid biceps brachii from restricting elbow extension.

ii. Posterior glide of the trochlea of the ulna and the radial head would cause decreased elbow extension PROM.

iii. The proximal aspect of the radial head and the trochlear surface of the ulna are concave surfaces. Based on the concave/convex theory of movement, a concave surface will glide in the same direction of movement as the bony segment it is a part of. The ulna and radius bone segments move in a posterior direction when the elbow is extended, therefore the concave articular surfaces will glide in a posterior direction.

Forearm Supination

i. Motion could be decreased at the superior radioulnar joint, the inferior radioulnar joint, and/or the humeroradial joint in the presence of decreased forearm supination PROM.

ii. The radial head spins on the capitulum when the forearm is supinated.

iii. Anterior glide of the radial head could be limited if forearm supination ROM is decreased.

iv. The radial head is a convex surface and the radial notch of the ulna is a concave surface. Based on the concave/convex theory of movement, a convex surface will glide in the opposite direction as the bone segment of which it is a part. The radius moves posteriorly and the radial head glides anteriorly when the forearm is supinated.

v. In full supination, the radius lies <u>alongside</u> the ulna.

Forearm Pronation

ii. Normal end feels for forearm pronation are hard or firm.

iii. A hard end feel for forearm pronation is the result of contact of the radius and the ulna. A firm end feel for forearm pronation results from tension in the quadrate ligament, the dorsal radioulnar ligament of the inferior radioulnar joint, the distal tract of the interosseous membrane, supinator and biceps brachii muscles with the elbow in extension.

iv. From full supination to full pronation, the radius <u>rotates</u> around the relatively <u>stationary</u> ulna.

5. Muscle Length Assessment and Measurement

Triceps

i. Origin[1]: Long head: infraglenoid tubercle of the scapula; Lateral head: posterolateral surface of the humerus between the radial groove and the insertion of teres minor; lateral intermuscular septum; Medial head: posterior surface of the humerus below the radial groove between the trochlea of the humerus and the insertion of teres major; medial and lateral intermuscular septum. Insertion[1]: Posteriorly on the proximal surface of the olecranon; some fibers continue distally to blend with the antebrachial fascia.

ii. Shoulder flexion and elbow flexion would place the triceps on stretch.

iii. A therapist would identify a <u>firm</u> end feel at the limit of <u>elbow flexion</u> PROM in the presence of a shortened triceps muscle.

6. Functional ROM at the Elbow and Forearm

A. i. a) In standing, it would not be possible to contact parts of the body proximal to the hips, and the posterolateral aspect of the contralateral hip with the elbow fixed in 0° extension.

b) In sitting, it would not be possible to contact parts of the body proximal to the mid-thigh level with the elbow fixed in 0° extension.

ii. Eating, drinking, brushing the teeth, combing or washing the hair, using the phone, dressing (i.e., doing up buttons, putting on a belt), and perineal hygiene would be impossible to perform with the elbow fixed in 0° extension.

B. i. a) If standing, it would be very difficult to contact areas distal to the mid-calf.

b) If sitting it would be very difficult to contact areas distal to the mid-calf.

ii. In most cases, all personal care ADL (i.e., feeding and personal hygiene) can be performed with the elbow fixed in a position of 90° flexion.[2,3]

C. The ROM requirements for ADL are influenced by the design of the furniture used, the placement of utensils, and the patient's posture. The start and the end positions and technique used to complete the activity also affect the ROM requirements. Therefore, the ROM values provided below are a guide only.

i. Drinking from a cup requires about 129°[4] of elbow flexion

ii. Holding the telephone to the ear requires about 136° to 140°[5,6] of elbow flexion

iii. Tying a shoe lace requires about 16°[5] of elbow flexion

iv. Combing the hair on the back of the head requires about 144°[5] of elbow flexion

v. Reaching for a wallet in a back pocket requires about 70°[5] of elbow flexion

D. i. Forearm pronation is required to pick up a small object from a table top.

ii. Forearm supination is required to receive change in the palm of the hand.

iii. Forearm pronation and forearm supination are required to eat with a fork.

iv. Forearm supination is required to reach a wallet in a back pocket.

v. Forearm supination is required to comb the hair on the vertex of the head.

E. According to Morrey et al.,[5] many self-care activities can be accomplished within the arc of movement from <u>30°</u> to <u>130°</u> elbow flexion and from <u>50°</u> of pronation to <u>50°</u> of supination.

References

1. Standring S, ed. *Gray's Anatomy: The Anatomical Basis of Clinical Practice*. 39th ed. London, UK: Elsevier Churchill Livingstone; 2005.
2. Vasen AP, Lacey SH, Keith MW, Shaffer JW. Functional range of motion of the elbow. *J Hand Surg Am*. 1995;20:288-292.
3. Nagy SM, Szabo RM, Sharkey NA. Unilateral elbow arthrodesis: the preferred position. *J South Orthop Assoc*. 1999;8(2): 80-85.
4. Safaee-Rad R, Shwedyk E, Quanbury AO, Cooper JE. Normal functional range of motion of upper limb joints during performance of three feeding activities. *Arch Phys Med Rehabil*. 1990;71:505-509.
5. Morrey BF, Askew LJ, An KN, Chao EY. A biomechanical study of normal functional elbow motion. *J Bone Joint Surg Am*. 1981;63:872-876.
6. Packer TL, Peat M, Wyss U, Sorbie C. Examining the elbow during functional activities. *Occup Ther J Res*. 1990;10:323-333.

Chapter 5: Wrist and Hand

1. Palpation

i. Styloid process of ulna: Wrist flexion and extension

ii. Distal palmar crease: Finger IP and MCP joint flexion (linear measurement of finger flexion to evaluate impairment of hand function)

iii. Third metacarpal bone: Wrist radial and ulnar deviation; MCP joint abduction of the middle finger; MCP joint flexion and extension of the middle finger.

iv. First carpometacarpal joint: Thumb CM joint flexion and extension

v. Capitate bone: Wrist radial and ulnar deviation

vi. Lateral aspect of the PIP joint line: PIP joint flexion and extension

2. Assessment Process

i. True

ii. False—PROM is used to determine an end feel

iii. True

iv. False—AROM can also be measured using a goniometer

3. Assessment of AROM at the Wrist and Hand Articulations

A. Make a fist: observe AROM of finger flexion, thumb flexion and adduction, and wrist extension. Open the hand, spread the fingers as far as possible and flex the wrist: observe AROM of finger extension and abduction, thumb extension, and wrist flexion.

B. i. Radiocarpal joint—the proximal surface of the proximal row of carpal bones (i.e., the scaphoid, lunate, triquetrum) is convex and articulates with the concave surface of the distal aspect of the radius and the articular disc of the inferior radioulnar joint.

Midcarpal joint—the proximal aspect of the distal row of carpal bones has a concave surface laterally (formed by the trapezoid and trapezium) and a convex surface medially (formed by the hamate and capitate). These surfaces articulate with the corresponding convex (formed by the scaphoid) and concave (formed by the scaphoid, lunate, and triquetrum) surfaces, respectively, on the distal aspect of the proximal row of carpal bones.

ii. The CM joint of the thumb is formed by the distal surface of the trapezium, which is concave anteroposteriorly and convex mediolaterally, that articulates with the corresponding reciprocal surface of the base of the first metacarpal.

iii. The MCP joints are each formed proximally by the convex head of the metacarpal articulating with the concave base of the adjacent proximal phalanx. The IP joints are each formed by the convex head of either the proximal or middle phalanx that articulates with the concave base of the middle or distal phalanx, respectively.

C. i. Wrist extension—movement of the hand in a posterior direction so that the posterior aspect of the hand moves toward the posterior aspect of the forearm; movement occurs in a sagittal plane around a frontal axis.

ii. Thumb abduction—the thumb moves in an anterior direction in a plane perpendicular to the palm of the hand; movement occurs in an oblique sagittal plane around an oblique frontal axis.

iii. Thumb extension at the CM joint—the thumb moves in the plane of the palm of the hand in a lateral direction away from the index finger; movement occurs in an oblique frontal plane around an oblique sagittal axis.

iv. Finger abduction—movement of the finger away from the midline of the hand (i.e., the third digit); movement occurs in the frontal plane around a sagittal axis.

v. Finger flexion at the PIP joint—bending of the finger so that the anterior aspect of the finger of the middle phalanx moves closer to the anterior aspect of the finger at the proximal phalanx; movement occurs in the sagittal plane around a frontal axis.

D. Ulnar deviation of the fingers, wrist flexion, or wrist extension are the substitute movements that may give the appearance of a greater range of wrist ulnar deviation than is actually present.

4. Assessment and Measurement of PROM at the Wrist and Hand

Wrist Ulnar Deviation

i. Firm

ii. Refer to Table 5-1.

iv. The goniometer is positioned on the posterior aspect of the wrist joint with the axis over the capitate bone.

v. False. The movable arm of the goniometer is aligned with the longitudinal axis of the third metacarpal. Maintaining this alignment prevents motion of the third finger at the MCP joint from being incorporated into the measurement for wrist ulnar deviation ROM.

Wrist Extension

i. An anterior glide of the proximal row of carpal bones at the radiocarpal joint could be decreased if wrist extension PROM is decreased.

ii. Based on the concave/convex theory of movement, a convex surface will glide in the opposite direction to the movement of the bony segment it is a part of. Therefore, during wrist extension, as the distal end of the bones that make up the proximal row of carpal bones move in a posterior direction, the convex surfaces of the proximal ends of the proximal row of carpal bones glide in the opposite direction (i.e., anteriorly) on the fixed concave surface of the distal radius and articular disc of the inferior radioulnar joint.

iii. The goniometer alignment for wrist extension is also used to assess wrist flexion and muscle length for the long finger flexors (flexor digitorum superficialis and profundus, flexor digiti minimi, and palmaris longus) and the long finger extensors (extensor digitorum communis, extensor indicis proprius, and extensor digiti minimi.

iv. When assessing wrist extension PROM, the fingers are relaxed and should be free to move into flexion to prevent stretch of the long finger flexors from limiting wrist extension PROM.

MCP Joint Extension of the Fingers and Thumb

i. In this case, the end feel occurred before the full normal PROM was reached, so the firm end feel would not be considered a normal end feel. A normal end feel exists when there is a full normal PROM at the joint and the normal anatomy at the joint stops movement.

ii. A posterior glide of the base of the proximal phalanx of the thumb would be decreased with decreased thumb MCP joint extension. Based on the concave/convex theory of movement, the concave surface of the base of the proximal phalanx will glide in the same direction as the movement of the proximal phalanx it is a part of. As the thumb extends, the proximal phalanx moves in a posterior direction and the concave base of the phalanx glides in a posterior direction.

iii. Flexion, extension is the capsular pattern at the MCP joints.

iv. The wrist is positioned in slight flexion to prevent stretch of the long finger flexors from restricting MCP joint extension ROM.

Finger MCP Joint Abduction

i. Firm

ii. Refer to Table 5-2.

Thumb CM Joint

i. Carpometacarpal flexion, extension, and abduction (opposition—using the ruler on the universal goniometer to take a linear measurement).

ii. Stabilize the trapezium, wrist, and forearm.

Ring Finger PIP Flexion

i. Hard/soft/firm

ii. Refer to Table 5-2.

Thumb Opposition

i. Opposition is a sequential movement that incorporates abduction, flexion, and adduction of the first metacarpal, with simultaneous rotation.[1]

ii. First CM Joint

5. Muscle Length Assessment and Measurement

Flexor Digitorum Superficialis, Flexor Digitorum Profundus, Flexor Digiti Minimi, and Palmaris Longus

i. Elbow extension; the elbow is held in this position to ensure full stretch is placed on the flexor digitorum superficialis and palmaris longus that have origins proximal to the elbow joint.

ii. If the length of the finger flexors is decreased, with the elbow extended, the forearm supinated and the fingers extended, wrist extension PROM will be restricted proportional to the decrease in muscle length. To assess this PROM restriction using a universal goniometer, the goniometer axis is placed at the level of the ulnar styloid process, the stationary arm is aligned parallel to the longitudinal axis of the ulna, and the movable arm is aligned parallel to the longitudinal axis of the fifth metacarpal. The therapist will note a firm end feel at the end of the restricted wrist PROM.

Lumbricales

i. The wrist is positioned in extension to place the flexor digitorum profundus on stretch, to assist in stabilizing the origin of the lumbricales on the tendons of the flexor digitorum profundus.

ii. If the length of the lumbricales is decreased, with the wrist in extension and the fingers flexed, MCP joint extension PROM will be restricted proportional to the degree of muscle shortness.

Extensor Digitorum Communis, Extensor Indicis Proprius, and Extensor Digiti Minimi

i. If the length of the long finger extensors is decreased, with the elbow extended, forearm pronated, and fingers flexed, wrist flexion PROM will be restricted proportional to the degree of muscle shortness.

6. Functional ROM at the Wrist and Hand

A. Wrist extension and ulnar deviation[2] are the two most important wrist positions or movements for ADL.

B. For feeding activities (i.e., drinking from a cup or glass, eating using a fork or spoon, and cutting using a knife), the ROM requirements are approximately underline{3°} wrist flexion to underline{35°} wrist extension[3,4] and from underline{20°} ulnar deviation to underline{5°} of radial deviation.[4]

C. The wrist optimizes the function of the hand to touch, grasp, or manipulate objects; positions the hand in space relative to the forearm[5]; serves to transmit load between the hand and forearm[5]; and serves to control the length–tension relations of the extrinsic muscles of the hand.

D. The functions of the hand are grasp, communication, manipulation of objects, receiving of sensory information from the environment.

E. underline{CM} joints. In the clinical setting, it is not possible to directly measure movements at the CM joints of the second through fifth metacarpals.

F. i. Wrist flexion—hooking a bra at the back, brushing one's teeth

ii. Wrist extension—writing, holding a glass

iii. Wrist radial deviation—hammering, painting a wall using long brush strokes

iv. Wrist ulnar deviation—hammering, opening a jar

v. Finger flexion—writing, turning a doorknob to open a door

vi. Finger extension—carrying a tray over one's shoulder with the wrist in extension, using the hand to push on the seat of a chair to stand from sitting.

vii. Thumb opposition—picking up the telephone receiver, threading a needle

G. Marked loss of wrist ROM may not significantly hinder a patient's ability to carry out ADL; however, activities of work or recreation were not included in Nelson's[6] study

H. The majority of ADL require flexion ROM at the MCP joints of the fingers and thumb.[8]

I. The functional ROM of the MCP joints is greatest on the ulnar side and least on the radial side of the hand.[7,9]

J. Bain and colleagues[9] reported finger PIP and DIP joint flexion ROM was required to perform 20 ADL as defined by the Sollerman test of hand grip function based on common hand grips used in ADL.

References

1. Levangie PK, Norkin CC. *Joint Structure and Function: A Comprehensive Analysis.* 3rd ed. Philadelphia, PA: FA Davis; 2001.

2. Ryu J, Cooney WP, Askew LJ, et al. Functional ranges of motion of the wrist joint. *J Hand Surg Am.* 1991;16:409-419.

3. Brumfield RH, Champoux JA. A biomechanical study of normal functional wrist motion. *Clin Orthop.* 1984;187:23-25.

4. Safaee-Rad R, Shwedyk E, Quanbury AO, Cooper JE. Normal functional range of motion of upper limb joints during performance of three feeding activities. *Arch Phys Med Rehabil.* 1990;71:505-509.

5. Nordin M, Frankel VH. *Basic Biomechanics of the Musculoskeletal System.* 3rd ed. Philadelphia, PA: Lippincott Williams & Wilkins; 2001.

6. Nelson DL. Functional wrist motion. *Hand Clin.* 1997; 13: 83–92.

7. Hayashi H, Shimizu H. Essential motion of metacarpophalangeal joints during activities of daily living. *J Hand Ther.* 2013;26:69-74.

8. Murai T, Uchiyama S, Nakamura K, Ido Y, Hata Y, Kato H. Functional range of motion in the metacarpophalangeal joints of the hand measured by single axis electric goniometers. *J Orthop Sci.* 2018;23:504-510.

9. Bain GI, Polites N, Higgs BG, Heptinstall RJ, McGrath AM. The functional range of motion of the finger joints. *J Hand Surg.* 2015;40E(4):406-411.

Chapter 6: Hip

1. Palpation

B. i. Hip flexion/extension; axis

 ii. Hip internal/external rotation; movable arm

 iii. Hip abduction/adduction; axis

 iv. Hip flexion/extension; movable arm

 v. Hip internal/external rotation; axis

C. i. Adductor magnus

 ii. Biceps femoris, semitendinosus, semimembranosus

2. Assessment of AROM at the Hip Joint

A. Acetabulum—concave shape; femoral head—convex shape

B. i. Hip extension: movement of the thigh in a posterior direction, in a sagittal plane about a frontal axis; reciprocal movement—flexion

 ii. Hip internal rotation: movement of the anterior surface of the thigh toward the midline of the body, in a transverse plane about a vertical/longitudinal axis; reciprocal movement—external rotation

 iii. Abduction: movement of the thigh away from the midline, in the frontal plane about a sagittal axis; reciprocal movement—adduction

C. i. See Figures 6-10 A and B and accompanying text.

 ii. See Figures 6-11 A and B and accompanying text.

D. Lumbar spine—flexion, extension, lateral flexion, rotation

Hip—flexion, extension, abduction, adduction, internal rotation, external rotation

Knee—flexion, extension

Ankle—dorsiflexion, plantarflexion, inversion, eversion

E. The patient must have the ability to bear full weight through the lower extremities, good balance, and adequate lower extremity muscle strength to support body weight in single-leg stance.

F. i. Hip flexion: Posterior pelvic tilt; lumbar spine flexion

 ii. Hip abduction: External rotation and flexion of the hip; hiking of the ipsilateral pelvis

 iii. Hip internal rotation: Lateral tilting of the pelvis; in sitting, shifting body weight to raise the pelvis and lift the buttocks off the sitting surface.

3. Assessment and Measurement of PROM at the Hip Joint

Hip Flexion

i. The knee was in flexion.

ii. The knee was in flexion to place the two-joint hamstring muscles on slack at the knee so that the length of the hamstrings would not limit the hip flexion ROM.

iii. The normal end feel for hip flexion is soft or firm.

iv. Refer to Table 6-1

Hip Extension

i. The knee was in extension on the test side.

ii. The knee was in extension to place the two-joint rectus femoris muscle on slack at the knee so that the length of the rectus femoris would not limit the hip flexion ROM.

iii. If stabilization was inadequate, <u>anterior pelvic tilt and extension of the lumbar spine</u> would result in erroneously large PROM values.

iv. Spin is the femoral head motion that could be decreased.

Hip Abduction

i. The leg(s) is/are perpendicular to an imaginary line drawn between the ASISs.

ii. Inferior glide could be restricted.

iii. The femoral head is a convex articular surface, and in accordance with the concave/convex theory of joint motion, the convex surface will move in the opposite direction to the movement of the bone, that moves in a superior direction. Thus, the convex articular surface moves in an inferior direction.

Hip Internal Rotation

i. Your partner's end feel would be considered normal if your partner had full PROM and a firm end feel.

ii. The normal limiting factors that create a normal end feel are tension in the ischiofemoral ligament, the posterior joint capsule, and the external rotator muscles of the hip.

iii. Start positions are sitting, supine, sit lying, and prone.

iv. The following femoral head glides could be limited: a posterior glide with the hip in anatomical position and an inferior glide with the hip in 90° flexion.

v. The femoral head is a convex articular surface, and in accordance with the concave/convex theory of joint motion, the convex surface will move in the opposite direction to the movement of the bone that moves in an anterior direction with the hip in anatomical position and a superior direction with the hip in 90° flexion. Thus, the convex articular surface of the femoral head will glide in a posterior direction with the hip in anatomical position or in an inferior direction with the hip in 90° flexion.

B. Capsular; a total joint reaction at the hip joint in which the entire joint capsule is affected.

4. Muscle Length Assessment and Measurement

Hamstrings

i. Posterior tilt position.

ii. extended beyond 20° knee flexion.

iii. The end feel is firm.

Hip Flexors

i. Iliacus, psoas major, tensor fascia latae, and rectus femoris are the muscles for which muscle length is being assessed.

ii. The nontest hip is held in flexion to flatten and stabilize the lumbar spine and pelvis in a neutral position and thus avoid the substitute motions of increased anterior pelvic tilt and lumbar lordosis from obscuring the presence of a hip flexion contracture.

iii. **Increased** lumbar lordosis can mask a hip flexion contracture.

iv. When assessing the hip flexor muscle length, the hip is positioned in abduction to place the tensor fascia latae on slack.

Tensor Fascia Latae

i. Origin[1]—Anterior aspect of the outer lip of the iliac crest; the outer surface and notch below the ASIS; and the deep surface of the fascia latae.

Insertion[1]—Via the iliotibial tract onto the lateral aspect of the lateral condyle of the tibia.

Hip adduction, hip extension, hip lateral rotation, and knee flexion are the positions that place maximal stretch on the simulated tensor fascia latae.

ii. The "Ober's Test: Trunk Prone" offers optimal stability of pelvis and lumbar spine.

5. Functional ROM at the Hip Joint

B. i. Riding a bicycle; sitting with the foot across the opposite thigh to tie a shoelace; stepping sideways past others to take one's seat in a theatre.

ii. Sitting with one thigh across the other; making an immediate turn in standing while pivoting on one leg and continuing the turn by adducting the contralateral leg; sitting with the legs outstretched and the legs crossed at the ankles.

iii. Mounting a bicycle; squatting to the floor to pick up an object; placing one's foot out of the car when getting out of the car; kicking a door closed with the lateral aspect of the foot when the knee is flexed.

iv. Examining the skin on the sole of the foot when performing foot hygiene activities; kicking a ball with the inside of the foot; sitting reaching down to tie a shoe on the floor.

C. i. The hip joint transmits forces between the ground and the pelvis to support body weight (e.g., standing; jumping) and acts as a fulcrum for the pelvis in single-leg stance (e.g., when lifting the foot up to ascend stairs). Hip movement moves the body closer to or farther from the ground (e.g., squatting to pick up an object from the ground; rising from sitting position), brings the foot closer to the body (e.g., to cut the toenails or pull on a sock), and positions the lower limb in space (e.g., moving the foot from the gas pedal to the brake; when stepping onto large stones to cross a creek).

ii. Common ADL can be accomplished in a normal manner with hip ROM of at least 20° flexion, 20° abduction, and 20° external rotation.[2]

References

1. Standring S, ed. *Gray's Anatomy: The Anatomical Basis of Clinical Practice*. 39th ed. London, UK: Elsevier Churchill Livingstone; 2005.
2. Johnston RC. Sonidt GL. Hip motion measurements for selected activities of daily living. *Clin Orthop Relat Res*. 1970;72:205-215.

Chapter 7: Knee

1. Palpation

i. Knee flexion/extension

Goniometer axis—lateral epicondyle of the femur

Stationary arm—greater trochanter of the femur

Moveable arm—lateral malleolus of the fibula

ii. Hamstrings or rectus femoris

Goniometer axis—lateral epicondyle of the femur

Stationary arm—greater trochanter of the femur

Moveable arm—lateral malleolus of the fibula

iii. True

2. Assessment Process

Records patient's history

Explains rationale and component parts of assessment

Observation

Assessment of AROM

Measurement of AROM, as required

Assessment of PROM

Measurement of PROM, as required

Assessment and measurement of muscle length, as required

Assessment of muscle strength

Application of other assessment techniques, as required

3. Assessment of AROM at the Knee Articulations

A. Femorotibial articulation: proximal components—convex femoral condyles; distal components—concave tibial condyles

Patellofemoral articulation: patellar surface—the surface is divided by a vertical ridge; the articular surface is flat or slightly convex mediolaterally and supero-inferiorly;[1] anterior surface of the femur—the surface is divided by the intercondylar groove; the articular surface is concave mediolaterally and convex superoinferiorly.[2]

B. Femorotibial joint movement: Knee flexion—bending of the knee so that the posterior surface of the calf moves toward the posterior surface of the thigh; Knee extension—straightening of the knee in the opposite direction to flexion. These movements occur around a frontal axis in the sagittal plane.

Internal tibial rotation—turning of the anterior surface of the tibia toward the midline of the body. External tibial rotation—turning of the anterior surface of the tibia away from the midline of the body. These movements occur around a longitudinal axis in the horizontal plane.

4. Assessment and Measurement of PROM at the Knee

Knee Flexion

i. A firm or soft end feel is normal.

iii. For normal limiting factors, refer to Table 7-1.

iv. If knee flexion ROM is assessed with the patient in prone lying, the rectus femoris would be stretched at the hip and could restrict knee flexion ROM.

Knee Extension

i. If knee extension ROM is assessed with the patient in sitting, the hamstring muscles would be stretched at the hip and could restrict knee extension ROM.

ii. Anterior glide would be decreased. The tibial condyles are concave surfaces. Based on the concave/convex theory of movement, a concave surface will glide in the same direction of movement as the bony segment it is a part of. When the knee is extended the tibia moves in an anterior direction; therefore, the concave articular surface of the tibia will glide in an anterior direction.

Tibial Rotation

i. Normal end feels are firm for tibial internal rotation and firm for tibial external rotation.

iii. Normal limiting factors—Tibial internal rotation: tension in the cruciate ligaments; tibial external rotation: tension in the collateral ligaments.[2]

Patellar Mobility

i. Patellar glides: distal glide, medial-lateral glide

ii. Normal vertical displacement: 8 cm[3]

iii. Normal PROM: 9.6 mm medially and 5.4 mm laterally[4]

5. Muscle Length Assessment and Measurement

Rectus Femoris

i. pelvis

iii. a) *Supine*: The patient's supine position and holding of the nontest hip in flexion stabilize the pelvis and lumbar spine. The therapist observes the anterior superior iliac spine (ASIS) to ensure there is no pelvic tilting.

b) *Prone*: Test position 1 (see Fig. 7-22): The patient's prone position (nontest leg over the side of the plinth, hip flexed, foot on floor) stabilizes the pelvis. A strap may also be placed over the buttocks to stabilize the pelvis.

Test position 2 (see Fig. 7-24): The patient's prone position helps to stabilize the pelvis. A strap may also be placed over the buttocks to stabilize the pelvis. The therapist observes the pelvis to ensure there is no anterior tilting of the pelvis.

6. Functional ROM at the Knee

A. The ROM requirements for ADL are influenced by the design of the furniture used, the placement of objects, and the patient's posture. The start and the end positions and technique used to complete the activity also affect the ROM requirements. Therefore, the ROM values provided below are a guide only.

i. About 117°[5] knee flexion

ii. About 93°[5] knee flexion

iii. About 106°[5] knee flexion

iv. About 83° to 105°[6] knee flexion

v. About 86° to 107°[6] knee flexion

B. Walking requires an ROM from about 0° of knee extension as the leg advances forward to make initial contact with the ground to a maximum of about 60° of knee flexion at initial swing so that the foot clears the ground as the extremity is advanced forward (from the Rancho Los Amigos gait analysis forms, as cited in Levangie and Norkin[7]).

C. Tibial rotation occurs in ADL that require:

i. movement into full knee extension (i.e., at the end of knee extension the tibia automatically rotates externally on the femur),

ii. movement of knee flexion from a position of full knee extension (i.e., at the beginning of knee flexion, the tibial automatically rotates internally on the femur),

iii. twisting movements of the body when the foot is planted on the ground.[8]

References

1. Levangie PK, Norkin CC. *Joint Structure and Function. A Comprehensive Analysis.* 4th ed. Philadelphia, PA: FA Davis, 2005.
2. Kapandji IA. *The Physiology of the Joints. Vol. 2.* 2nd ed. New York, NY: Churchill Livingstone; 1982.
3. Soderberg GL. *Kinesiology: Application to Pathological Motion.* 2nd ed. Baltimore, MD: Williams & Wilkins; 1997.
4. Skalley TC, Terry GC, Teitge RA. The quantitative measurement of normal passive medial and lateral patellar motion limits. *Am J Sports Med.* 1993;21:728-732.
5. Laubenthal KN, Smidt GL, Kettlekamp DB. A quantitative analysis of knee motion during activities of daily living. *Phys Ther.* 1972;52:34-42.
6. Livingston LA, Stevenson JM, Olney SJ. Stairclimbing kinematics on stairs of differing dimensions. *Arch Phys Med Rehabil.* 1991;72:398-402.
7. Levangie PK, Norkin CC. *Joint Structure and Function. A Comprehensive Analysis.* 3rd ed. Philadelphia, PA: FA Davis; 2001.
8. Smith LK, Weiss EL, Lehmkuhl LD. *Brunnstrom's Clinical Kinesiology.* 5th ed. Philadelphia, PA: FA Davis; 1996

Chapter 8: Ankle and Foot

1. Palpation

A. i. Great toe: MTP joint abduction/adduction (moveable arm)
        MTP joint flexion/extension (moveable arm)
        IP joint flexion/extension (stationary arm)
    ii. Subtalar joint inversion/eversion (axis)
    iii. Ankle dorsiflexion/plantarflexion (stationary arm)

2. Assessment Process

i. True
ii. True
iii. True
iv. False-if ROM is WNL the therapist may not measure the PROM

3. Assessment of AROM at the Ankle and Foot

i. Ankle joint—dorsiflexion/plantarflexion (oblique sagittal plane/oblique frontal axis).

Subtalar joint—inversion/eversion (oblique frontal plane/oblique sagittal axis).

IP joints—flexion/extension (sagittal plane/frontal axis).

4. Assessment and Measurement of PROM at the Ankle and Foot

Ankle Dorsiflexion

i. Normal end feel is firm/hard.
ii. The knee is flexed 20° to 30° to place the gastrocnemius on slack and prevent shortness of gastrocnemius from restricting ankle dorsiflexion PROM.

iii. *Ankle joint*—The proximal concave articulating surface of the joint, commonly referred to as the ankle mortise, is formed by the medial aspect of the lateral malleolus, the distal tibia, and the lateral aspect of the medial malleolus. This concave surface is mated with the convex surface of the body of the talus.

Ankle Plantarflexion

i. The forefoot is mobile and the hindfoot is immobile; therefore, the therapist would align the moveable arm of the goniometer with the hindfoot, more specifically parallel to the sole of the heel to eliminate substitute forefoot movement from the measurement.

ii. During ankle plantarflexion, the convex surface of the body of the talus glides anteriorly on the fixed ankle mortise.

iii. Normal limiting factors: Tension in the anterior joint capsule, anterior portion of the deltoid ligament, anterior talofibular ligaments, and the ankle dorsiflexors; contact between the talus and the tibia. These structures create a firm or a hard end feel.

Subtalar inversion

i. Lateral glide of the posterior facet of the calcaneus would be limited.

ii. Medial glide of the anterior and middle facets would be limited.

iii. The posterior facet of the calcaneus is a convex articular surface, and in accordance with the concave/convex theory of joint motion, the convex surface will move in the opposite direction to the movement of the bone. Therefore, when the calcaneus moves in a medial direction, the convex articular surface moves in a lateral direction on the fixed concave surface of the talus.

The anterior articular surfaces of the calcaneus are concave, and in accordance with the concave/convex theory of joint motion, the concave surface will move in the same direction as the movement of the bone. Therefore, when the calcaneus moves in a medial direction, the concave articular surfaces also move in a medial direction.

Great Toe MTP Joint Extension

i. The firm end feel would not be a normal end feel because the structures that produce the end feel restrict the PROM before the full PROM is achieved.

ii. Dorsal glide would be restricted because the articular surface of the base of the proximal phalanx of the great toe is concave, and in accordance with the concave/convex theory of joint motion, the concave surface will move in the same direction as the movement of the proximal phalanx, i.e., in a dorsal direction with great toe MTP joint extension.

iii. The pattern of movement restriction at the first MTP joint in the presence of a capsular pattern would be extension, flexion.

5. Muscle Length Assessment and Measurement

Gastrocnemius

i. *Origin*[1]: Medial head: proximal and posterior aspect of the medial condyle of the femur posterior to the adductor tubercle; lateral head: lateral and posterior aspect of the lateral condyle of the femur; lower part of the supracondylar line.

Insertion[1]: Via the Achilles tendon into the calcaneus.

ii. Knee extension and ankle dorsiflexion would place the muscle on stretch.

iii. A firm end feel would be noted if the gastrocnemius were shortened.

6. Functional ROM at the Ankle and Foot

A. 10° ankle dorsiflexion; 20° plantarflexion (from the Rancho Los Amigos gait analysis forms as cited in Levangie and Norkin[2])

B. i. *Ankle dorsiflexion*—descending stairs, rising from sitting, squatting to pick up an object from the floor

ii. *Ankle plantarflexion*—reaching for an object on a high shelf, depressing the accelerator of a car, ascending stairs

iii. *Toe extension*—reaching for an object on a high shelf, walking, squatting to pick up an object from the floor

C. The ROM requirements for ADL are influenced by the design of the furniture used, the height of the step, and the patient's height. The start and the end positions and technique used to complete the activity also affect the ROM requirements. Therefore, these ROM values are a guide only.

i. Rise from sitting on a standard-height chair: 28°[3] ankle dorsiflexion.

ii. Descend a standard-height step: 21° to 36°[4] ankle dorsiflexion.

References

1. Soames RW. Skeletal system. In: Salmons S, ed. *Muscle. Gray's Anatomy*. 38th ed. New York, NY: Churchill Livingstone; 1995.
2. Levangie PK, Norkin CC. *Joint Structure & Function: A Comprehensive Analysis*. 3rd ed. Philadelphia, PA: FA Davis; 2001.
3. Ikeda ER, Schenkman ML, Riley PO, Hodge WA. Influence of age on dynamics of rising from a chair. *Phys Ther*. 1991;71:473-481.
4. Livingston LA, Stevenson JM, Olney SJ. Stairclimbing kinematics on stairs of differing dimensions. *Arch Phys Med Rehabil*. 1991;72:398-402.

Chapter 9: Head, Neck, and Trunk

1. Palpation

A. i. Landmarks: tip of the chin, suprasternal notch; other movements: neck extension

ii. Landmarks: mastoid process, lateral aspect of the acromion process; other movements: none

iii. Landmarks: spines of C7 and S2; or the suprasternal notch (with the patient in prone); other movements: thoracolumbar spine flexion (C7 and S2)

iv. Landmarks: spine of S2; point 15 cm proximal to the spine of S2; other movements: lumbar spine extension

v. Landmarks: lateral aspect of the acromion process; the uppermost point of the iliac crest at the midaxillary line or the superior aspect of the greater trochanter; other movements: none

B. i. Landmarks: vertex of the head, spine of T1 or spine of the scapula; other movements: neck flexion, neck lateral flexion.

ii. Landmarks: spines of C7 and S2; other movements: thoracolumbar spine flexion

iii. Landmarks: spine of S2; point 15 cm proximal to the spine of S2; other movements: lumbar spine extension

iv. Landmarks: spines of T1 and S2; other movements: none

v. Landmarks: spines of T1 and T12; other movements: none

C. It is not necessary to identify any surface anatomy locations when using the CROM to assess neck ROM.

2. Assessment and Measurement of ARom

TMJ Movements

i. Jaw movements: Depression (mouth opening), occlusion (mouth closing), protraction, retraction, and lateral deviation.

ii. The proximal joint surface consists of the concave mandibular fossa, and the convex temporal articular eminence that lies anterior to the fossa. The proximal joint surface articulates with the reciprocally shaped superior surface of the articular disc that is anteroposteriorly concavoconvex. The inferior surface of the articular disc is concave and is mated with the convex condyle of the mandible to form the lower compartment of the TMJ.

iii. TMJ movements that can be measured using a rule are mandibular depression, lateral deviation, and protrusion.

iv. Functional ROM is determined for mouth opening by placing two or three flexed proximal interphalangeal joints between the upper and lower central incisor teeth.[1] The fingers represent a distance of about 35 to 50 mm.[1]

Neck Extension

Neck extension ROM will be underestimated if the mouth is open during the tape measurement; therefore, the mouth should be closed when assessing neck ROM.

Neck Left Lateral Flexion

Substitute movements to be avoided: Elevation of the shoulder girdle to approximate the ear, ipsilateral trunk lateral flexion

Neck Right Rotation

i. Start position: The patient is in supine with the head and neck in anatomical position.

ii. The inclinometer is positioned in the midline at the base of the forehead.

Thoracolumbar Spine Flexion

Thoracolumbar spine flexion can be measured using inclinometers positioned at C7 and S2.

Lumbar Spine Flexion

Lumbar spine extension can also be measured using a tape measure and the same anatomical landmarks (i.e., spine of S2 and a point 15 cm above S2).

Thoracolumbar Spine Extension (Prone Press-up)

Factors that may result in inaccurate ROM measurements: If the upper extremities are weak, the patient may not be able to move the trunk through the full available trunk extension ROM; the pelvis being raised from the plinth during the test motion; the tape measure not being perpendicular to the plinth.

Thoracolumbar Spine Rotation

The anatomic landmarks: lateral aspect of the acromion process; the uppermost point of the iliac crest at the midaxillary line, or the superior aspect of the greater trochanter.

Thoracolumbar Spine Lateral Flexion

i. Substitute movements to avoid: trunk flexion, trunk extension, ipsilateral hip and knee flexion, raising the contralateral or ipsilateral foot from the floor.

ii. Thoracolumbar spine lateral flexion AROM can be measured using inclinometers. One inclinometer is placed midline at the level of the PSIS (i.e., over the S2 spinous process) and a second inclinometer is placed over the C7 spinous process.

3. Muscle Length Assessment and Measurement

Toe-Touch Test

i. False

ii. False

iii. True

4. Functional ROM at the Head, Neck, and Trunk

A. i. *Thoracolumbar flexion*: Squatting to pick up an object from the floor; sitting; placing dishes in a dishwasher.

ii. *Thoracolumbar extension*: Looking at or reaching for a book on a high shelf situated directly in front of you; lying prone on the elbows to read a book; throwing a ball.

iii. *Cervical spine rotation*: Looking both ways to cross the street; indicating a negative response to a question; looking behind when backing up a car.

iv. *Cervical spine lateral flexion*: Sitting and looking under the table for a dropped object; tilting the head to remove water from one's ear; moving one's head to the side when styling the hair using a blow dryer.

B. Trunk motions or movements of the feet to reposition the body are strategies that could be used to increase the field of vision.

C. i. *Sitting and tying a shoe with the foot flat on the floor*: Cervical spine extension, thoracic and lumbar spine flexion.

ii. *Combing the hair on the back of one's head*: Cervical spine rotation; may also include cervical spine extension and lateral flexion.

iii. *Brushing one's teeth*: TMJ depression (i.e., mouth opening).

iv. *Reaching for a wallet in a back pocket*: Thoracic and lumbar spine flexion and rotation.

Reference

1. Magee DJ. *Orthopedic Physical Assessment*. 4th ed. Philadelphia, PA: Saunders; 2002.

Note: Page numbers followed by *f* denote figures; those followed by *t* denote tables.